Aging

Geroscience as the New Public Health Frontier

SECOND EDITION

A subject collection from *Cold Spring Harbor Perspectives in Medicine*

Aging

Geroscience as the New Public Health Frontier

SECOND EDITION

A subject collection from *Cold Spring Harbor Perspectives in Medicine*

EDITED BY

James L. Kirkland
Mayo Clinic

S. Jay Olshansky
University of Illinois at Chicago

George M. Martin
University of Washington

COLD SPRING HARBOR LABORATORY PRESS
Cold Spring Harbor, New York • www.cshlpress.org

Aging: Geroscience as the New Public Health Frontier, Second Edition
A subject collection from *Cold Spring Harbor Perspectives in Medicine*
Articles online at www.perspectivesinmedicine.org

Executive Editor	Richard Sever
Project Supervisor	Barbara Acosta
Permissions Administrator	Carol Brown
Production Editor	Diane Schubach
Production Manager/Cover Designer	Denise Weiss
Publisher	John Inglis

Front cover artwork: Image from iStock.com/George Peters.

Library of Congress Cataloging-in-Publication Data

Names: Kirkland, James (James L.), editor. | Olshansky, Stuart Jay, 1954-editor. | Martin, George M., 1927-2022, editor.
Title: Aging : geroscience as the new public health frontier/edited by James L. Kirkland, Mayo Clinic, S. Jay Olshansky, University of Illinois at Chicago, and George M. Martin, University of Washington.
Description: Second edition. | Cold Spring Harbor, New York : Cold Spring Harbor Laboratory Press, [2024] | A subject collection from Cold Spring Harbor Perspectives in Medicine. | Includes bibliographical references and index. |
Summary: "Aging is a contributing factor in cancer, Alzheimer's and numerous other conditions. This new edition updates our understanding of the biological processes involved and potential approaches to address clinical problems associated with aging"-- Provided by publisher.
Identifiers: LCCN 2023029721 (print) | LCCN 2023029722 (ebook) | ISBN 9781621824312 (cloth) | ISBN 9781621824329 (epub)
Subjects: LCSH: Aging--Physiological aspects. | Longevity--Physiological aspects. | Aging--Molecular aspects.
Classification: LCC QP86 .A3757 2024 (print) | LCC QP86 (ebook) | DDC 612.6/7–dc23/eng/20230921
LC record available at https://lccn.loc.gov/2023029721
LC ebook record available at https://lccn.loc.gov/2023029722

10 9 8 7 6 5 4 3 2 1

For a complete catalog of all Cold Spring Harbor Laboratory Press publications, visit our website at www.cshlpress.org.

Contents

Contents

In Memoriam: George M. Martin (1927–2022)

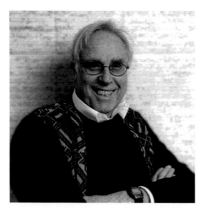

GEORGE M. MARTIN, A CO-EDITOR OF THIS VOLUME, passed away during its final stages of completion. George was a pioneer in, and beloved long-time contributor to, what today we call geroscience, as well as any number of allied biomedical disciplines.

Son of a New York City policeman, George received both his BS degree in Chemistry and his MD at the University of Washington. After an internship at the Montreal General Hospital and residency at the University of Chicago, he joined the faculty of the University of Washington in 1957 and remained on that faculty until his death in December 2022 at the age of 95.

The breadth of his scientific contributions is stunning. Much of his research focused on somatic cell genetics and how the corruption of gene activity with age contributed to degenerative phenotypes. He was an early investigator of the biology of replicative life span of cultured fibroblasts and the link between cell culture models and the aging of whole organisms. As early as 1965, he noted with colleagues Charles Epstein and Arnold Motulsky how the Werner's syndrome (WS) caricatured many aspects of accelerated aging, including early death, and three decades later was involved in identifying the mutant gene that caused that syndrome. Characteristically, he also connected his observations of cellular replicative senescence and WS by investigating whether fibroblasts from people with WS exhibited reduced life span. They did—as did fibroblasts from people with other genetic syndromes that mimicked aspects of accelerated aging such as Down's and Hutchinson–Gilford syndromes. George also had a knack for coining new terminology. Some of my favorites that are still with us were "proliferative homeostasis" and "epigenetic drift." The genetic syndromes that caricatured accelerated aging he called "segmental progeroid syndromes," another term that has stuck. His interest in these syndromes also stuck. He was still publishing on WS in 2022.

George also contributed to Alzheimer's disease research, where he published dozens of papers and was involved in the discovery of the gene encoding Presenilin 1, mutations in which are responsible for the most common inherited form of the disease. He recognized early on the importance of epigenetics in regulating genes involved in aging and he was an early thinker interpreting medical discoveries associated with aging in an evolutionary context. When I did a sabbatical in George's laboratory in 2001–2002, we spent as much time discussing evolutionary biology as we did discussing oxidative damage to bird cells, the project we were working on together.

Fittingly, his research was recognized with numerous honors and awards, including the Pruzanski award from the American College of Medical Genetics, the World Alzheimer Congress Lifetime Achievement award, the Brookdale and Kleemeier awards from the Gerontological Society of America, the Allied-Signal Corporation award, the Irving S. Wright award from the American Federation for Aging Research, and the American Aging Association's Research Medal and Distinguished Scientist award. In 1992, he was elected to the Institute of Medicine (now the National Academy of Medicine) of the National Academy of Sciences.

He also held over the course of his career a range of leadership positions. He served on the National Institute of Aging's National Advisory Council and Board of Scientific Counselors, was President of the Tissue Culture Society and the Gerontological Society of America, held the position of Scientific Director of the American Federation for Aging Research for almost a decade, and served on the Scientific Advisory Board of the Glenn Foundation for Medical Research and the Ellison Medical Foundation during its entire 16-year history.

George's impact on the field was even more extensive than one might guess from this abbreviated list of his research accomplishments and leadership positions. He was also a mentor *par excellence*, both officially to his students, postdocs, and junior faculty, but unofficially to many more, including me. I will always be grateful for his wise advice and encouragement when I stumbled into the field from the rather unusual direction of field ecology and evolutionary biology.

Finally, George never lost his broad intellectual curiosity or his appreciation of the joys of life and that made him an always engaging dinner companion and friend. He had a subtly mischievous sense of humor, which I particularly appreciated and which is on display in the eye-catching title of an "idea" paper he wrote the early 1970s. That title, "On Immortality: An Interim Solution," is pure George Martin.

STEVEN N. AUSTAD
University of Alabama at Birmingham

Foreword

WHEN THE TERM "GEROSCIENCE" FIRST appeared in the literature 10 years ago, in a paper by Ron Kohanski and me (Sierra and Kohanski 2013), we knew the concept was solid and had the potential to bring together many aspects of biomedical research. After all, the concept was simple, and based on a universally understood and accepted concept: aging is the major risk factor for diseases. What had changed—and the opportunity we seized—was that the previous decade had shown enormous advances in our understanding of the molecular and cellular underpinnings of aging (López-Otín et al. 2013; Kennedy et al. 2014). As a result, there was a yet-to-be-defined, but plausible opportunity to use that knowledge as a new way of improving the quality of life for old people. We just needed a catchy term, geroscience, and that was provided by my friend Gordon Lithgow from the Buck Institute for Aging Research.

Yet we could not imagine at the time that the concept would attract so much attention and flourish in so many different directions. This book addresses the many aspects in which geroscience has grown to be relevant, from its inception on the role of basic aging biology as a driver of major diseases, to the role of geroscience in health itself (not just the absence of disease) and the downstream economic and social consequences that successful application of geroscience principles would force humanity to contemplate.

It is bittersweet that the late George Martin is an editor of this compendium. George was one of the earliest adherents to the then new concept of geroscience, as he enthusiastically told me at a Gordon Conference shortly after the first paper was published and as we were preparing to hold the first Geroscience Summit at the National Institute on Aging (NIA). Subsequently, and while the field was still young, I had the good fortune of being asked to edit a book called *Advances in Geroscience*. Like this one, that volume had contributions from many top scientists, and I had the audacity of asking George to write its preface. Luckily, he agreed, and I cherish the honor of his words. It is therefore bittersweet, as mentioned, that I should now be writing the preface to a book with George as an editor.

FELIPE SIERRA
Hevolution Foundation

REFERENCES

Sierra F, Kohanski R. 2013. Geroscience offers a new model for investigating the links between aging biology and susceptibility to aging-related chronic diseases. *Public Policy & Aging Report* **23:** 7–11.

López-Otín C, Blasco MA, Partridge L, Serrano M, Kroemer G. 2013. The hallmarks of aging. *Cell* **153:** 1194–1217.

Kennedy BK, Berger SL, Brunet A, Campisi J, Cuervo AM, Epel ES, Franceschi C, Lithgow GJ, Morimoto RI, Pessin JE, et al. 2014. Aging: a common driver of chronic diseases and a target for novel interventions. *Cell* **159:** 709–713.

Preface

The sun rises and sets, seasons change, leaves fall to the ground, the Earth revolves around the Sun, the North Star always points north, and creatures like humans, dogs, mice, and elephants are born, grow up, grow old, and eventually die. The laws of nature that drive the biological functioning of our bodies operate with regularity, like clocks ticking in the background or the beat of our heart beneath our chest.

— *A Measured Breath of Life*
Olshansky and Carnes (2013)

T HE QUESTION OF HOW LONG HUMANS CAN live and whether humanity can influence the processes that contribute to the duration and quality of our lives is a foundational question in science. This is not a new inquiry. When Michelangelo painted the *Creation of Adam* on the ceiling of the Sistine Chapel in Rome in the sixteenth century, he portrayed humanity as having been molded by the hand of its creator, in his image, as a "perfect" physical specimen—with alleged 900+ year life spans according to the Old Testament. Biblical scholars suggest that a fall from this idealized notion of "perfection" is the reason the life spans of humans have grown shorter. By contrast, Darwin's theory of evolution in the late nineteenth century emphasized the opposite message by focusing on the imperfections in the anatomic structures and functions of humans and other living things as the strongest evidence for his theory. Alfred Russell Wallace, in the time of Darwin, suggested that aging and death are programmed as a way to remove the old to make way for the young.

As familiar as Michelangelo and Darwin may be to us today, speculation about human longevity and health dates back millennia. Aristotle speculated that aging is caused by the loss of an innate moisture in the body, and that the loss of functioning was nature's ingenious way of preparing us for death—as if aging was an organized and purposeful phenomenon. Galen from the second century AD and Avicenna from the eleventh century AD both believed that aging was an inevitable and natural part of the order of the universe, which led them to believe that the daily pursuit of a healthy life was a far more productive way of living rather than engaging in a constant battle against death. Fatalists dominated early thinking about why we live as long as we do.

Others were not so fatalistic. The Chinese philosopher Ko Hung advocated for the use of Taoist methods of extending life through controlling one's breath—with immortality as the ultimate goal. Roger Bacon from the thirteenth century and Luigi Cornaro from the fifteenth century believed that life-prolonging chemicals, foods, other substances, and even caloric restriction would enable humanity to achieve much longer life spans. Perhaps most relevant to today was the view from French zoologist Georges Buffon, who suggested that "physical laws" regulate the duration of life in humans and other species. These laws, according to Buffon, link the biological clocks that govern growth and development to similar clocks that he thought influenced duration of life. Buffon argued that the duration of life of species is calibrated, as a ratio, to the timing and length of each species' reproductive window—as if a biological clock is ticking for one set of events early in the life course, but which has an inadvertent influence on the timing of death and the diseases that precede it. This should sound familiar to evolutionary biologists familiar with twentieth century concepts of antagonistic pleiotropy, mutation accumulation, and disposable soma and to demographers familiar with the "law of mortality" first discussed by British actuary Benjamin Gompertz in 1825.

It appears that most of these historical figures who considered life span determination were each right in their own way. The artistic-like perfection of the human body is exemplified by the near flawless maintenance and repair mechanisms of our nuclear DNA, and the perpetuation of the immortal germ line through sexual reproduction. Public health and modern medicine have made it possible for most people born today to survive to older ages, allowing humanity to experience the aging of our bodies for the first time with great regularity. However, our extended lives came with a Faustian bargain.

Our bodies are a complex web of pulleys, pumps, levers, and hinges, woven together by a living, breathing, suite of anatomic structures and functions that deliver nutrients to and remove waste products from every cell in the body—every moment of every day in our lives. When our bodies are used beyond what may be thought of as their biological or Darwinian warranty period (e.g., beyond the end of the reproductive window), the diseases and disorders now commonly associated with aging or senescence appear with clock-like regularity—governing the duration of our lives in the absence of genetic programs to make them operate. The variation observed in disease expression and length of life is expected in a world in which inherited and acquired risk factors dominate longevity determination, but, overall, the age pattern of death in humans has stayed remarkably constant since vital statistics were first collected more than 200 years ago.

Humanity achieved its goal of life span extension for most people during the public health revolution of the twentieth century, although disparities remain and are a central focus of public health today. Now we are left to deal with the consequences of our success. Using the poetic words of Sir Peter Medawar, aging is revealed "only by the most unnatural experiment of prolonging an animal's life by sheltering it from the hazards of its ordinary existence." Now that we live these unnaturally long lives and our aging bodies are experiencing more health challenges than we bargained for, what's next?

The approach that our modern world has taken to the gift of long life and its accompanying aging-related diseases is a natural response: attack them with the same sense of purpose adopted more than a century ago when communicable diseases dominated the longevity landscape, one at a time, as they arise. This disease-specific model has been successful, but a new Faustian bargain has presented itself in the modern era—and it is not nearly as appealing as the first bargain we agreed to in the middle of the nineteenth century when declining early age mortality was exchanged for longer lives and aging-related diseases. Success today in attacking the diseases of aging leaves behind a suite of less appealing health challenges that are more resistant to traditional interventions because the biological process of aging—which is uninfluenced by changes in the risk of disease—marches on in the background, unaltered by changes in behavioral risk factors and modern medicine.

People reaching older ages may yearn for "extended warranties" on our body parts that wear with time and use, but modern medicine is not delivering like it used to. Instead, we are receiving a continuous flow of band aids that yield short-term benefits, but which may inadvertently deliver the one thing we fear most—an extension of frailty and disability instead of the health span extension we desire. This is likely to happen if we make ourselves live longer without ensuring that the added survival time is accompanied by good health.

The good news is that human ingenuity has once again presented us with a suite of alternative "fixes" designed to attack the underlying source of the maladies associated with survival to older ages—the biological process of aging itself. The rise of "geroscience," or what was first called the "longevity dividend," is a new public health effort designed specifically to address the Faustian bargain of biological aging emerging as the primary risk factor for disease and death. Geroscience is a paradigm shift in the way in which medicine, science, and public health think about and treat the maladies that are present in aging bodies. Geroscience was a fanciful theoretical idea when first presented a half century ago—it is theoretical no more.

In 2015, the three editors of this volume published the first book ever written on the rise of geroscience, its importance to public health, and the various approaches that scientists were taking at the time to advance this nascent field. Thousands of books and scientific articles have since flooded the scientific literature. We are now beyond the nascent stage of this new field—trying to figure out what we have created, its potential impact on health and longevity, how to fund the science, which pathways to pursue, how to measure and demonstrate safety and efficacy, what happens if we succeed or fail, and, perhaps most important to many, how to communicate what this all means to people not familiar with the promise of geroscience.

Our first book summarized the logic used to support the rise of geroscience, and some of the initiatives pursued at the time that looked most promising. A lot has happened in the last 8 years. The pursuit of health span over life span has become a meme within the vibrant geroscience community, and advances have occurred along multiple fronts. In this new updated volume, we take you with us on the journey this new field is taking as we navigate our way through the initial stages of a major new movement in public health.

The book begins with a dedication to our third editor—Dr. George Martin—who unfortunately passed away in late 2022 after a very long and distinguished career in aging science. While George will be missed as this field progresses, his presence will endure through the powerful influence he has already had on the entire field and the majority of the scientists now pursuing the goals outlined in this book. This volume is dedicated to Dr. Martin.

In a Foreword written by one of the fathers of the modern geroscience initiative—Dr. Felipe Sierra—the logic and background behind this new movement is presented to those less familiar with the field. The heart of the book is the next section, devoted to many, but certainly not all, of the various pathways that researchers are pursuing to modulate the biological process of aging for the purpose of extending health span.

Driving the development of the latest science in the field is a more thorough understanding of the health and economic consequences if geroscience is successful. There have only been a few papers ever written on this topic, but the importance of understanding what will happen to national economies and personal health care costs, if successful, is at the heart of geroscience's appeal to many.

One of the more interesting stories that has developed regarding the rise of geroscience is how the science is being funded. In today's world where deep pockets abound, influence is sought, and profits associated with the development of perhaps one of the most valuable commodities that can exist (interventions that manufacture healthy life) are clearly visible. You will learn here how geroscience is coming to life in nontraditional ways.

In the final analysis, this book chronicles a fascinating journey into the launch of something that is rarely seen in public health and medicine—an intervention that has global health and economic consequences that can and will influence most people alive today and all future generations. The scientists that wrote the articles in this book are central figures in this movement—but there are many more who are part of the story and working feverishly to bring this movement to life. We would encourage readers to stay updated on developments in this field because of its potential global impact—this volume is an excellent way to catch up on advances that have occurred within just the last 8 years.

James L. Kirkland
S. Jay Olshansky
George M. Martin

From Life Span to Health Span: Declaring "Victory" in the Pursuit of Human Longevity

S. Jay Olshansky

School of Public Health, University of Illinois at Chicago, Chicago, Illinois 60612, USA
Correspondence: sjayo@uic.edu

A difficult dilemma has presented itself in the current era. Modern medicine and advances in the medical sciences are tightly focused on a quest to find ways to extend life—without considering either the consequences of success or the best way to pursue it. From the perspective of physicians treating their patients, it makes sense to help them overcome immediate health challenges, but further life extension in increasingly more aged bodies will expose the saved population to an elevated risk of even more disabling health conditions associated with aging. Extended survival brought forth by innovations designed to treat diseases will likely push more people into a "red zone"—a later phase in life when the risk of frailty and disability rises exponentially. The inescapable conclusion from these observations is that life extension should no longer be the primary goal of medicine when applied to long-lived populations. The principal outcome and most important metric of success should be the extension of health span, and the technological advances described herein that are most likely to make the extension of healthy life possible.

ON THE ORIGIN OF LIFE SPAN

How long people live as individuals, the expected duration of life of people of any age based on current death rates in a national population, and the demographic aging of national populations (e.g., proportion of the population aged 65 and older), are simple metrics that are colloquially understood as reflective of health and longevity. Someone that lives for 100 years had a life span of a century, and a life expectancy at birth of 80 years for men in the United States means that male babies born today will live to an average of 80 years if death rates at all ages today prevail throughout the life of the cohort. When life expectancy rises or declines, that is interpreted as an improvement or worsening of public health. These demographic and statistical metrics are reflective measurement tools only—they disclose little about why they change or vary, they reveal nothing about why they exist at all, and they are indirect and imprecise measures of the health of a population.

Understanding why there is a species-specific life span to begin with and what forces influence its presence, level, and the dynamics of variation and change (collectively referred to here as "life span determination") is critical to comprehending why the topic (e.g., the longevity dividend and geroscience) is now so important, why claims about forthcoming radical life extension are misguided positions of advocacy, why victory can now be declared in humanity's pursuit of longevity, and why biomedical research and modern medicine should now be focused on extending health span rather than exclusively trying to make us live longer.

WHY DO SPECIES-SPECIFIC LIFE SPANS EXIST?

This question was first asked and then answered in the nineteenth century by French physiologist Pierre Flourens who asked a simple question in his book *Human Longevity and the Amount of Life upon the Globe*—"What is the natural, usual, and normal duration of the life of man?" (Flourens 1855). This question was not new since the greatest thinkers of every era throughout history speculated about the human life span and devised what they believed were methods of modifying how long people are capable of living (Gruman 1966), but it was Flourens who provided a biological answer more than two centuries before the evolutionary theory of senescence laid down the principal answer to this question.

Questions of this sort are not esoteric—how long we live as individuals and populations has important public policy implications. For example, the future solvency of age-entitlement programs (such as those involving retirement and health) are heavily dependent on how many people live to retirement age and how long they draw benefits from such programs once they begin doing so. Current and future demands on health care resources are fundamentally influenced by length of life; planning for retirement and how long to remain in the labor force are all influenced by an answer to this seemingly simple question. As such, understanding the human life span has taken on new and important roles in the modern public policy arena.

To answer this question, I will draw on first principles from the field of evolutionary biology based on a famous quote from the geneticist Theodosius Dobzhansky (1973) who once stated, "… nothing in biology makes sense except in the light of evolution" (Dobzhansky 1973). To appreciate the first principles behind the human life span, consider the Renaissance view of humankind that was present for centuries before

Flourens, evolutionary biology, and other biological sciences emerged. According to this view, humans are "perfect" physical specimens molded by the hand of a creator—with a life span potential purported to be close to 1000 years if the Old Testament is to be taken literally. The imagery that best exemplifies this view of humanity's perfection is Michelangelo's painting *The Creation of Adam* on the ceiling of the Sistine Chapel.

By contrast, the underlying principle of Darwin's theory of evolution was not the Renaissance view of perfection, but rather the exact opposite. Darwin's view of evolution originated with imperfections in the anatomic structures and functions of the human body that led to evolutionary change across long time periods, sexual reproduction as a means to maintain the immortality of the germ line, a "disposable" soma, and, ultimately, an explanation for why humans live as long as we do.

A case can be made that both Michelangelo and Darwin were right. On the one hand, there is an artistic-like perfection of the human body exemplified by the near flawless maintenance and repair mechanisms of nuclear DNA (Kirkwood 2005; Maynard et al. 2015). It is difficult to fathom that each cell in the human body confronts more than 10,000 potentially damaging chemical and radiation-based hits every day (Ames et al. 1993)—and yet the DNA contained within the 3.72×10^{13} cells in our bodies (Bianconi et al. 2013) is maintained and repaired continuously, 24/7, with *close to* flawless perfection. In this regard, it is hard to argue with Michelangelo's view of humanity's perfection.

Yet, Darwin focused on the minutia—the *close to* part of humanity's "perfect" DNA repair story—the tiny imperfections that make their way through from one generation to the next (rather than the level of perfection present), as the basis upon which evolution takes place. According to both Darwin and Stephen J. Gould (1977), evolution takes places in fits and starts rather than gradually, which means eons of evolutionarily quiescent time is punctuated by rapid evolutionary events. Over time, sexual reproduction evolved as a mechanism through which DNA has become immortalized. As Dawkins

Cite this article as *Cold Spring Harb Perspect Med* doi: 10.1101/cshperspect.a041480

(2016) eloquently stated with his selfish gene hypothesis, somas (our bodies) are the vehicles through which DNA achieved immortality. This also means that somas, the vehicles that transport genes across time, are eventually disposable (Kirkwood 1977). The subsequent "discarding" of the soma (which is a passive, not an active process—and the timing with which it occurs), is why there is a life span.

Details of the evolutionary theory of senescence are contained in detail in the literature, so there is no need to engage that line of reasoning any further here. Suffice it to say that the price paid for the immortality of the germ line is a suite of anatomic structures and functions within our bodies that, when used beyond what may be thought of as their biological or Darwinian warranty period (Olshansky et al. 2001a; Carnes et al. 2003), leads to many of the diseases and disorders now commonly associated with aging or senescence. The divergent but intimately linked views of Michelangelo and Darwin exemplify the importance of a biological perspective on aging, the diseases that accompany it, and, ultimately, the forces that influence and limit the life span of our species.

ARE THERE TICKING BIOLOGICAL TIME BOMBS IN OUR BODIES?

Given the consistent message that death eventually comes to all living things, and the highly predictable timing with which it occurs for every species, it would be easy to conclude that a clock is ticking in each of us that measures biological time from conception, and which directly causes us to age and eventually die. Yet, if aging is indeed an inadvertent byproduct of genetically fixed programs for growth, development, and reproduction, then there can be neither death genes nor longevity genes that evolved under the direct force of natural selection. Why is that?

Death programs cannot exist as a direct product of evolution because the end result would be the systematic demise of all living things at an age beyond which almost every member of a species would ordinarily be expected to live. Aging programs cannot exist for the same reason. A bio-

logical time bomb driven by genes designed exclusively to kill at older ages is equivalent to automobile manufacturers building in an explosive device that is set off only when the car reaches 1 million miles. Since cars are not ordinarily driven that far, such a death program would rarely if ever be triggered—rendering it useless. In humans and other living things, genetically fixed life span programs that cause aging or death would be equally useless—and for the exact same reason. There is no point in building (or having natural selection expend precious biological resources) in a genetic program that would rarely if ever be used under normal conditions.

Does the absence of aging and death programs mean humans can live forever, or at least much longer than we do now as some claim? (Wilmoth 1998; Oeppen and Vaupel 2002). As it turns out, this question about a "limit" to life or finite amount of measured survival time is one of the most misunderstood topics in the field of aging today. Let us clear up this issue once and for all.

There is a limit to life; it is fundamentally rooted in biology, and, provided in the next section, is a simple explanation for why this is so. In fact, it is more than a bit surprising that anyone would question the presence of a human life span or "limit to life" given the ubiquitous presence of death all around us. If the wrong tools of science are used it becomes easy to believe that radical life extension or immortality are almost within the grasp of science's hand.

WHAT IS THE HUMAN LIFE SPAN?

As a reminder, *life expectancy* is a demographic term used to represent the expected remaining years of life based on a current life table—it is a population statistic that takes into account observed death rates at all ages in a given country in a calendar year. Life expectancy can be calculated for people of any age, but it is most often reported at birth. *Life span* is the observed duration of life of an individual. *Maximum life span* is the observed duration of life of the longest-lived member of the species—defined by how long one person lived. Life expectancy and maximum life span are often used interchangeably, but they are vastly different numbers. The term "life expectancy" is defined here as "period life expectancy at birth."

One of the best and earliest explanations of why there are species-specific life spans comes from French naturalist Georges Buffon (1747). He speculated that every person has the same allotment of time from birth to death, and that duration of life depends not on our habits, customs, or quality of food, but rather on physical laws that regulate the number of our years. This concept of a physical law regulating duration of life is nearly identical to Gompertz's (1872) view about physical laws governing what he called the Law of Mortality. However, Buffon was not aware of the importance of genetic heterogeneity in the eighteenth century, so his view of equal allotments of time for everyone was misguided. Buffon further stated that each species possesses a suite of fixed biological attributes (e.g., gestation period, age patterns of growth, and constant physical form), so if all biological phenomena conform to fixed laws like those governing the timing of gestation and sexual maturity, then duration of life must also be fixed accordingly.

Buffon's language about a linkage between reproduction and the timing of death preceded the evolutionary theory of senescence by more than two centuries and Gompertz's Law of Mortality by more than one century. Buffon's interest in life span was based on an extensive database of life history characteristics that he collected for a variety of species (e.g., dogs, cats, rabbits, humans, etc.). Based on these data, Buffon reasoned that a species' life span is a product of interconnected chains of functional relationships between biological attributes. He envisioned a fixed duration of gestation giving rise to a fixed duration of growth, which, in turn, leads to a fixed duration of life. Thus, Buffon was the first to articulate that life span is calibrated to the onset and length of a species' reproductive window. He went on to suggest that the life span (e.g., life expectancy) of a species is consistently six to seven times greater than the time required to reach puberty. In humans, this would be ~85 years.

The maximum life expectancy of humans has often been associated with the number 85 in the scientific literature. For example, Fries (1980) speculated that the upper limit to human life ex-

pectancy at birth is 85 years based on an extension of historical trends in life expectancy at birth and at older ages where they converge on or about age 85. Olshansky et al. (1990) used complete life tables for the U.S. population, and later included data from other countries (Olshansky et al. 2001b) to demonstrate that the metric of life expectancy at birth becomes less sensitive to declining mortality the higher it rises. Once it reaches 85 (82 for men and 85 for women), the magnitude of the decline in mortality required to nudge life expectancy higher becomes particularly onerous, although not impossible. This line of reasoning was further supported by arguments about how the anatomical structures of the human body make it difficult to justify life expectancies for national populations much beyond 85 since components of the body consistently wear out over time, and not all of them can be repaired or replaced by medical intervention (Olshansky et al. 2001a, 2007). A far more detailed look into the proximate biological forces that influence duration of life in humans (Carnes et al. 2013) supported the same conclusion that Buffon came to in the eighteenth century—that life expectancy at birth is unlikely to exceed about 85 for men and women combined any time soon—unless technological advances occur that slow the biological rate of aging.

With regard to the human life span, there is theoretical, empirical, and biological justification to conclude that the human life span is about 85 years for men and women combined and maximum life span is currently 122 (Robine et al. 2019)—but this maximum might increase slightly in the coming decades with larger cohorts moving through the age structure (de Beer et al. 2017). There is empirical evidence to suggest that it will continue to be rare to have humans live beyond the age of 115 (Dong et al. 2016).

As originally stated by Olshansky et al. (1990), this life expectancy limit should be viewed as a glass ceiling that can be broken through with the use of technological advances that modify the rate at which biological aging occurs. While efforts are underway now to do just that, currently there are no biomedical interventions that have been documented to extend life beyond the limits described here. How far humanity can raise the life expectancy ceiling beyond the current limit is unknown.

ARGUMENTS FOR AND AGAINST RADICAL LIFE EXTENSION

Scientists who speculate on forthcoming radical increases in human longevity have generated a range of views from the promise of immortality to modest increases in this century. Four unique arguments have formed along these lines. The first is the "One More Day of Life" argument set forth by Wilmoth (1997) where the case was made that there are no biological or demographic constraints on generating one more day of life indefinitely. The central question asked was how death rates or life expectancy would behave if a limit to life was being approached. If the expected statistical behavior is not observed using the tools at his disposal, he reasoned, then the hypothesized limit must be too far beyond the observed longevity horizon to be detected.

The evidence presented by Wilmoth includes (1) data from Sweden for the period 1851–1990 that, despite a high degree of variation in the age of the longest-lived person, exhibit an increasing trend over this time period (based on data from one man and one woman from Sweden in each calendar year); (2) the hypothesis that a limited life span requires death rates to rise exponentially throughout the entire age structure—a pattern of mortality he suggested does not appear in humans (some evidence indicates otherwise) (Gavrilov and Gavrilova 2011); (3) the hypothesis that a decrease in the variability of death rates at older ages is not sufficient proof of a limit to life; and (4) the suggestion that the absence of a positive correlation between mortality level and the pace of mortality decline in some countries means a lower limit to the hazard function cannot be detected using demographic methods. The conclusion drawn from this analysis was that demographic/statistical/biological evidence for a limit to life could not be detected—even though there was no measure of any biological force of longevity determination in this analysis.

Wilmoth (1998) then carried his line of reasoning significantly further by concluding that "over sufficiently long time periods, it is not at all unusual for death rates to decline by half or more," and therefore "there is simply no convincing evidence (demographic, biological, or otherwise) of a lower bound on death rates other than zero." Wilmoth used a purely demographic tool to declare that immortality is plausible—there was no biology in this assessment. Wilmoth's reasoning is predicated on the assumption that demographic/statistical conditions are legitimate guideposts that can be used to reveal proximity to a limit to life. However, there are no a priori reasons why death rates must rise exponentially for a limit to be observed, or that mortality has to compress into a narrower age range, or that a positive correlation between level of mortality and pace of mortality decline is a defining characteristic of limits. Wilmoth declared those defining limits himself.

The obstacle to this line of reasoning is the consistent message imposed by the force of mortality. Even when annual death rates of 50% are applied to a hardy group of survivors to extreme old age, everyone in every birth cohort eventually dies within a short time frame, even though statistical reasoning might lead some to believe otherwise. Very few people survive past age 115 and most deaths in any given cohort occur at highly regular ages that are tightly compressed within a few decades between ages 60 and 90.

A simple analogy reveals the serious flaw in this argument. Consider the world record for the one-mile run—which is currently 3 min 43 sec. This record has declined steadily, in linear fashion since the middle of the nineteenth century when it was 4 min 28 sec (it is worth noting that this running record has not changed since it was last broken in 1999). Using Wilmoth's line of reasoning, it may be argued that there are no demonstrable reasons why one more second cannot always be shaved off this record—leading to the statistically logical but biologically untenable forecast that someone will eventually run one mile instantaneously. This argument could even be bolstered by a well-known biological fact—there is no genetic program in humans that precludes shaving time from the world record for the one-mile run. Yet, we need nothing more than common sense to inform us that the human body design will not allow this to happen

(Olshansky et al. 1990). In similar fashion, while Wilmoth is correct in assuming that there is no genetic program that precludes the indefinite addition of one more day of life, in identical fashion, the biomechanics of the human body will not allow this to happen.

The biology of life and death was disregarded in this purely quantitative analysis and the resulting conclusion was that demographic/statistical evidence for a limit to life cannot be detected using observed demographic data—and therefore such limits must not exist. The reason proponents of this view cannot see a life span limit is because demographic/statistical reasoning is not where the evidence for life span limits resides. This argument is akin to claiming that air does not exist because it cannot be seen directly with the naked eye; evidence for a limit to life is contained outside the statistical analysis of mortality events observed in just a handful of people.

A second line of reasoning used to support infinite or dramatically higher life spans was set forth by de Gray (2005a) where the argument was made that *everything* that goes wrong with the human body can be repaired continuously, to perfection, indefinitely, by rapidly approaching technology that, in fact, does not yet exist. These so-called rejuvenation technologies are predicted to occur with "90% confidence" sometime between 2015 and 2040 with a massive funding effort. The mathematical logic behind this notion of radical life extension is derived from a concept invented by de Gray called "actuarial escape velocity" (AEV)—which is described as a scenario where "mortality rates fall so fast that people's remaining (not merely total) life expectancy increases with time." That is, remaining life expectancy gets longer the older one gets. The audacious claim using this line of reasoning is that at the oldest ages (past age 105) where annual conditional probabilities of death have consistently remained in the range of 50%, the probability of death will "…fall to 5% or lower, and mostly to below 1%…" (De Gray 2005b).

This argument lacks empirical evidence or validity—which is a kind way of saying the survival probabilities and resulting life expectancy estimates were made up. In fact, the notion of AEV is so far from reality that this author views it as "voodoo demography." It is worth noting that about 5 years after this prediction was made by de Gray, life expectancy began stagnating or declining in most parts of the developed world; that is, life expectancy began heading in the exact opposite direction as that predicted using AEV (more on this point later) (Case and Deaton 2015). The suggestion that death rates at extreme old age will decline from 50% to mostly below 1%, is at best derisory.

A third argument in favor of both radical life extension and immortality comes from Kurzweil and Grossman (2005). They argue that there are three bridges to eternal life. The first bridge is represented by an estimated 20 years the authors claim will be added to life expectancy with the use of nutritional supplements; but just like AEV, there is no empirical evidence to support the claim of an additional 20 years. Bridge two technologies are anticipated biomedical advances like stem cell therapy and genetic engineering that are thought to add another 20 years to life expectancy (a number provided by the author without empirical support); and the third bridge is nanotechnology, which the authors claim will be able to repair everything that goes wrong in the body, indefinitely, yielding eternal life. The bridge analogy is appealing at one level because many of these technological advances are likely. The problem is that it is difficult at best to estimate life expectancy benefits for technologies that do not yet exist.

The last argument favoring radical life extension is appealing to some because the case is made that the phenomenon of greatly extended lives is already here (Oeppen and Vaupel 2002; Vaupel et al. 2021). In this case, the authors do not bother with biology, they do not mention any new technological advances that are forthcoming with hypothetical life expectancy gains, and they do not even come up with concepts like AEV. Instead, they simply declare that half the babies born today will live to 100, and base this on an extrapolation of the historical trend in "best practice" life expectancy. For those who do not know what this is, take the annual world record for longevity in all national populations and plot them on a graph from the past into the present, pull out a ruler to extend this into the next century, and then simply declare that there is empirical evidence supporting the claim that radical life extension is already here. This is analogous to declaring that half the babies born today in the United States will be able to run a 3-min mile in their lifetime because a handful of people beat a 4-min mile running record each year since the middle of the twentieth century.

The bottom line is that all of the arguments advocating for radical life extension with the claim that large increases in life span are forthcoming or are already here lack theoretical, biological, and empirical support. These resemble positions of advocacy rather than science-based estimates of human life expectancy.

DECLARING VICTORY IN HUMANITY'S QUEST FOR LONGEVITY

Reductions in childhood diseases can occur only once for a population; once such gains are achieved, the only outlets for further significant gains in life expectancy must come from extending the lives of older people (Olshansky 2018). Given that multiple fatal conditions accrue in older people because of biological aging (e.g., a fundamental and inevitable risk that occurs independent of conventional behavioral risk factors for diseases) and once survival past age 65 years becomes common in a country, life expectancy gains must decelerate, even if medical advances and improved lifestyles continue to occur (Olshansky et al. 1990). Although unsupported claims have been made that the historic rise in life expectancy has been steady and has continued to the present (Vaupel et al. 2021), data from the *Human Mortality Database* demonstrate definitively that the rise in life expectancy at birth in most developed nations has been decelerating (mortality.org) as predicted (Olshansky et al. 1990).

In fact, trends in life expectancy in many developed nations since 2010 have shown a deceleration in the rate of increase, a stagnation, or even a decline (Ho and Hendi 2018). The COVID pandemic exacerbated this recent trend in life expectancy stagnation with extremely large drops observed in 2020–2021 (Mazzuco and Campostrini 2022; Stephenson 2022), but these are likely to be anomalies and some bounce back improvement in life expectancy is expected in the coming years.

Because the point of diminishing returns on life expectancy (∼85 years for men and women combined) has been approached in many parts of the world, and because the change in life expectancy at birth is decelerating and approaching or has already reached a point of diminishing returns, there is reason to conclude that the goal of life extension for the human species has largely been achieved. The time has arrived to declare victory in humanity's quest to combat the scourges of mortality that precluded extended survival for the vast majority of our species throughout history. Now that most people born in the modern era have an excellent chance of survival past the age of 65, and, among these survivors, many will survive to ages 85 and older, the goal of life extension has been accomplished.

Do not interpret this declaration as justification to relax efforts to combat the plentiful causes of early mortality due to harmful behavioral risk factors such as smoking, obesity, lack of exercise, avoidance of life saving vaccines, drug use, violence, etc. Declines in death rates and additional gains in life expectancy from gaining control over these causes of death remain a high priority in public health. It is just that inroads against these causes of death will no longer yield significant gains in life expectancy for national populations—certainly nothing on the order of claims that radical life extension is forthcoming.

THE TIME HAS ARRIVED TO TARGET AGING

A rather difficult dilemma has presented itself in the modern era, and, in the final analysis, that is what this entire collection is all about. Modern medicine and advances in the medical sciences are laser focused on a constant quest for finding ways to extend people's lives—without considering either the consequences of success or the best way to pursue it. At one level—from the angle of the physician treating their patient—this makes perfect sense as their objective is to help their patients overcome the immediate health challenges they face. The current focus of most of modern medicine is on chronic, fatal age-related diseases, in much the same way infectious diseases were confronted more than a century ago (i.e., one at a time as if independent of each other). Even though there have been many successes in efforts to combat aging-related diseases, further life extension in an aging world will expose the saved population to an elevated risk for all other aging-related diseases. That is, with extended survival brought forth by a suite of innovations designed to treat diseases that present themselves in older bodies, more people will survive into what may be thought of as a "red zone"—a later phase in life when the risk of frailty and disability rise exponentially—especially among those saved from dying at earlier ages as a byproduct of medical interventions (Fig. 1).

Keep in mind that the biological processes of aging force human bodies to become ever more susceptible to fatal and disabling conditions as survival extends further into the red zone; so unwanted health conditions emerge with greater frequency not so much because of how life has been lived (although harmful lifestyles can accelerate their emergence and progression) but because of how long life has already been lived.

Time becomes the greatest challenge in aging bodies, so the target of medicine and public health should begin shifting to biological time (the aging process that gives rise to disease) rather than byproducts of aging—the diseases that modern medicine focuses on.

With death inevitable, the modern attempt to counteract aging-related diseases reveals a phenomenon known as competing risks. When the risk of death from one disease decreases, the risk of death from other diseases increases or becomes more apparent. With advancing age, the period between the emergence of competing diseases shortens and rises exponentially with advancing age. The hazard in old age is not so much that one disease displaces another, but that the new diseases are often much more debilitating. For example, finding a cure for cancer may cause an unintended increase in the prevalence of Alzheimer disease.

The inescapable conclusion from these observations is that life extension should no longer be the primary goal of medicine when applied to long-lived populations. Pushing out the blue line may yield some modest increases in life expectancy, but the price paid for success could very well

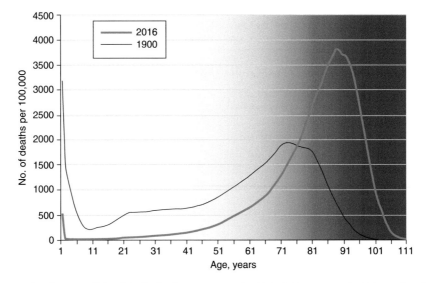

Figure 1. Age distribution of life table deaths for women in the United States, per 100,000 people, 1900–2016. (Source: Olshansky et al. 2020). The red zone represents a period in life when the risk of frailty and disability begins to increase rapidly. The goal of modern medicine is to push out the envelope of survival and extend the blue line to later ages. The goal of aging science, by contrast, is to delay and compress the red zone, which has the goal of extending the period of healthy life. The data used to generate this figure comes from the *Human Mortality Database* (mortality.org).

Cite this article as *Cold Spring Harb Perspect Med* doi: 10.1101/cshperspect.a041480

be an expansion of morbidity. The principal outcome and most important metric of success, therefore, should be the extension of health span, and the technological advances that make the extension of a healthy life possible. The recommendation from this line of reasoning is that delaying and compressing the red zone should become the primary target of medicine and aging science.

While it is likely that an extended health span will be accompanied by an extension of life span, the primary metric of success in medicine and biology should be on what it takes to help humanity live healthier lives on the heels of a declared success in our effort to combat the challenges to extended survival faced by our ancestors.

WHAT IS HEALTH SPAN?

The conceptual formulation and measurement of health span in humans is not new. Sanders (1964) laid the conceptual groundwork for the idea behind measuring health span; Chiang (1965) developed the first mathematical models that measured the health of populations beyond those derived from vital statistics; Sullivan (1966) outlined the problems associated with the creation of a single index that combined measurements of health and mortality; and Moriyama (1968) further elaborated on the importance and measurement of population health rather than just mortality. These measurement issues were subsequently resolved, and Sullivan (1971) provided the first calculations of healthy life expectancy based on measures of survival time both free from disability and with disability.

The logic behind the use of health span is straightforward. Vital statistics such as death rates and resulting life tables used to estimate period life expectancy at birth and older ages, are indirect measures of a population's health. From Sanders to Sullivan, it was acknowledged that a more direct metric is required that combines measures of both health and mortality, into a single life table estimate that more accurately reflects the health of populations.

Interest in measuring health span gained considerable interest in the ensuing decades as researchers from across the globe grappled with the difficulty in securing common methods of data and measurement metrics that would allow for valid comparisons across time and population subgroups. Excellent summaries of the history behind health span—including measurement issues and trends in national populations —may be found in Crimmins (2015) and Robine and Saito (2003). The metric of health span is now globally accepted, measured, and used routinely by the Global Burden of Disease Project and World Health Organization (GBD 2019 Demographics Collaborators 2020).

The use of a health span metric has now become central to the goals of geroscience because a successful effort to extend healthy life must be measured using standardized tools of science that have already been established in humans. Two main articles (Goldman et al. 2013; Scott et al. 2021) document the health and economic gains associated with successful efforts to slow aging and extend health span as a primary target and demonstrate that the absolute number of frail older individuals would be far fewer by midcentury (relative to byproducts of conventional disease-oriented treatments), accompanied by billions of dollars of health savings, with just a small successful effort to slow aging in people. A clarion call for a switch to health span extension over life span extension is now common in the various fields that inform aging science (Miller 2002; Fontana et al. 2010; Burch et al. 2014; Sierra et al. 2021; Olshansky et al. 2022).

A conceptual framework and detailed discussion of measurement and data issues involving health span metrics in animal models has been described by Seals and Melov (2014). The importance of this work in translational geroscience is that before clinical trials of geroprotective therapeutics can be tested in humans, animal models are required that mimic the effects of purported interventions on both length and quality of life. The image provided from the Seals and Melov paper (Fig. 2) conveys the conceptual model for health span extension involving both animal and human models of intervention.

CONCLUSIONS

The metrics of life span and health span are central to our understanding of human health.

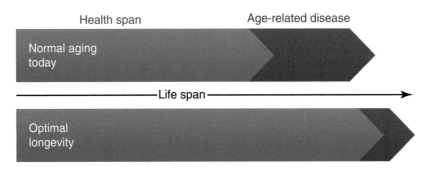

Figure 2. Increasing health span and optimal longevity. Comparisons versus ideal health span. Extending health span is a critical component of achieving optimal longevity, defined as living long but with good health, function, productivity, and independence.

During the last two centuries, humanity experienced dramatic health changes that offered wonderful opportunities to explore later regions of the life span in ways never before experienced by previous generations. The benefits of life extension combined with demographic shifts that caused population aging have been so profound that scientists contend that a new map of life is warranted (Carstensen 2011). Figuring out how to navigate our way through the gift of additional survival time has led to wonderful new opportunities to explore life in ways rarely experienced by anyone in history (Rowe 2015).

However, life extension and population aging arrived with an equally difficult set of challenges. The medical cost of extended survival has skyrocketed as survival has extended into older regions of the life span where the cost of care and the avoidance of death is extremely high (Dieleman et al. 2020). Humanity has yet to come to terms with the inevitability of death and when to turn off or dampen the expensive medical machines that often end up yielding little more than additional weeks or months of life at an extremely high cost (Emanuel et al. 2002). Living up to one-third of life in retirement or some version of it is something that few are prepared to handle financially (Olshansky et al. 2020).

The modern medical machine is still centrally focused on a disease model that has been with us since public health began the battle with communicable diseases nearly two centuries ago. The question raised here is whether this disease model is still applicable in an aging world where there is reason to declare victory in humanity's effort to extend life. The literature will continue to zero in on the various pathways that scientists in the field of aging are pursuing to modulate biological time as a new method of primary prevention. There is reason for great optimism.

REFERENCES

Ames BN, Shigenaga MK, Hagen TM. 1993. Oxidants, antioxidants, and the degenerative diseases of aging. *Proc Natl Acad Sci* **90:** 7915–7922. doi:10.1073/pnas.90.17.7915

Bianconi E, Piovesan A, Facchin F, Beraudi A, Casadei R, Frabetti F, Vitale L, Pelleri MC, Tassani S, Piva F, et al. 2013. An estimation of the number of cells in the human body. *Ann Hum Biol* **40:** 463–471. doi:10.3109/03014460.2013.807878

Buffon GLL. 1747. *Histoire naturelle: générale et particulière des crustacés et des insectes.* Wentworth Press, Paris.

Burch J, Augustine AD, Frieden LA, Hadley E, Howcroft TK, Johnson R, Khalsa PS, Kohanski RA, Li XL, Macchiarini F, et al. 2014. Advances in geroscience: impact on healthspan and chronic disease. *J Gerontol A Biol Sci Med Sci* **69:** S1–S3. doi:10.1093/gerona/glu041

Carnes BA, Olshansky SJ, Grahn D. 2003. Biological evidence for limits to the duration of life. *Biogerontology* **4:** 31–45. doi:10.1023/A:1022425317536

Carnes BA, Olshansky SJ, Hayflick L. 2013. Can human biology allow most of us to become centenarians? *J Gerontol A Biol Sci Med Sci* **68:** 136–142. doi:10.1093/gerona/gls142

Carstensen L. 2011. *A long bright future.* Perseus, New York.

Case A, Deaton A. 2015. Rising morbidity and mortality in midlife among white non-Hispanic Americans in the 21st century. *Proc Natl Acad Sci* **112:** 15078–15083. doi:10.1073/pnas.1518393112

Chiang CL. 1965. *An index of health: mathematical models.* PHS Publication No. 1000, Series 2, No. 5. U.S. Government Printing Office, Washington, DC.

Cite this article as *Cold Spring Harb Perspect Med* doi: 10.1101/cshperspect.a041480

Crimmins EM. 2015. Lifespan and healthspan: past, present, and promise. *Gerontologist* **55:** 901–911. doi:10.1093/geront/gnv130

Dawkins R. 2016. *The selfish gene*, 4th ed. Oxford University Press, Oxford.

de Beer J, Bardoutsos A, Janssen F. 2017. Maximum human lifespan may increase to 125 years. *Nature* **546:** E16–E17. doi:10.1038/nature22792

De Gray ADNJ. 2005a. Foreseeable and more distant rejuvenation therapies. In *Ageing interventions and therapies* (ed. Rattan SIS), pp. 379–395. World Scientific, Singapore.

De Gray ADNJ. 2005b. Foreseeable and more distant rejuvenation therapies. In *Ageing interventions and therapies* (ed. Rattan SIS), p. 393. World Scientific, Singapore.

Dieleman JL, Cao J, Chapin A, Chen C, Li Z, Liu A, Horst C, Kaldjian A, Matyasz T, Scott KW, et al. 2020. US health care spending by payer and health condition, 1996–2016. *JAMA* **323:** 863–884. doi:10.1001/jama.2020.0734

Dobzhansky T. 1973. Nothing in biology makes sense except in the light of evolution. *Am Biol Teach* **35:** 125–129. doi:10.2307/4444260

Dong X, Milholland B, Vijg J. 2016. Evidence for a limit to human lifespan. *Nature* **538:** 257–259. doi:10.1038/nature19793

Emanuel EJ, Ash A, Yu W, Gazelle G, Levinsky NG, Saynina O, McClellan M, Moskowitz M. 2002. Managed care, hospice use, site of death, and medical expenditures in the last year of life. *Arch Intern Med* **162:** 1722–1728. doi:10.1001/archinte.162.15.1722

Flourens P. 1855. *Human longevity and the amount of life upon the globe*. H. Balliere, London.

Fontana L, Partridge L, Longo VD. 2010. Extending healthy life span—from yeast to humans. *Science* **328:** 321–326. doi:10.1126/science.1172539

Fries JF. 1980. Aging, natural death, and the compression of morbidity. *N Engl J Med* **303:** 130–135. doi:10.1056/NEJM198007173030304

Gavrilov LA, Gavrilova NS. 2011. Mortality measurement at advanced ages: a study of the social security administration death master file. *North Am Actuar J* **15:** 432–447. doi:10.1080/10920277.2011.10597629

GBD 2019 Demographics Collaborators. 2020. Global age-sex-specific fertility, mortality, healthy life expectancy (HALE), and population estimates in 204 countries and territories, 1950–2019: A comprehensive demographic analysis for the global burden of disease study 2019. *Lancet* **396:** 1160–1203. doi:10.1016/S0140-6736(20)30977-6

Goldman DP, Cutler D, Rowe JW, Michaud PC, Sullivan J, Peneva D, Olshansky SJ. 2013. Substantial health and economic returns from delayed aging may warrant a new focus for medical research. *Health Aff (Millwood)* **32:** 1698–1705. doi:10.1377/hlthaff.2013.0052

Gompertz B. 1872. On one uniform law of mortality from birth to extreme old age, and on the law of sickness. *J Inst Actuar* **16:** 329–344.

Gould SJ. 1977. *Ever since Darwin*. W.W. Norton, New York.

Gruman GJ. 1966. A history of ideas about the prolongation of life: the evolution of prolongevity hypotheses to 1800. *Trans Am Philos Soc* **56:** 1–102. doi:10.2307/1006096

Ho JY, Hendi AS. 2018. Recent trends in life expectancy across high income countries: retrospective observational study. *BMJ* **362:** k2562.

Kirkwood TBL. 1977. Evolution of aging. *Nature* **270:** 301–304. doi:10.1038/270301a0

Kirkwood TB. 2005. Understanding the odd science of aging. *Cell* **120:** 437–447. doi:10.1016/j.cell.2005.01.027

Kurzweil R, Grossman T. 2005. *Fantastic voyage*. Plume, New York.

Maynard S, Fang EF, Scheibye-Knudsen M, Croteau DL, Bohr VA. 2015. DNA damage, DNA repair, aging, and neurodegeneration. *Cold Spring Harb Perspect Med* **5:** a025130. doi:10.1101/cshperspect.a025130

Mazzuco S, Campostrini S. 2022. Life expectancy drop in 2020. estimates based on human mortality database. *PLoS ONE* **17:** e0262846. doi:10.1371/journal.pone.0262846

Miller RA. 2002. Extending life: Scientific prospects and political obstacles. *Milbank Q* **80:** 155–174. doi:10.1111/1468-0009.00006

Moriyama IM. 1968. Problems in the measurement of health status. In *Indicators of social change* (ed. Sheldon EB, Moore WE), Chap. 11, pp. 573–600. Russell Sage Foundation, New York.

Oeppen J, Vaupel JW. 2002. Demography. broken limits to life expectancy. *Science* **296:** 1029–1031. doi:10.1126/science.1069675

Olshansky SJ. 2018. From lifespan to healthspan. *JAMA* **320:** 1323–1324. doi:10.1001/jama.2018.12621

Olshansky SJ, Carnes BA, Cassel C. 1990. In search of Methuselah: estimating the upper limits to human longevity. *Science* **250:** 634–640. doi:10.1126/science.2237414

Olshansky SJ, Carnes BA, Butler RN. 2001a. If humans were built to last. *Sci Am* **284:** 50–55. doi:10.1038/scientificamerican0301-50

Olshansky SJ, Carnes BA, Désesquelles A. 2001b. Prospects for human longevity. *Science* **291:** 1491–1492. doi:10.1126/science.291.5508.1491

Olshansky SJ, Butler RN, Carnes BA. 2007. Re-engineering humans. *Scientist* **21:** 28–31.

Olshansky SJ, Ashburn K, Stuckey J. 2020. *Pursuing wealthspan: How science is revolutionizing wealth management*. Methuselah, Buffalo Grove, IL.

Olshansky SJ, Martin G, Kirkland J. 2022. *Aging: the longevity dividend*. Cold Spring Harbor Laboratory Press, Cold Spring Harbor, NY.

Robine JM, Saito Y. 2003. Survival beyond age 100: the case of Japan. *Popul Dev Rev* **29:** 208–228.

Robine JM, Allard M, Herrmann FR, Jeune B. 2019. The real facts supporting Jeanne Calment as the oldest ever human. *J Gerontol A Biol Sci Med Sci* **74:** S13–S20. doi:10.1093/gerona/glz198

Rowe JW. 2015. Successful aging of societies. *Daedalus* **144:** 5–12. doi:10.1162/DAED_a_00325

Sanders BS. 1964. Measuring community health levels. *Amer J Public Health* **54:** 1063–1070. doi:10.2105/AJPH.54.7.1063

Scott AJ, Ellison M, Sinclair DA. 2021. The economic value of targeting aging. *Nat Aging* **1:** 616–623. doi:10.1038/s43587-021-00080-0

Seals DR, Melov S. 2014. Translational geroscience: emphasizing function to achieve optimal longevity. *Aging* **6:** 718–730. doi:10.18632/aging.100694

Sierra F, Caspi A, Fortinsky RH, Haynes L, Lithgow GJ, Moffitt TE, Olshansky SJ, Perry D, Verdin E, Kuchel GA. 2021. Moving geroscience from the bench to clinical care and health policy. *J Am Geriatr Soc* **69:** 2455–2463. doi:10.1111/jgs.17301

Stephenson J. 2022. COVID-19 deaths helped drive largest drop in US life expectancy in more than 75 years. *JAMA Health Forum* **3:** e215286. doi:10.1001/jamahealthforum.2021.5286

Sullivan DF. 1966. *Conceptual problems in developing an index of health.* PHS Publication, No. 1000, Series 2, No. 17. U.S. Government Printing Office, Washington, DC.

Sullivan DF. 1971. A single index of mortality and morbidity. *HSMHA Health Rep* **86:** 347–354. doi:10.2307/4594169

Vaupel JW, Villavicencio F, Bergeron-Boucher MP. 2021. Demographic perspectives on the rise of longevity. *Proc Natl Acad Sci* **118:** e2019536118. doi:10.1073/pnas.2019536118

Wilmoth JW. 1997. In search of limits. In *Between Zeus and the salmon* (ed. Wachter K, Finch C), pp. 38–64. National Research Council, Washington, DC.

Wilmoth JR. 1998. The future of human longevity: a demographer's perspective. *Science* **280:** 395–397. doi:10.1126/science.280.5362.395

Cite this article as *Cold Spring Harb Perspect Med* doi: 10.1101/cshperspect.a041480

Past and Future Directions for Research on Cellular Senescence

Yi Zhu,[1,2] Zacharias P. Anastasiadis,[3] Jair Machado Espindola Netto,[2] Tamara Evans,[2] Tamar Tchkonia,[1,2] and James L. Kirkland[1,4]

[1]Department of Physiology and Biomedical Engineering; [2]Robert and Arlene Kogod Center on Aging; [3]Department of Biochemistry and Molecular Biology; [4]Division of General Internal Medicine, Department of Medicine, Mayo Clinic, Rochester, Minnesota 55905, USA

Correspondence: kirkland.james@mayo.edu

Cellular senescence was initially described in the early 1960s by Hayflick and Moorehead. They noted sustained cell-cycle arrest after repeated subculturing of human primary cells. Over half a century later, cellular senescence has become recognized as one of the fundamental pillars of aging. Developing senotherapeutics, interventions that selectively eliminate or target senescent cells, has emerged as a key focus in health research. In this article, we note major milestones in cellular senescence research, discuss current challenges, and point to future directions for this rapidly growing field.

The increase in numbers of older individuals (age > 65) to more than 20% of the population has created a global challenge in ensuring that health systems can meet the needs of older patients and foster healthier life in old age. Aging is a multifactorial and complex process that can begin even before conception (e.g., in Down syndrome [Meharena et al. 2022]), which over time leads to reduced resistance to multiple diseases, probability of survival, and capacity for self-regulation, repair, and adaptation to environmental insults (López-Otin et al. 2013; Cohen 2018). A deeper understanding of the fundamental mechanisms of aging processes is necessary to discover interventions that promote health span, the period during life free of disability, pain, cognitive impairment, and loss of independence.

The aging process is both characterized and driven by shared cellular and molecular mechanisms termed the pillars or hallmarks of aging. These include genomic instability, telomeric dysfunction, epigenetic alterations and other DNA changes, loss of proteostasis, dysregulated nutrient-sensing, mitochondrial dysfunction, progenitor ("stem") cell dysfunction, altered intercellular communication, and cellular senescence, among others (López-Otin et al. 2023). These fundamental aging mechanisms progress at the molecular, cellular, tissue, and systemic levels and largely account for older age being the leading risk factor for multiple acute and chronic disorders and diseases. These include, among many others, cardiovascular diseases, cancers, osteoarthritis, diabetes, lung, liver, kidney, skin, and eye diseases, and neurodegenerative diseases such as Alzheimer's disease (AD) and Parkinson's disease (PD) (Niccoli and Partridge 2012; Hou et al. 2019). Given that aging is a shared underlying risk factor for multiple conditions, the geroscience hypothesis holds that manipulating fundamental aging mechanisms could delay, prevent, alleviate, or treat multiple disorders and diseases.

Cellular senescence, a cell fate that entails essentially stable growth arrest and resistance to apoptosis in response to cellular damage and stress, has been implicated as a mechanism contributing to development of many diseases and age-related conditions (Tchkonia et al. 2013). Senescent cells can develop at any point during life, tend to accumulate with aging (particularly in the context of dysfunction), and can appear at sites of pathology in multiple chronic as well as acute diseases, even in younger individuals. It appears that most other fundamental aging processes can induce cellular senescence, suggesting it might be widely involved in the genesis of aging phenotypes and multiple disorders and diseases. Consequently, targeting cellular senescence may provide protection against many pathologies and perhaps even attenuate or delay declines in health span in older individuals or younger people with cellular senescence-related disorders.

THE DISCOVERY OF CELLULAR SENESCENCE

In the early 1960s, Leonard Hayflick and Paul Moorhead reported that primary human fibroblasts isolated from embryonic lung tissue fail to further proliferate after a limited number of population doublings and thereafter exhibit a characteristic flattened and enlarged morphology (Hayflick and Moorhead 1961). This phenomenon of a maximum proliferative cellular life span in noncancerous cells is recognized as the Hayflick limit, and the replicatively exhausted cells were termed senescent, from Latin "senex" meaning "old." Since then, the original

definition of cellular senescence has expanded and become relevant in multiple other contexts, including aging in vivo and diseases.

INDUCTION OF CELLULAR SENESCENCE

Cellular senescence can be triggered in response to various intrinsic and extrinsic stimuli as well as developmental signals (Kumari and Jat 2021). The most frequent senescence inducers are replicative exhaustion, ionizing and nonionizing radiation, oncogene activation, genotoxic drugs, oxidative stress, metabolic dysfunction, demethylating and acetylating agents, mechanical or shear stresses, infections, and inflammation (Hernandez-Segura et al. 2018). Senescence is a highly dynamic and orchestrated process during which the properties of senescent cells continuously change and vary depending on their microenvironmental context (Kumari and Jat 2021). The different types of inducing stimuli prompt different types of senescence, such as telomere-dependent replicative senescence, developmentally programmed senescence, or nontelomeric stress-induced premature senescence, including oncogene-induced senescence (OIS), therapy-induced senescence (TIS), unresolved DNA damage-induced senescence, epigenetically induced senescence, and mitochondrial dysfunction-associated senescence (Kumari and Jat 2021).

The cell-cycle exit during development of senescence occurs at defined cell-cycle checkpoints. Briefly considering these checkpoints provides context for use of several senescence "markers," including $p16^{INK4a}$, $p21^{CIP1/WAF1}$, cyclin-dependent kinase inhibitor 1A (P21, Cip1), and p53 (Blagosklonny and Pardee 2002). The first is the G_1/S checkpoint, also known as the restriction point. Retinoblastoma protein, Rb, is a primary regulator of the G_1 phase of the cell cycle and an important tumor suppressor. The active form of Rb is the un- or hypophosphorylated form. During the normal progression of G_1, the CDK4/cycD complex catalyzes the initial monophosphorylation of Rb and then CDK2/cycE hyperphosphorylates and inactivates Rb to release the transcription factor, E2F. E2F is itself a transcription factor for cycE. Hence, phosphorylation of Rb reinforces its inactivation through a CDK2/cycE-mediated hyperphosphorylation feedback loop. E2F then activates the transcription of genes facilitating S phase progression.

Alternatively, when a cell does not pass the restriction point, p16^{INK4A} prevents the inactivation of Rb by inhibiting CDK4/cycD and preventing the initial Rb monophosphorylation. Active Rb recruits HDAC, a histone deacetylase, which causes chromatin compaction and thereby blocks binding sites that would have been activated by the E2F transcription factors, resulting in continued repression of E2F-controlled genes and cell-cycle arrest. This can be further reinforced and stabilized in response to DNA damage by p53-mediated activation of p21$^{CIP1/WAF1}$, which inhibits the G to S phase transition by inhibiting CDK2/cycE. Under sustained stress, such as persistent DNA damage signaling or hypoxia, this temporary cell-cycle arrest can turn into permanent senescence.

The next major checkpoint is the G$_2$/M DNA damage checkpoint. The critical target of this checkpoint is CDK1/cycB, which can be inhibited in response to DNA damage by p21$^{CIP1/WAF1}$ through p53-dependent p21$^{CIP1/WAF1}$ up-regulation. Normally, CDK1/cycB activates Cdc25. Cdc25 is a phosphatase that dephosphorylates and thereby deactivates CDK1/cycB inhibitors such as Wee1. But in the event of DNA damage, p21$^{CIP1/WAF1}$ inhibition of CDK1/cycB ensures Cdc25 is not activated and Wee1 is not inhibited, further stabilizing the inhibition of CDK1/cycB by p21$^{CIP1/WAF1}$. In this way, p53 and p21$^{CIP1/WAF1}$ regulate both the G$_2$/M DNA damage checkpoint and the G$_1$/S checkpoint.

HALLMARKS OF SENESCENCE

Cellular senescence is associated with multiple phenotypic and molecular changes that can help to distinguish senescent cells from quiescent or terminally differentiated cells. In the mid-1990s, an increased lysosomal β-galactosidase activity (SA-βgal) at pH 6.0 was reported by Dimri et al. (1995) as a biomarker of cellular senescence both in situ and in vitro. Nowadays, either chemogenic or fluorescent probes can be used to detect SA-βgal by staining or flow cytometry. However, increased SA-βgal activity is neither fully sensitive (not all types of senescent cells express it) nor specific to senescent cells. It can be detected in macrophages and multiple types of postmitotic cells, such as neurons (de Mera-Rodríguez et al. 2021). Despite this, due to its technical simplicity, SA-βgal remains a commonly used assay for estimating senescent cell abundance in vivo and in vitro. Senescent cells not only have increased SA-βgal but also increased size and number of lysosomes, which result in the enhanced granularity that is sometimes used as another morphologic feature for identifying senescent cells (Robbins et al. 1970; Gorgoulis et al. 2019).

Major alterations occur not only in lysosomes but the nucleus as well. Heterochromatin reorganization occurs during progression of senescence. The heterochromatin associated with this process is most prominent among domains of facultative heterochromatin that often form in senescent human cells, termed senescence-associated heterochromatin foci (SAHF) (Narita et al. 2003). DNA segments with chromatin alterations reinforcing senescence (DNA-SCARS) are other markers indicative of senescence (Rodier et al. 2011). DNA-SCARS are dynamically formed, unique chromatin structures that functionally regulate multiple aspects of the senescent phenotype.

Dysfunctional telomeres, which are ordinarily protective structures at the ends of linear DNA comprised of specific repeated DNA elements, is another feature of senescence. Cell stresses such as hypoxia or DNA damage trigger a DNA damage response (DDR). The activation of the DDR at telomeres results in the formation of telomere-associated DDR foci (TAFs) or telomere-induced DNA damage foci (TIFs), which are sites of DNA damage that normal DNA repair mechanisms cannot repair. Thereafter, persistent DNA damage signaling initiates the senescence process. Cellular TAFs and TIFs, which are among the more sensitive and specific markers for senescence, can be quantified in cell cultures and tissues.

As discussed previously, another feature of cellular senescence is certain process-associated pathways. In response to cellular stress, diverse effector programs, including those related to cell cycling, DNA repair, and cell death, are activated to mitigate cellular and tissue damage. If the stress or damage cannot be resolved, the cellular senescence program can be initiated and regulated by the p16^{INK4a}/Rb and/or p53/p21$^{CIP1/WAF1}$ tumor suppressor pathways. They simultaneously or independently maintain the senescent state by inducing widespread changes in gene expression, since p53 and pRb are master transcriptional regulators. The p53/p21$^{CIP1/WAF1}$ and the p16^{INK4a}/Rb pathways interact with and influence each other through multiple cross-talk mechanisms. p21$^{WAF1/CIP1}$ acts downstream of p53, whereas p16^{INK4a} acts upstream of pRb. They are crucial cyclin-dependent kinase inhibitors (CDKIs) and act as negative regulators of cell-cycle progression. Thus, p16^{INK4a} and/or p21$^{CIP1/WAF1}$ are frequently, but not always, increased in senescent cells.

Cytoplasmic DNA, such as mtDNA released from stressed mitochondria or cytoplasmic chromatin fragments (CCFs) released from damaged nuclei, trigger inflammation response in senescent cells (Miller et al. 2021). Recently, the activation of endogenous retrotransposable elements, line 1 elements, and the ensuing activation of an IFN-I response, have been reported in late-stage senescent cells (De Cecco et al. 2019; Gorbunova et al. 2021).

THE SENESCENCE-ASSOCIATED SECRETORY PHENOTYPE

A functional output of senescent cells is the senescence-associated secretory phenotype, or SASP, which encompasses a variety of secreted bioactive factors that can include cytokines, chemokines, growth factors, proteases, profibrotic factors, prothrombotic factors, lipids and other metabolites and bioactive small molecules, miRNAs, other noncoding nucleotides, and extracellular vesicles (Zhu et al. 2014; Basisty et al. 2020). The SASP was initially characterized using antibody arrays in human fibroblasts and epithelial cells (Coppé et al. 2008). Given the complexity of senescence induction and differences in the cell types that become senescent, senescent cell functional output is highly diverse and context-dependent. Many stress response pathways are involved in establishing and maintaining the SASP. These pathways can also be interlinked, leading to pro-

longed activation, such as in the cases of the p38MAPK (Freund et al. 2011), mTOR/nutrient sensing (Laberge et al. 2021), JAK/STAT (Xu et al. 2016; Kandhaya-Pillai et al. 2022), NF-κB (Salminen et al. 2012), and cGAS-STING (Yang et al. 2017) pathways.

The effects of the SASP can be pleiotropic and complex. The SASP can be tissue damaging and proinflammatory or can promote tissue regeneration, and the extent of expression of different elements of the SASP depends on the type of cell that became senescent, the inducer of senescence, how long the cell has been senescent, and the microenvironment (Tripathi et al. 2021a). For example, SARS-CoV-2 S-antigen can accentuate release of tissue-damaging SASP factors (Camell et al. 2021; Tripathi et al. 2021b; Kandhaya-Pillai et al. 2022; Schmitt et al. 2023). The SASP appears to be important for many biological processes, such as embryogenesis, immune surveillance, and, in some cases, wound repair. Wound or tissue repair occurs highly dynamically and throughout life, and it involves extensive cellular communication orchestrated by cytokines, chemokines, growth factors, and components of the extracellular milieu. The SASP might sometimes be needed for new tissue formation and tissue remodeling during the wound-healing process, although there are situations in which generation of senescent cells actually impedes acute wound repair (Dańczak-Pazdrowska et al. 2023) (e.g., in muscle [Moiseeva et al. 2023] or chronic skin wounds [Wyles et al. 2023]). During embryonic development, the SASP recruits immune cells to fine-tune the embryogenesis process and enhances plasticity and stemness in surrounding cells to promote tissue regeneration (Muñoz-Espin and Serrano 2014). In addition, senescent cells can play a role in immune surveillance. They can attract, anchor, and activate immune cells at sites of damage through the SASP and act as immunogenic targets for immune clearance (Prata et al. 2018).

The SASP is an example of antagonistic pleiotropy, the evolutionary hypothesis that a trait advantageous early in life, when natural selection pressure is highest, can be selected for despite deleterious consequences of the same trait in old age. Despite the beneficial physiological functions of the SASP, persistent senescence or unresolvable senescent cell accumulation can be detrimental. Given the detrimental effects of accumulated senescent cells and the SASP (in those cases when it is tissue-damaging), senescent cells are likely causally implicated in multiple phenotypes and pathologies such as osteoarthritis-like phenotypes, frailty, impaired metabolic function, and shortened health span. In the past few years, there have been extensive studies to elucidate the role of senescence in the onset of multiple pathologies and diseases. For instance, despite cellular senescence being initiated as a protective mechanism against cancer, senescence markers have been observed in numerous human cancers. They are linked to an increased risk of recurrence and poor survival outcomes. The SASP was identified as a driver of cell growth, promoting tumorigenesis in the tumor microenvironment through a paracrine route (Gonzalez-Meljem et al. 2018) —the proteases and matrix-modifying enzymes of the SASP can alter the microenvironment, resulting in tumor progression (Coppé et al. 2010; Liu et al. 2022). Furthermore, certain cytokines released by senescent cells or that are produced by immune cells as a consequence of the presence of senescent cells such as IL-17, IL-21, and IL-23, appear to further modulate the immune response, especially adaptive T-cell subtypes, and predispose to cancers, cardiac dysfunction, neurodegeneration, infection, and frailty. In addition to the SASP factors directly released by senescent cells, tissue-damaging or disease-promoting factors such as these that are released by immune or other cell types in response to senescent cells could serve as useful gerodiagnostics (see below).

Extracellular matrix (ECM) production can be another effect of the SASP. The ECM is crucial in maintaining normal tissue structure and cell-to-cell communication, and many pathological conditions arise from dysregulated ECM remodeling because of aging or damage (Coppé et al. 2010; Blokland et al. 2020). The SASP can drive pathological increases in ECM deposition and remodeling, resulting in tissue fibrosis (Blokland et al. 2020). Additionally, the SASP can impair the functionality of progenitor cells by altering the ECM, which progenitor cells depend upon for maintaining self-renewal capability and capacity for differentiating into specialized cell types. SASP proinflammatory factors and growth factors can cause progenitor cells to lose multipotency (or "stemness") by causing sustained mitotic stimulation.

Multiple diseases and disorders involve senescent cells, and the abundance of senescent cells correlates with the onset of pathologies, including idiopathic pulmonary fibrosis (IPF), neurodegenerative diseases, liver diseases, kidney-related diseases, and cardiovascular diseases. The high burden of senescent cells in multiple metabolic and endocrine tissues was found to be associated with disease progression and dysregulated glucose homeostasis in type 2 diabetes. Removal of accumulated senescent cells increased health span in murine models, suggesting that the SASP can play a deleterious role in age-related multimorbidity. The SASP can disrupt tissue homeostasis by promoting chronic inflammation, fibrosis, and progenitor cell dysfunction. Chronic inflammation is associated with the dysfunction that can develop with aging, and the SASP can directly initiate chronic inflammation in surrounding tissues or indirectly induce secondary inflammation through chronic activation of immune cells and spread of senescence locally and systemically (Prata et al. 2018; Xu et al. 2018; Schmitt et al. 2023). Emerging evidence suggests that proinflammatory SASP factors can be amplified, potentially contributing to the high susceptibility to hyperinflammation frequently observed in the elderly in the course of multiple pathological conditions, such as infectious diseases (e.g., COVID-19 [Camell et al. 2021; Tripathi et al. 2021b]). Collectively, this evidence highlights that targeting senescent cells and/or the SASP using "senotherapeutics" might be a strategy for delaying, preventing, alleviating, or treating multiple disorders and diseases across the life span (Fig. 1).

THE GROWING FIELD OF SENOLYTICS

Given that cellular senescence is a stable cell growth arrest that often entails enhanced expression of $p21^{CIP1/WAF1}$, $p16^{INK4a}$, both (or sometimes neither), a genetic senescent cell ablation method of fusing the $p16^{INK4A}$ or $p21^{CIP1/WAF1}$ promoter region with apoptosis machinery was

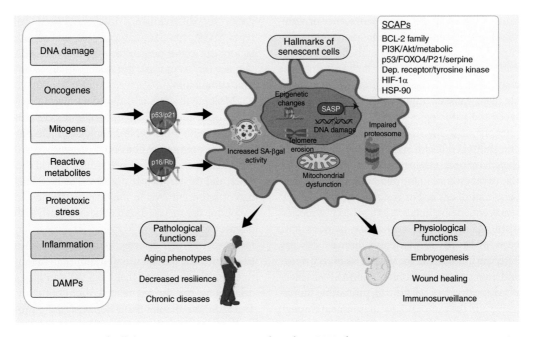

Figure 1. Features of cellular senescence. Various stimuli such as DNA damage, oncogenes, mitogens, reactive metabilites, proteotoxic stress, inflammation, and DAMPs (damage associated molecular patterns) can induce cellular senescence across the life span. Senescent cells and their senescence-associated secretory phenotype (SASP) exert both physiological and pathological roles in age-related dysfunction and multiple diseases. (Figure created with BioRender.com.)

used to target senescent cells in tissues (Baker et al. 2011; Demaria et al. 2014; Wang et al. 2022). As those senescent cells with a proapoptotic SASP rely on one or more senescent cell antiapoptotic pathways (SCAPs) to evade cell death, a hypothesis-driven and mechanism-based drug discovery approach was used to seek small molecules that selectively induce apoptosis in the senescent cells that are tissue-damaging by deactivating these SCAPs. Based on this approach, the first senolytic drugs discovered, dasatinib (D) and quercetin (Q), target key nodes of the SCAP network, including ephrins/dependence receptors, PI3Kδ/Akt/metabolic factors, and Bcl-xL; p21$^{CIP1/WAF1}$/serpines (PAI-1/PAI-2). The combination of D + Q has been used to test the effectiveness of senolytic treatment across multiple conditions (Zhu et al. 2015; Wissler Gerdes et al. 2020).

Following the initial discovery via RNA interference approaches that the BCL-2 family is a prosurvival pathway in certain types of senescent cells (Zhu et al. 2015), the Bcl-2/Bcl-xL inhibitors

navitoclax, A-1331852, and A-1155463 were confirmed to be senolytic in many but not all senescent cell types (Zhu et al. 2016, 2017). However, off-target effects of Bcl-2 family inhibitors on platelets and neutrophils limit their translational potential. Later, multiple senolytic compounds targeting different SCAPs were developed, including HSP90 inhibitors (Fuhrmann-Stroissnigg et al. 2017), FOXO4-p53 inhibitors (Baar et al. 2017), and Na$^+$/K$^+$-ATPase inhibitors (Triana-Martínez et al. 2019). In addition, natural flavonoids and related compounds such as fisetin, piperlongumine, curcumin, and procyanidin C1 showed certain senolytic activities, although their exact molecular mechanisms of action are not yet fully clear in all cases (Wang et al. 2016; Zhu et al. 2016; Yousefzadeh et al. 2018; Li et al. 2019; Xu et al. 2021).

Another approach for eliminating senescent cells is to use proteolysis-targeting chimeras (PROTACs): fused molecules comprising a ligand specific to a target protein and a ligand capable of recruiting an E3 ubiquitin ligase (Sakamoto et al. 2001). PROTACs can recognize and degrade targeted SCAP proteins through the ubiquitin–proteasome system, which induces cell death in the senescent cells that rely on those particular SCAPs. Despite the potential to reduce off-target effects using PROTACs, they are large molecules comprising fused ligands and further pharmacokinetic and pharmacodynamic studies will be needed to enable efficient delivery in vivo (He et al. 2020).

Senomorphics, also known as senostatics, reduce SASP factor release without inducing senescent cell death. Given the complexity of senescence induction, the SASP can be blunted by interfering in one or multiple SASP regulatory pathways, such as p38-MAPK inhibitors, NF-κB inhibitors, mTOR inhibitors, and JAK/STAT3 inhibitors. Alternately, senomorphic effects may be achieved through specific neutralizing antibodies against individual SASP factors, such as IL-1α, IL-8, Activin A, or IL-6 (Zhang et al. 2023). Senomorphics may not only attenuate release of tissue-damaging SASP factors, but also delay or prevent senescence induction due to the spread of senescence caused by certain SASP factors. Maintaining the effects of senomorphics can entail a need for more continuous administration than senolytics to achieve SASP-inhibiting blood levels, which might be problematic due to the lack of specificity for senescent cells of some senomorphic drugs (Wissler Gerdes et al. 2020; Zhang et al. 2023).

Recently, other novel senotherapeutic strategies have been devised based on the modulating immune system. Surveillance by senescent cells can activate immune cell responses and recruit particular classes of immune cells (Kale et al. 2020; Chen et al. 2023), such as macrophages, natural killer (NK) cells, or cytotoxic T cells. Aging or tissue damage can impede immune cell function through a separate, non-cell-cycle-based process, immunosenescence, partly explaining the accumulation of senescent cells in tissues with aging. Developing immunotherapies targeting senescent cells might be a tractable senotherapeutic strategy. For example, the chimeric antigen receptor T (CART)-cell therapy approach was developed to specifically target senescent cells through a senescent cell-specific surface marker, urokinase-type

plasminogen activator receptor (uPAR), and may be of benefit for treating liver adenocarcinoma and liver fibrosis in preclinical models (Amor et al. 2020). DPP4 (dipeptidyl-peptidase 4) is another potential senescent cell-surface target expressed by certain types of senescent cells (Kim et al. 2017). Anti-DPP4 antibodies have been used to recognize DPP4-positive senescent cells and lead to their preferential elimination by NK cells (Kim et al. 2017). Other immunotherapies were subsequently developed based on senescent cell-surface markers, including B2M, CD9 receptor, NOTCH receptors (Yoshioka et al. 2021), and others (Rossi and Abdelmohsen 2021). Vaccination is another potential approach: mice were immunized against the antigen, glycoprotein nonmetastatic melanoma protein B (GPNMB), a senescent cell-surface marker (Suda et al. 2022). Although immune clearance of senescent cells has potentially promising outcomes, a deeper understanding of the interplay between senescent cells and the immune system is critical, warranting more studies to achieve insight relevant for designing immune cell–based interventions to treat age-related dysfunction and chronic diseases. Also, methods need to be developed for stopping continued senescent cell removal due to immune therapy–mediated interventions should senescent cells be needed (e.g., during pregnancy for placental mediation of parturition).

HUMAN STUDIES

The first in situ evidence that senescent cells present and accumulate with age in human skin tissues was reported in 2009 by taking advantage of increased SA-βgal activity (Dimri et al. 1995). Since then, many senescence hallmarks have been used to identify senescent cells across human tissues and organs, not only during the aging process but also related to multiple diseases (Tuttle et al. 2021). Indeed, senescent cell accumulation with aging in healthy individuals is sometimes slight: those older individuals with frailty and multimorbidity may have a higher senescent cell burden than healthy older individuals. Greater expression of the senescence markers, γH2AX, p16^{INK4A}, p21$^{CIP1/WAF1}$, and p53, was observed in glial cells, progenitor cells, and damaged neurons with tau tangles in humans with neurodegenerative diseases than those without (Jurk et al. 2012; Shanbhag et al. 2019; Vazquez-Villasenor et al. 2020). These markers were also present in the context of eye pathologies, and some, not all, of these markers are associated with specific stages of eye diseases, including endothelial corneal dystrophy, glaucoma, cataracts, and retinal microaneurysms (Lee et al. 2021a; López-Otin et al. 2023). p16^{INK4A} was increased in the human livers with fibrosis, and p16^{INK4A} correlated with histological stages of fibrosis (Wandrer et al. 2018). Other senescent cell markers, including telomeric dysfunction (Amsellem et al. 2011), SASP regulators (Houssaini et al. 2018), and Lamin B1 (Saito et al. 2019), have been used to track senescent cell abundance in lung tissues from patients with chronic obstructive pulmonary disease (COPD). Recently, patients with SARS-CoV-2 infection were shown to have senescence markers in their airway mucosa and increased circulating SASP factors (Lee et al. 2021b). Despite extensive evidence for increased senescent cell burden in human tissues in multiple disorders and diseases, the use of robust and universal senescence markers to precisely characterize the dynamics and function of senescent cells in situ remains challenging due to the heterogeneous nature of senescent cells across tissues and disease states.

To extend successful preclinical findings to humans, more than 20 clinical trials of senolytic therapies have been initiated and some of them have been completed. Although much is known about side effects of the senolytic agents in these trials from experience during their use over many years for treating other conditions or their being natural products, much remains to be learned about them in the context of being administered as senolytics, especially potential long-term side effects. To explore their efficiency and effectiveness, pilot clinical trials have proceeded in patients with serious conditions, such as diabetic kidney disease, AD, advanced frailty, and IPF. The results of the first-in-human, single-arm, open-label clinical trial of senolytics (D + Q) were reported in 2019 (Justice et al. 2019). Fourteen subjects with IPF, a senescence-associated disease, showed improved physical performance 5 days after nine doses of D + Q over 3 weeks (Cope 1986; Justice et al. 2019). However, as this study was not placebo-controlled and was small, a phase 2 trial is necessary before firm conclusions can be drawn. Intriguingly, a post hoc analysis of a continuation of this study involving 20 subjects showed increased urine levels of the geroprotective factor α-Klotho after compared to before senolytic treatment (Zhu et al. 2022).

The first evidence for senescent cell clearance by senolytics in humans was reported in an open-label phase 1 pilot study in which nine subjects with diabetic kidney disease were recruited and administered 3 days of D + Q (Hickson et al. 2019). A significant reduction of p16^{INK4A} and p21$^{CIP1/WAF1}$ highly expressing senescent cells and SA-βgal-positive cells was observed in adipose tissue. Circulating SASP factors, including IL-1α, IL-6, and matrix metalloproteinases (MMPs), were decreased after compared to before senolytic administration. Given encouraging preclinical results of senolytics in AD mouse models, an open-label pilot trial (SToMP-AD) tested safety, feasibility, and efficacy of D + Q in five subjects with early-stage AD (Gonzales et al. 2022). This pilot study was completed recently, and preliminary results are about to be published. Not all initial studies of senolytics have been successful: a pilot human trial by a biotech company reported that treatment with an MDM2 inhibitor-based senolytic compound, UBX101, in patients with osteoarthritis failed to meet its primary end point. It needs to be anticipated that many trials will fail, adding to the imperative to view current trials as initial steps along a potentially long path, particularly before senolytics are considered for preventing conditions in relatively healthy individuals. The pilot clinical trials have provided valuable data about the feasibility of testing senolytics in future larger randomized controlled trials for serious senescence-related diseases. Growing numbers of clinical studies are underway or planned to examine the effectiveness of senolytics for senescence-associated conditions, including COVID-19, age-related skeletal health, frailty in cancer survivors, diabetic macular edema, neovascular age-related macular degeneration, and others (Table 1).

Table 1. Examples of ongoing clinical trials of senolytics

ClinicalTrials.gov number	Trial title	Current status	Diseases	Senolytics	Phase
NCT04785300	ALSENLITE: senolytics for Alzheimer's disease	Enrolling by invitation	Mild cognitive impairment; Alzheimer's disease	Dasatinib + quercetin	Phases 1 and 2 (PMID:34366147)
NCT04733534	An open-label intervention trial to reduce senescence and improve frailty in adult survivors of childhood cancer	Recruiting	Frailty; childhood cancer	Dasatinib + quercetin; fisetin	Phase 2
NCT04537299	COVID-FIS: pilot in COVID-19 (SARS-CoV-2) of fisetin in older adults in nursing homes	Enrolling by invitation	Covid19; SARS-CoV infection	Fisetin	Phase 2 (PMID:34375437)
NCT04476953	COVID-FISETIN: pilot in SARS-CoV-2 of fisetin to alleviate dysfunction and inflammation	Enrolling by invitation	Covid19	Fisetin	Phase 2
NCT04771611	COVFIS-HOME: COVID-19 pilot study of fisetin to alleviate dysfunction and decrease complications	Completed	Covid19	Fisetin	Phase 2
NCT04313634	Targeting cellular senescence with senolytics to improve skeletal health in older humans	Recruiting	Healthy	Dasatinib + quercetin; fisetin	Phase 2
NCT04063124	Senolytic therapy to modulate progression of Alzheimer's disease	Completed	Alzheimer's disease	Dasatinib + quercetin	Phases 1 and 2 (PMID:34687726)
NCT03675724	Alleviation by fisetin of frailty, inflammation, and related measures in older adults	Recruiting	Frail elderly syndrome	Fisetin	Phase 2
NCT03430037	Alleviation by fisetin of frailty, inflammation, and related measures in older women	Recruiting	Frail elderly syndrome	Fisetin	Phase 2
NCT03325322	Inflammation and stem cells in diabetic and chronic kidney disease	Enrolling by invitation	Chronic kidney diseases; diabetic nephropathies	Fisetin	Phase 2
NCT02874989	Targeting proinflammatory cells in idiopathic pulmonary fibrosis: a human trial	Completed	Idiopathic pulmonary fibrosis	Dasatinib + quercetin	Phase 1 (PMID:30616998)
NCT02848131	Senescence in chronic kidney disease	Enrolling by invitation	Chronic kidney disease	Dasatinib + quercetin	Phase 2 (PMID:31542391)
NCT02652052	Hematopoietic Stem Cell Transplant Survivors Study (HTSS)	Recruiting	Stem cell transplant	Dasatinib + quercetin	Not applicable

Continued

Table 1. *Continued*

ClinicalTrials.gov number	Trial title	Current status	Diseases	Senolytics	Phase
NCT04771611	COVFIS-HOME: COVID-19 pilot study of fisetin to alleviate dysfunction and decrease complications	Enrolling by invitation	Covid19; coronavirus infection	Fisetin	Phase 2
NCT04685590	Senolytic therapy to modulate the progression of Alzheimer's disease (SToMP-AD) study	Recruiting	Alzheimer's disease; early onset of mild cognitive impairment	Dasatinib + quercetin	Phase 2 (PMID:34366147; 34687726)
NCT04210986	Senolytic drugs attenuate osteoarthritis-related articular cartilage degeneration: a clinical trial	Active, not recruiting	Osteoarthritis	Dasatinib + quercetin	Phases 1 and 2
NCT05416515	A study of fisetin to treat carpal tunnel syndrome	Recruiting	Carpal tunnel syndrome	Fisetin	Phase 2
NCT05593588	Senolytics treatment of interstitial lung disease in common variable immunodeficiency	Not yet recruiting	Common variable immunodeficiency	Fisetin	Phase 2
NCT05595499	Treatment of frailty with fisetin (TROFFi) in breast cancer survivors	Recruiting	Breast cancer	Fisetin	Phase 2

Cite this article as *Cold Spring Harb Perspect Med* doi: 10.1101/cshperspect.a041205

TRANSLATIONAL GEROSCIENCE NETWORK

The Translational Geroscience Network (TGN) was established to accelerate testing the geroscience hypothesis that targeting fundamental aging mechanisms, including cellular senescence, can delay, prevent, alleviate, or treat multiple diseases and disabilities in humans. Envisioning a time- and cost-efficient approach to conducting geroscience-guided trials targeting the biology of aging, the national TGN collaborative was initiated by eight U.S. research institutes—Mayo Clinic, Harvard, John Hopkins, Wake Forest, Universities of Minnesota, Michigan, and Connecticut, and University of Texas Health Sciences Center at San Antonio—with additional collaborators at Northwestern University, St. Jude Children's Cancer Center, City of Hope, the Steadman Philippon Clinic, and others (Fig. 2).

The TGN provides expertise, infrastructure, and coordination needed for geroscience-based studies to be conducted in parallel and with comparable designs, as well as sharing data generated by these studies. It is hoped this will accelerate the discovery and translation of interventions targeting fundamental aging mechanisms into clinical application. Beyond fundamental scientific and regulatory support for the trials, the TGN also created both a Facility for Geroscience Analysis (FGA), which assays >150 factors in body fluids and other biospecimens across the trials, and a biobank to facilitate reverse translation from bedside to bench to fuel discovery science. The FGA is developing, standardizing, and implementing sensitive, reproducible, and reliable methods to measure candidate gerodiagnostics and composites of tests that assay all of the pillars of aging, predict which interventions to use and when, follow responses to geroscience interventions, and predict clinical improvement (Fig. 3). The TGN has a subcommittee that manages data acquisition, analysis, and development of predictive algorithms. The

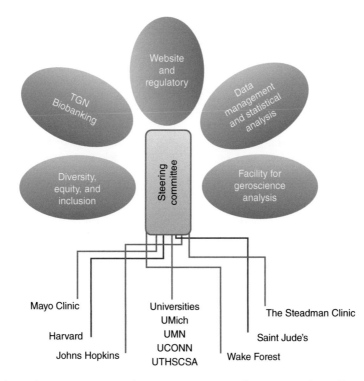

Figure 2. Translational Geroscience Network structure, partners, and governance. (UMich) University of Michigan, (UMN) University of Minnesota, (UCONN) University of Connecticut, (UTHSCSA) University of Texas Health Sciences Center at San Antonio.

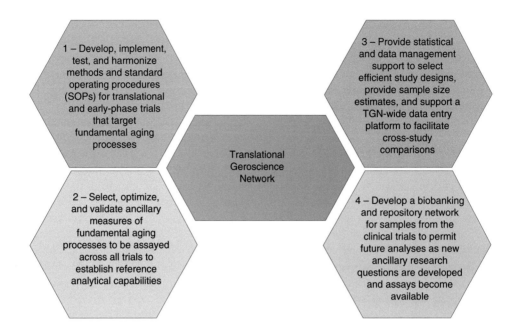

Figure 3. Translational Geroscience Network (TGN) activities for facilitating geroscience-focused clinical trials.

TGN may help to accelerate exploration of the translational potential of senotherapeutics for challenging diseases and disorders across the life span.

CONCLUDING REMARKS AND FUTURE PERSPECTIVES

The rapidly growing field of cellular senescence has opened up many challenging yet unsettled questions. First, the most widely used senescence markers, SA-βgal and the cell-cycle inhibitors, p16^{INK4A} and p21$^{CIP1/WAF1}$, are neither fully sensitive nor specific for identifying senescent cells. Given that the dynamics of senescent cell occurrence and accumulation are cell origin-, causation-, stage-, and physiological context–dependent, it may be difficult to pinpoint a single universal marker for detecting all senescent cells. There is a need to identify and characterize different types of senescent cells across organs, various health conditions, and the life span. Delineating biological functions and consequences of different types of senescent cells will require precise spatial and temporal information about senescent cells and their changes in response to interventions in humans. Advances in single-

cell technologies provide opportunities to profile features of DNA methylation, chromatin accessibility, mRNA, and protein expression at single-cell resolution. Integrative single-cell multiomics analysis holds potential for characterizing senescent cell subtypes, possibly offering new insights into their function and pathophysiological processes. Importantly, these technologies open an avenue for identifying novel factors that can potentially be used for developing new mouse models to study the biology of cellular senescence and identify additional senolytic targets. Application of artificial intelligence algorithms to integrative single-cell multiomics analysis may also be useful in identifying new interventions.

A threshold hypothesis about senescent cell accumulation has been proposed (Chaib et al. 2022). This posits that accumulation of whole-body senescent cell burden results in paracrine and endocrine spread of senescence that outpaces the capacity of the immune system to clear them, resulting in accumulation. This triggers and accelerates pathogenic changes. Importantly, accelerated accumulation of persistent senescent cells may predispose to multiple age-related phenotypes and diseases, perhaps contributing to age-related multimorbidity. Despite the detrimental roles of senescent cells, they also have necessary physiological functions. Carefully distinguishing physiological or "beneficial" from pathological accumulation of senescent cells and developing interventions specifically targeting detrimental cells could be of benefit.

Genome instability, inflammation, low NAD$^+$, mitochondrial dysfunction, oxidative stress, protein aggregates, and lipotoxicity can induce cellular senescence. Conversely, senescent cells appear to causally contribute to and exacerbate many of other fundamental aging processes, such as inflammation, fibrosis, NAD$^+$ depletion, decreased α-Klotho, accumulation of aggregated and misfolded proteins, progenitor cell dysfunction, adaptive immune cell dysfunction, and others. Hence, fundamental aging processes appear to be interlinked, supporting a "unitary theory of targeting fundamental aging mechanisms": that targeting one fundamental aging mechanism may alleviate many or most of the others. This may explain in part why targeting a single fundamental aging mechanism, such as cellular senescence, can delay, prevent, or alleviate multiple age-related phenotypes as a group. If the unitary theory is correct, it will be critical to test whether combining individual interventions targeting different aging mechanisms results in less-than-additive, additive, or synergistic effects. More needs to be understood about nondividing, differentiated cell types, such as neurons, adipocytes, osteocytes, or cardiomyocytes, which can acquire a senescent-like state, and the SASP of such cells. Whether and how such cells contribute to tissue dysfunction and to what extent these cells should be eliminated is as yet unclear.

There has been initial success in very small, early human pilot trials of senolytics. However, the impact of senescent cell clearance needs much further study in double-blind, placebo-controlled clinical trials, including for repurposed agents or natural products with safety profiles already known in other contexts. Unless such trials show target engagement, minimal short- and long-term adverse events, and clinical utility, in our view these interventions should not be prescribed in routine clinical practice or used over-the-counter by the general public. Given that cellular senescence is a common contributing factor to multiple diseases and disorders, future clinical trials combining senolytics with disease-specific interventions hold additional potential for treating currently incurable diseases such as many neurodegenerative diseases and cancers.

REFERENCES

Amor C, Feucht J, Leibold J, Ho YJ, Zhu C, Alonso-Curbelo D, Mansilla-Soto J, Boyer JA, Li X, Giavridis T, et al. 2020. Senolytic CAR T cells reverse senescence-associated pathologies. *Nature* 583: 127–132. doi:10.1038/s41586-020-2403-9

Amsellem V, Gary-Bobo G, Marcos E, Maitre B, Chaar V, Validire P, Stern JB, Noureddine H, Sapin E, Rideau D, et al. 2011. Telomere dysfunction causes sustained inflammation in chronic obstructive pulmonary disease. *Am J Respir Crit Care Med* 184: 1358–1366. doi:10.1164/rccm.201105-0802OC

Baar MP, Brandt RMC, Putavet DA, Klein JDD, Derks KWJ, Bourgeois BRM, Stryeck S, Rijksen Y, van Willigenburg H, Feijtel DA, et al. 2017. Targeted apoptosis of senescent cells restores tissue homeostasis in response to chemotoxicity and aging. *Cell* 169: 132–147.e16. doi:10.1016/j.cell.2017.02.031

Baker DJ, Wijshake T, Tchkonia T, LeBrasseur NK, Childs BG, van de Sluis B, Kirkland JL, van Deursen JM. 2011. Clearance of p16Ink4a-positive senescent cells delays ageing-associated disorders. *Nature* 479: 232–236. doi:10.1038/nature10600

Basisty N, Kale A, Jeon OH, Kuehnemann C, Payne T, Rao C, Holtz A, Shah S, Sharma V, Ferrucci L, et al. 2020. A proteomic atlas of senescence-associated secretomes for aging biomarker development. *PLoS Biol* 18: e3000599. doi:10.1371/journal.pbio.3000599

Blagosklonny MV, Pardee AB. 2002. The restriction point of the cell cycle. *Cell Cycle* 1: 103–110. doi:10.4161/cc.1.2.108

Blokland KEC, Pouwels SD, Schuliga M, Knight DA, Burgess JK. 2020. Regulation of cellular senescence by extracellular matrix during chronic fibrotic diseases. *Clin Sci (Lond)* 134: 2681–2706. doi:10.1042/CS20190893

Camell CD, Yousefzadeh MJ, Zhu Y, Prata L, Huggins MA, Pierson M, Zhang L, O'Kelly RD, Pirtskhalava T, Xun P, et al. 2021. Senolytics reduce coronavirus-related mortality in old mice. *Science* 373: eabe4832. doi:10.1126/science.abe4832

Chaib S, Tchkonia T, Kirkland JL. 2022. Cellular senescence and senolytics: the path to the clinic. *Nat Med* 28: 1556–1568. doi:10.1038/s41591-022-01923-y

Chen HA, Ho YJ, Mezzadra R, Adrover JM, Smolkin R, Zhu C, Woess K, Bernstein N, Schmitt SG, Fong L, et al. 2023. Senescence rewires microenvironment sensing to facilitate antitumor immunity. *Cancer Discov* 13: 432–453. doi:10.1158/2159-8290.CD-22-0528

Cohen AA. 2018. Aging across the tree of life: the importance of a comparative perspective for the use of animal models in aging. *Biochim Biophys Acta Mol Basis Dis* **1864:** 2680–2689. doi:10.1016/j.bbadis.2017.05.028

Cope C. 1986. Minipuncture angiography. *Radiol Clin North Am* **24:** 359–367. doi:10.1016/S0033-8389(22)00842-9

Coppé JP, Patil CK, Rodier F, Sun Y, Muñoz DP, Goldstein J, Nelson PS, Desprez PY, Campisi J. 2008. Senescence-associated secretory phenotypes reveal cell-nonautonomous functions of oncogenic RAS and the p53 tumor suppressor. *PLoS Biol* **6:** 2853–2868. doi:10.1371/journal.pbio.0060301

Coppé JP, Desprez PY, Krtolica A, Campisi J. 2010. The senescence-associated secretory phenotype: the dark side of tumor suppression. *Annu Rev Pathol* **5:** 99–118. doi:10.1146/annurev-pathol-121808-102144

Dańczak-Pazdrowska A, Gornowicz-Porowska J, Polańska A, Krajka-Kuźniak V, Stawny M, Gostyńska A, Rubiś B, Nourredine S, Ashiqueali S, Schneider A, et al. 2023. Cellular senescence in skin-related research: targeted signaling pathways and naturally occurring therapeutic agents. *Aging Cell* **22:** e13845. doi:10.1111/acel.13845

De Cecco M, Ito T, Petrashen AP, Elias AE, Skvir NJ, Criscione SW, Caligiana A, Broccoli G, Adney EM, Boeke JD, et al. 2019. L1 drives IFN in senescent cells and promotes age-associated inflammation. *Nature* **566:** 73–78. doi:10.1038/s41586-018-0784-9

Demaria M, Ohtani N, Youssef SA, Rodier F, Toussaint W, Mitchell JR, Laberge RM, Vijg J, Van Steeg H, Dollé ME, et al. 2014. An essential role for senescent cells in optimal wound healing through secretion of PDGF-AA. *Dev Cell* **31:** 722–733. doi:10.1016/j.devcel.2014.11.012

de Mera-Rodríguez JA, Álvarez-Hernán G, Gañan Y, Martín-Partido G, Rodríguez-León J, Francisco-Morcillo J. 2021. Is senescence-associated β-galactosidase a reliable in vivo marker of cellular senescence during embryonic development? *Front Cell Dev Biol* **9:** 623175. doi:10.3389/fcell.2021.623175

Dimri GP, Lee X, Basile G, Acosta M, Scott G, Roskelley C, Medrano EE, Linskens M, Rubelj I, Pereira-Smith O, et al. 1995. A biomarker that identifies senescent human cells in culture and in aging skin in vivo. *Proc Natl Acad Sci* **92:** 9363–9367. doi:10.1073/pnas.92.20.9363

Freund A, Patil CK, Campisi J. 2011. p38MAPK is a novel DNA damage response-independent regulator of the senescence-associated secretory phenotype. *EMBO J* **30:** 1536–1548. doi:10.1038/emboj.2011.69

Fuhrmann-Stroissnigg H, Ling YY, Zhao J, McGowan SJ, Zhu Y, Brooks RW, Grassi D, Gregg SQ, Stripay JL, Dorronsoro A, et al. 2017. Identification of HSP90 inhibitors as a novel class of senolytics. *Nat Commun* **8:** 422. doi:10.1038/s41467-017-00314-z

Gonzales MM, Garbarino VR, Marques Zilli E, Petersen RC, Kirkland JL, Tchkonia T, Musi N, Seshadri S, Craft S, Orr ME. 2022. Senolytic therapy to modulate the progression of Alzheimer's disease (SToMP-AD): a pilot clinical trial. *J Prev Alzheimers Dis* **9:** 22–29. doi:10.14283/jpad.2021.62

Gonzalez-Meljem JM, Apps JR, Fraser HC, Martinez-Barbera JP. 2018. Paracrine roles of cellular senescence in promoting tumourigenesis. *Br J Cancer* **118:** 1283–1288. doi:10.1038/s41416-018-0066-1

Gorbunova V, Seluanov A, Mita P, McKerrow W, Fenyö D, Boeke JD, Linker SB, Gage FH, Kreiling JA, Petrashen AP, et al. 2021. The role of retrotransposable elements in ageing and age-associated diseases. *Nature* **596:** 43–53. doi:10.1038/s41586-021-03542-y

Gorgoulis V, Adams PD, Alimonti A, Bennett DC, Bischof O, Bishop C, Campisi J, Collado M, Evangelou K, Ferbeyre G, et al. 2019. Cellular senescence: defining a path forward. *Cell* **179:** 813–827. doi:10.1016/j.cell.2019.10.005

Hayflick L, Moorhead PS. 1961. The serial cultivation of human diploid cell strains. *Exp Cell Res* **25:** 585–621. doi:10.1016/0014-4827(61)90192-6

He Y, Zhang X, Chang J, Kim HN, Zhang P, Wang Y, Khan S, Liu X, Zhang X, Lv D, et al. 2020. Using proteolysis-targeting chimera technology to reduce navitoclax platelet toxicity and improve its senolytic activity. *Nat Commun* **11:** 1996. doi:10.1038/s41467-020-15838-0

Hernandez-Segura A, Brandenburg S, Demaria M. 2018. Induction and validation of cellular senescence in primary human cells. *J Vis Exp.* doi:10.3791/57782-v

Hickson LJ, Langhi Prata LGP, Bobart SA, Evans TK, Giorgadze N, Hashmi SK, Herrmann SM, Jensen MD, Jia Q, Jordan KL, et al. 2019. Senolytics decrease senescent cells in humans: preliminary report from a clinical trial of dasatinib plus quercetin in individuals with diabetic kidney disease. *EBioMedicine* **47:** 446–456. doi:10.1016/j.ebiom.2019.08.069

Hou Y, Dan X, Babbar M, Wei Y, Hasselbalch SG, Croteau DL, Bohr VA. 2019. Ageing as a risk factor for neurodegenerative disease. *Nat Rev Neurol* **15:** 565–581. doi:10.1038/s41582-019-0244-7

Houssaini A, Breau M, Kebe K, Abid S, Marcos E, Lipskaia L, Rideau D, Parpaleix A, Huang J, Amsellem V, et al. 2018. mTOR pathway activation drives lung cell senescence and emphysema. *JCI Insight* **3:** e93203. doi:10.1172/jci.insight.93203

Jurk D, Wang C, Miwa S, Maddick M, Korolchuk V, Tsolou A, Gonos ES, Thrasivoulou C, Saffrey MJ, Cameron K, et al. 2012. Postmitotic neurons develop a p21-dependent senescence-like phenotype driven by a DNA damage response. *Aging Cell* **11:** 996–1004. doi:10.1111/j.1474-9726.2012.00870.x

Justice JN, Nambiar AM, Tchkonia T, LeBrasseur NK, Pascual R, Hashmi SK, Prata L, Masternak MM, Kritchevsky SB, Musi N, et al. 2019. Senolytics in idiopathic pulmonary fibrosis: results from a first-in-human, open-label, pilot study. *EBioMedicine* **40:** 554–563. doi:10.1016/j.ebiom.2018.12.052

Kale A, Sharma A, Stolzing A, Desprez PY, Campisi J. 2020. Role of immune cells in the removal of deleterious senescent cells. *Immun Ageing* **17:** 16. doi:10.1186/s12979-020-00187-9

Kandhaya-Pillai R, Yang X, Tchkonia T, Martin GM, Kirkland JL, Oshima J. 2022. TNF-α/IFN-γ synergy amplifies senescence-associated inflammation and SARS-CoV-2 receptor expression via hyper-activated JAK/STAT1. *Aging Cell* **21:** e13646. doi:10.1111/acel.13646

Kim KM, Noh JH, Bodogai M, Martindale JL, Yang X, Indig FE, Basu SK, Ohnuma K, Morimoto C, Johnson PF, et al. 2017. Identification of senescent cell surface targetable

protein DPP4. *Genes Dev* **31:** 1529–1534. doi:10.1101/gad
.302570.117

Kumari R, Jat P. 2021. Mechanisms of cellular senescence:
cell cycle arrest and senescence associated secretory phenotype. *Front Cell Dev Biol* **9:** 645593. doi:10.3389/fcell
.2021.645593

Laberge RM, Sun Y, Orjalo AV, Patil CK, Freund A, Zhou L,
Curran SC, Davalos AR, Wilson-Edell KA, Liu S, et al.
2021. Author correction: MTOR regulates the pro-tumor-
igenic senescence-associated secretory phenotype by promoting IL1A translation. *Nat Cell Biol* **23:** 564–565.
doi:10.1038/s41556-021-00655-4

Lee KS, Lin S, Copland DA, Dick AD, Liu J. 2021a. Cellular
senescence in the aging retina and developments of seno-
therapies for age-related macular degeneration. *J Neuroinflammation* **18:** 32. doi:10.1186/s12974-021-02088-0

Lee S, Yu Y, Trimpert J, Benthani F, Mairhofer M, Richter-
Pechanska P, Wyler E, Belenki D, Kaltenbrunner S,
Pammer M, et al. 2021b. Virus-induced senescence is a
driver and therapeutic target in COVID-19. *Nature* **599:**
283–289. doi:10.1038/s41586-021-03995-1

Li W, He Y, Zhang R, Zheng G, Zhou D. 2019. The curcumin
analog EF24 is a novel senolytic agent. *Aging (Albany NY)*
11: 771–782. doi:10.18632/aging.101787

Liu H, Zhao H, Sun Y. 2022. Tumor microenvironment and
cellular senescence: understanding therapeutic resistance
and harnessing strategies. *Semin Cancer Biol* **86:** 769–781.
doi:10.1016/j.semcancer.2021.11.004

López-Otín C, Blasco MA, Partridge L, Serrano M, Kroemer
G. 2013. The hallmarks of aging. *Cell* **153:** 1194–1217.
doi:10.1016/j.cell.2013.05.039

López-Otín C, Blasco MA, Partridge L, Serrano M, Kroemer
G. 2023. Hallmarks of aging: An expanding universe. *Cell*
186: 243–278. doi:10.1016/j.cell.2022.11.001

Meharena HS, Marco A, Dileep V, Lockshin ER, Akatsu GY,
Mullahoo J, Watson LA, Ko T, Guerin LN, Abdurrob F, et
al. 2022. Down-syndrome-induced senescence disrupts
the nuclear architecture of neural progenitors. *Cell Stem
Cell* **29:** 116–130 e7. doi:10.1016/j.stem.2021.12.002

Miller KN, Victorelli SG, Salmonowicz H, Dasgupta N,
Liu T, Passos JF, Adams PD. 2021. Cytoplasmic DNA:
sources, sensing, and role in aging and disease. *Cell* **184:**
5506–5526. doi:10.1016/j.cell.2021.09.034

Moiseeva V, Cisneros A, Sica V, Deryagin O, Lai Y, Jung S,
Andrés E, An J, Segalés J, Ortet L, et al. 2023. Senescence
atlas reveals an aged-like inflamed niche that blunts muscle regeneration. *Nature* **613:** 169–178. doi:10.1038/
s41586-022-05535-x

Muñoz-Espin D, Serrano M. 2014. Cellular senescence: from
physiology to pathology. *Nat Rev Mol Cell Biol* **15:** 482–
496. doi:10.1038/nrm3823

Narita M, Nuñez S, Heard E, Narita M, Lin AW, Hearn SA,
Spector DL, Hannon GJ, Lowe SW. 2003. Rb-mediated
heterochromatin formation and silencing of E2F target
genes during cellular senescence. *Cell* **113:** 703–716.
doi:10.1016/S0092-8674(03)00401-X

Niccoli T, Partridge L. 2012. Ageing as a risk factor for disease. *Curr Biol* **22:** R741–R752. doi:10.1016/j.cub.2012.07
.024

Prata L, Ovsyannikova IG, Tchkonia T, Kirkland JL. 2018.
Senescent cell clearance by the immune system: emerging

therapeutic opportunities. *Semin Immunol* **40:** 101275.
doi:10.1016/j.smim.2019.04.003

Robbins E, Levine EM, Eagle H. 1970. Morphologic changes
accompanying senescence of cultured human diploid
cells. *J Exp Med* **131:** 1211–1222. doi:10.1084/jem.131.6
.1211

Rodier F, Muñoz DP, Teachenor R, Chu V, Le O, Bhaumik D,
Coppé JP, Campeau E, Beauséjour CM, Kim SH, et al.
2011. DNA-SCARS: distinct nuclear structures that sustain damage-induced senescence growth arrest and inflammatory cytokine secretion. *J Cell Sci* **124:** 68–81.
doi:10.1242/jcs.071340

Rossi M, Abdelmohsen K. 2021. The emergence of senescent
surface biomarkers as senotherapeutic targets. *Cells* **10:**
1740. doi:10.3390/cells10071740

Saito N, Araya J, Ito S, Tsubouchi K, Minagawa S, Hara H, Ito
A, Nakano T, Hosaka Y, Ichikawa A, et al. 2019. Involvement of lamin B1 reduction in accelerated cellular senescence during chronic obstructive pulmonary disease
pathogenesis. *J Immunol* **202:** 1428–1440. doi:10.4049/
jimmunol.1801293

Sakamoto KM, Kim KB, Kumagai A, Mercurio F, Crews CM,
Deshaies RJ. 2001. Protacs: chimeric molecules that target
proteins to the Skp1-Cullin-F box complex for ubiquitination and degradation. *Proc Natl Acad Sci* **98:** 8554–
8559. doi:10.1073/pnas.141230798

Salminen A, Kauppinen A, Kaarniranta K. 2012. Emerging
role of NF-κB signaling in the induction of senescence-
associated secretory phenotype (SASP). *Cell Signal* **24:**
835–845. doi:10.1016/j.cellsig.2011.12.006

Schmitt CA, Tchkonia T, Niedernhofer LJ, Robbins PD,
Kirkland JL, Lee S. 2023. COVID-19 and cellular senescence. *Nat Rev Immunol* **23:** 251–263. doi:10.1038/
s41577-022-00785-2

Shanbhag NM, Evans MD, Mao W, Nana AL, Seeley WW,
Adame A, Rissman RA, Masliah E, Mucke L. 2019. Early
neuronal accumulation of DNA double strand breaks in
Alzheimer's disease. *Acta Neuropathol Commun* **7:** 77.
doi:10.1186/s40478-019-0723-5

Suda M, Shimizu I, Katsuumi G, Hsiao CL, Yoshida Y, Matsumoto N, Yoshida Y, Katayama A, Wada J, Seki M, et al.
2022. Glycoprotein nonmetastatic melanoma protein B
regulates lysosomal integrity and lifespan of senescent
cells. *Sci Rep* **12:** 6522. doi:10.1038/s41598-022-10522-3

Tchkonia T, Zhu Y, van Deursen J, Campisi J, Kirkland JL.
2013. Cellular senescence and the senescent secretory
phenotype: therapeutic opportunities. *J Clin Invest* **123:**
966–972. doi:10.1172/JCI64098

Triana-Martínez F, Picallos-Rabina P, Da Silva-Álvarez S,
Pietrocola F, Llanos S, Rodilla V, Soprano E, Pedrosa P,
Ferreirós A, Barradas M, et al. 2019. Identification and
characterization of cardiac glycosides as senolytic compounds. *Nat Commun* **10:** 4731. doi:10.1038/s41467-019-
12888-x

Tripathi U, Misra A, Tchkonia T, Kirkland JL. 2021a. Impact
of senescent cell subtypes on tissue dysfunction and repair: importance and research questions. *Mech Ageing
Dev* **198:** 111548. doi:10.1016/j.mad.2021.111548

Tripathi U, Nchioua R, Prata L, Zhu Y, Gerdes EOW, Giorgadze N, Pirtskhalava T, Parker E, Xue A, Espindola-
Netto JM, et al. 2021b. SARS-CoV-2 causes senescence
in human cells and exacerbates the senescence-associated

secretory phenotype through TLR-3. *Aging (Albany NY)* **13:** 21838–21854. doi:10.18632/aging.203560

Tuttle CSL, Luesken SWM, Waaijer MEC, Maier AB. 2021. Senescence in tissue samples of humans with age-related diseases: a systematic review. *Ageing Res Rev* **68:** 101334. doi:10.1016/j.arr.2021.101334

Vazquez-Villasenor I, Garwood CJ, Heath PR, Simpson JE, Ince PG, Wharton SB. 2020. Expression of p16 and p21 in the frontal association cortex of ALS/MND brains suggests neuronal cell cycle dysregulation and astrocyte senescence in early stages of the disease. *Neuropathol Appl Neurobiol* **46:** 171–185. doi:10.1111/nan.12559

Wandrer F, Han B, Liebig S, Schlue J, Manns MP, Schulze-Osthoff K, Bantel H. 2018. Senescence mirrors the extent of liver fibrosis in chronic hepatitis C virus infection. *Aliment Pharmacol Ther* **48:** 270–280. doi:10.1111/apt.14802

Wang Y, Chang J, Liu X, Zhang X, Zhang S, Zhang X, Zhou D, Zheng G. 2016. Discovery of piperlongumine as a potential novel lead for the development of senolytic agents. *Aging (Albany NY)* **8:** 2915–2926. doi:10.18632/aging.101100

Wang L, Wang B, Gasek NS, Zhou Y, Cohn RL, Martin DE, Zuo W, Flynn WF, Guo C, Jellison ER, et al. 2022. Targeting p21(Cip1) highly expressing cells in adipose tissue alleviates insulin resistance in obesity. *Cell Metab* **34:** 186. doi:10.1016/j.cmet.2021.12.014

Wissler Gerdes EO, Zhu Y, Tchkonia T, Kirkland JL. 2020. Discovery, development, and future application of senolytics: theories and predictions. *FEBS J* **287:** 2418–2427. doi:10.1111/febs.15264

Wyles SP, Dashti P, Pirtskhalava T, Tekin B, Inman C, Gomez LS, Lagnado AB, Prata L, Jurk D, Passos JF, et al. 2023. A chronic wound model to investigate skin cellular senescence. *Aging (Albany NY)* **15:** 2852–2862. doi:10.18632/aging.204667

Xu M, Tchkonia T, Kirkland JL. 2016. Perspective: targeting the JAK/STAT pathway to fight age-related dysfunction. *Pharmacol Res* **111:** 152–154. doi:10.1016/j.phrs.2016.05.015

Xu M, Pirtskhalava T, Farr JN, Weigand BM, Palmer AK, Weivoda MM, Inman CL, Ogrodnik MB, Hachfeld CM, Fraser DG, et al. 2018. Senolytics improve physical function and increase lifespan in old age. *Nat Med* **24:** 1246–1256. doi:10.1038/s41591-018-0092-9

Xu Q, Fu Q, Li Z, Liu H, Wang Y, Lin X, He R, Zhang X, Ju Z, Campisi J, et al. 2021. The flavonoid procyanidin C1 has

senotherapeutic activity and increases lifespan in mice. *Nat Metab* **3:** 1706–1726. doi:10.1038/s42255-021-00491-8

Yang H, Wang H, Ren J, Chen Q, Chen ZJ. 2017. cGAS is essential for cellular senescence. *Proc Natl Acad Sci* **114:** E4612–E4620. doi:10.1073/pnas.1705499114

Yoshioka H, Yamada T, Hasegawa S, Miyachi K, Ishii Y, Hasebe Y, Inoue Y, Tanaka H, Iwata Y, Arima M, et al. 2021. Senescent cell removal via JAG1-NOTCH1 signalling in the epidermis. *Exp Dermatol* **30:** 1268–1278. doi:10.1111/exd.14361

Yousefzadeh MJ, Zhu Y, McGowan SJ, Angelini L, Fuhrmann-Stroissnigg H, Xu M, Ling YY, Melos KI, Pirtskhalava T, Inman CL, et al. 2018. Fisetin is a senotherapeutic that extends health and lifespan. *EBioMedicine* **36:** 18–28. doi:10.1016/j.ebiom.2018.09.015

Zhang L, Pitcher LE, Prahalad V, Niedernhofer LJ, Robbins PD. 2023. Targeting cellular senescence with senotherapeutics: senolytics and senomorphics. *FEBS J* **290:** 1362–1383. doi:10.1111/febs.16350

Zhu Y, Armstrong JL, Tchkonia T, Kirkland JL. 2014. Cellular senescence and the senescent secretory phenotype in age-related chronic diseases. *Curr Opin Clin Nutr Metab Care* **17:** 324–328. doi:10.1097/MCO.0000000000000065

Zhu Y, Tchkonia T, Pirtskhalava T, Gower AC, Ding H, Giorgadze N, Palmer AK, Ikeno Y, Hubbard GB, Lenburg M, et al. 2015. The Achilles' heel of senescent cells: from transcriptome to senolytic drugs. *Aging Cell* **14:** 644–658. doi:10.1111/acel.12344

Zhu Y, Tchkonia T, Fuhrmann-Stroissnigg H, Dai HM, Ling YY, Stout MB, Pirtskhalava T, Giorgadze N, Johnson KO, Giles CB, et al. 2016. Identification of a novel senolytic agent, navitoclax, targeting the Bcl-2 family of anti-apoptotic factors. *Aging Cell* **15:** 428–435. doi:10.1111/acel.12445

Zhu Y, Doornebal EJ, Pirtskhalava T, Giorgadze N, Wentworth M, Fuhrmann-Stroissnigg H, Niedernhofer LJ, Robbins PD, Tchkonia T, Kirkland JL. 2017. New agents that target senescent cells: the flavone, fisetin, and the BCL-X(L) inhibitors, A1331852 and A1155463. *Aging (Albany NY)* **9:** 955–963. doi:10.18632/aging.101202

Zhu Y, Prata L, Gerdes EOW, Netto JME, Pirtskhalava T, Giorgadze N, Tripathi U, Inman CL, Johnson KO, Xue A, et al. 2022. Orally active, clinically translatable senolytics restore α-Klotho in mice and humans. *EBioMedicine* **77:** 103912. doi:10.1016/j.ebiom.2022.103912

Roles of NAD$^+$ in Health and Aging

Sofie Lautrup,[1,6] Yujun Hou,[2,6] Evandro F. Fang,[1,3] and Vilhelm A. Bohr[4,5]

[1]Department of Clinical Molecular Biology, University of Oslo and Akershus University Hospital, 1478 Lørenskog, Norway

[2]Institute for Regenerative Medicine, Shanghai East Hospital, Frontier Science Center for Stem Cell Research, Shanghai Key Laboratory of Signaling and Disease Research, School of Life Sciences and Technology, Tongji University, Shanghai 200092, China

[3]The Norwegian Centre on Healthy Ageing (NO-Age), Oslo, Norway

[4]DNA Repair Section, National Institute on Aging, National Institutes of Health, Baltimore, Maryland 21224, USA

[5]Danish Center for Healthy Aging, University of Copenhagen, 2200 Copenhagen, Denmark

Correspondence: e.f.fang@medisin.no; vbohr@sund.ku.dk

NAD$^+$, the essential metabolite involved in multiple reactions such as the regulation of cellular metabolism, energy production, DNA repair, mitophagy and autophagy, inflammation, and neuronal function, has been the subject of intense research in the field of aging and disease over the last decade. NAD$^+$ levels decline with aging and in some age-related diseases, and reduction in NAD$^+$ affects all the hallmarks of aging. Here, we present an overview of the discovery of NAD$^+$, the cellular pathways of producing and consuming NAD$^+$, and discuss how imbalances in the production rate and cellular request of NAD$^+$ likely contribute to aging and age-related diseases including neurodegeneration. Preclinical studies have revealed great potential for NAD$^+$ precursors in promotion of healthy aging and improvement of neurodegeneration. This has led to the initiation of several clinical trials with NAD$^+$ precursors to treat accelerated aging, age-associated dysfunctions, and diseases including Alzheimer's and Parkinson's. NAD supplementation has great future potential clinically, and these studies will also provide insight into the mechanisms of aging.

THE DISCOVERY OF NAD$^+$

Nicotinamide adenine dinucleotide (NAD) can exist in two forms, the oxidized form, NAD$^+$, and the reduced form, NADH, which are coupled together and known as a "redox couple." While they are chemically similar, here we mainly focus on NAD$^+$. NAD$^+$ is an essential metabolite for life and health, as it participates in dozens of known cellular reactions that affect redox status, energy production, and metabolic homeostasis, in addition to having anti-inflammatory properties, and assisting in stem cell rejuvenation, autophagy/mitophagy, nuclear–mitochondrial communication, and cellular resilience and survival (Verdin 2015; Fang et al. 2016a,b; Lautrup

---

[6]Co-first authors.

Cite this article as *Cold Spring Harb Perspect Med* doi: 10.1101/cshperspect.a041193

et al. 2019). NAD$^+$ (named "cozymase" at that time) was purified by Arthur Harden and William John Young in 1906 (Harden and Young 1906) as an essential component in fermentation (Harden and Young 1906). Hans von Euler-Chelpin continued the work initiated by Harden and Young, reporting that the structure of NAD$^+$ is made up of two nucleotides. Combined, Harden, Young, and Euler-Chelpin showed that fermentation depends on NAD$^+$, and, in 1929, Arthur Harden and Hans von Euler-Chelpin were awarded the Nobel Prize. Dr. Hans von Euler-Chelpin stated in his Nobel lecture that "cozymase [NAD$^+$] is one of the most widespread and biologically important activators within the plant and animal world" (Euler 1930). Simultaneously, Otto Heinrich Warburg discovered the redox abilities of NAD$^+$ and NADH and their necessity for fermentation (Warburg and Christian 1936). In the 1940s, Arthur Kornberg discovered the reaction in which the precursor nicotinamide mononucleotide (NMN) is converted to NAD$^+$, and via this he found NAD synthetase (Kornberg 1948). He was awarded the Nobel Prize for his findings in 1950.

The investigations of the disease pellagra, now known to be caused by NAD$^+$ precursor deficiency, also contributed significantly to the knowledge about NAD$^+$ that we have today. Dr. Joseph Goldberger initially described pellagra as a nutritional deficiency, with dermatitis, diarrhea, dementia, and consequently death as the central characteristics of the disease. Conrad A. Elvehjem and C.K. Koehn conducted controlled experiments in dogs, which led to their discovery that nicotinic acid (NA), initially termed "anti-black tongue factor," was the mitigating factor in pellagra (Elvehjem et al. 1974). Later, Jack Preiss and Philip Handler connected NA to NAD$^+$ by clarifying the steps and enzymes in what is now referred to as the Preiss–Handler pathway, in which NA is metabolized by a three-step process to NAD$^+$ (Preiss and Handler 1958a,b).

Our current understanding of NAD$^+$ and its roles in cellular bioenergetics really began in the 1960s and 1970s with the identification of NAD$^+$-dependent reactions and proteins. Chambon, Weill, and Mandel described the process of poly ADP-ribosylation (PARP) as an NAD$^+$-dependent reaction (Chambon et al. 1963), initiating the field of PARP studies. Additionally, the identification of yeast SIR2 as NAD$^+$-dependent deacetylates by Guarente and colleagues revealed an additional group of NAD$^+$ consumers (Imai et al. 2000). In 2004, Brenner and colleagues identified the NAD$^+$ precursor nicotinamide riboside (NR) and uncovered the two-step process from NR to NAD$^+$ (Bieganowski and Brenner 2004). In recent years, interest in NAD$^+$ and its bioavailable precursors, including NR, NMN, and nicotinamide (NAM), has spiked. This review will summarize the knowledge gained from preclinical and clinical studies on the decline of NAD$^+$ during aging and the reasons for and consequences of reduced NAD. Furthermore, the identification and purification of NAD$^+$ precursors have opened the door to discovery of methods that can boost the level of intracellular and organismal NAD$^+$ levels, which will also be discussed here.

NAD$^+$-CONSUMING ENZYMES, BIOSYNTHETIC PATHWAYS, AND METABOLISM

NAD$^+$ is highly compartmentalized in different subcellular organelles, including in the nucleus, cytoplasm, and mitochondria. Mitochondria contain the largest subcellular pools of NAD$^+$ (Berger et al. 2005; Dölle et al. 2010; Nikiforov et al. 2011). While NAD$^+$ might be transported from cytoplasm to other subcellular organs (like mitochondria), it is generally believed that each pool of NAD$^+$ is independently regulated, involving subcellular specific localization of proteins involved in NAD$^+$ production and consumption (Berger et al. 2005; Gilley and Coleman 2010; Mayer et al. 2010).

NAD$^+$ is a fundamental molecule for several metabolic and cellular processes. It works as a redox coenzyme, because the conversion of NAD$^+$ to NADH is necessary for the citric acid cycle, β-oxidation, and glycolysis. Simultaneously, the oxidation of NADH to NAD$^+$ by complex I in the mitochondrial electron transport chain participates in ATP production and other essential metabolic processes. Major NAD$^+$-synthetic pathways, including the salvage pathway (including extracellular recycling and the newly discovered NADH pathway), the kynurenine pathway (de novo), and the Preiss–Handler pathway are discussed below.

The Four Classes of NAD$^+$-Consuming Proteins

NAD$^+$ is a cosubstrate for at least four main classes of enzymes producing NAM as a byproduct of their consumption of NAD$^+$. These known NAD$^+$-consuming proteins include PARPs, the class III histone deacetylases sirtuins (SIRTs), ADP ribosyl-cyclases (CD38, CD73), and NADase sterile α and TIR motif-containing 1 (SARM1) (Lautrup et al. 2019; Covarrubias et al. 2021).

A central family of NAD$^+$ consumers are the PARPs, with PARP1 constituting the main PARP activity related to DNA damage (Rouleau et al. 2010; Fang et al. 2014). PARP1 is a key protein in the DNA damage response, locating sites with damaged DNA and using NAD$^+$ to generate long PAR chains (PARylation) on itself and on histones and other proteins, which acts as a scaffold to facilitate DNA repair (Fang et al. 2016a,b; Ray Chaudhuri and Nussenzweig 2017; Wilson et al. 2023a). PARP-mediated NAD$^+$ consumption has also been linked to the process of aging, pathological aging, and age-related diseases (more details below). The second class of NAD$^+$ consumers are the SIRTs. The mammalian SIRT family consists of seven mammalian SIRT proteins, which regulate many cellular processes including neuronal survival, metabolism, stress responses, and aging (Chalkiadaki and Guarente 2015; Covarrubias et al. 2021). Both the NAD$^+$-consuming PARPs and SIRTs are hyperactive in autophagy-deficient cells, and NAD$^+$ depletion contributes to death of autophagy-/mitophagy-deficient cells (Kataura et al. 2022). The past decade of research has revealed that NAD$^+$-consuming enzymes can directly regulate autophagy in cells, from early transcription events to late-stage autophagosome–lysosome fusion events (Wilson et al. 2023b).

The third group of NAD$^+$ consumers contains the ADP ribosyl-cyclases CD38/CD157, which convert NAD$^+$ to cyclic ADP ribose (cADPR) and adenine diphosphate ribose (ADPR) under neutral pH conditions; in acidic conditions, they convert NAD$^+$ to nicotinamide adenine dinucleotide phosphate (NADP), and then to NA adenine dinucleotide phosphate (NAADP) (Reiten et al. 2021). CD38 and CD157 play important roles in the regulation of social behavior, calcium homeostasis, immune function, mitochondrial function, metabolism, and hormone secretion (Jin et al. 2007; Liu et al. 2008, 2017; Camacho-Pereira et al. 2016). Similarly, SARM1 has NADase properties, and produces NAM, cADPR, and ADPR while consuming NAD$^+$. SARM1 is primarily expressed in neurons where SARM1-mediated NAD$^+$ degradation promotes axon degeneration exclusively in damaged axons, as well as during neuronal morphogenesis and inflammation (Gerdts et al. 2015; Essuman et al. 2017; Murata et al. 2018; Figley and DiAntonio 2020). SARM1 functions as a metabolic sensor, which is activated by a large change in the NMN-to-NAD$^+$ ratio, and binding of NMN is required for injury-induced SARM1 activation and axon destruction (Figley et al. 2021). SARM1 is also expressed in immune cells (Panneerselvam et al. 2013; Gürtler et al. 2014; Zhao et al. 2019), but the underlying mechanism that SARM1 uses to regulate immunity is largely unexplored. Collectively, our current understanding of NAD$^+$ and its consuming enzymes highlights the vital importance of NAD$^+$ in life and health.

The Salvage Pathway and Related NAD$^+$ Precursors

The salvage pathway generates NAD$^+$ from the precursor NAM or the upstream precursors NR or NMN as summarized in Figure 1A. The precursor NAM is produced during the degradation and consumption of NAD$^+$, and exogenous NAM, in addition to NR and NMN, arrive from a variety of foods including fruits, vegetables, milk, and meat (Chi and Sauve 2013; Mills et al. 2016; Fang et al. 2017; Covarrubias et al. 2021). The route of cell entry for NAD and the precursors mentioned here are still not completely understood. In specific cell types and conditions, NAD$^+$ can be transported into the cell via the transporter connexin 43 (Cx43) (Billington et al. 2008; Liu et al. 2018), whereas the smaller precursors, such as NAM, NMN, and NR, can enter the

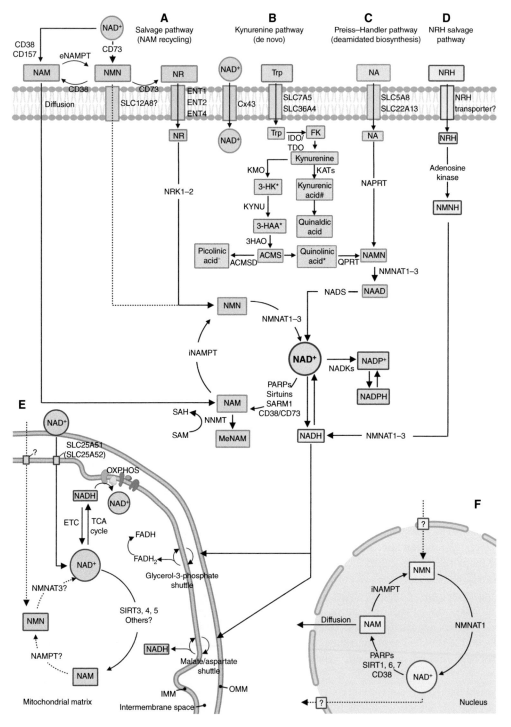

Figure 1. NAD$^+$ biosynthetic pathways and subcellular interactions. The biosynthesis of NAD$^+$ includes four pathways: the salvage pathway (*A*), the kynurenine pathway (*B*), the Preiss–Handler pathway (*C*), and the newly proposed dihydronicotinamide riboside (NRH) salvage pathway (*D*). The salvage pathway synthesizes NAD$^+$ from intracellular nicotinamide (NAM), extracellular NAD$^+$ and related metabolites (NAM, nicotinamide riboside [NR], nicotinamide mononucleotide [NMN]). Within the cell, NR is phosphorylated by nicotinamide riboside kinases (NRK1–2) to NMN. NMN is also produced from NAM by the intracellular NAMPT (iNAMPT). NAD$^+$ is generated from NMN through NMNAT1–3. (*Legend continues on following page.*)

Cite this article as *Cold Spring Harb Perspect Med* doi: 10.1101/cshperspect.a041193

cell via direct diffusion (NAM) or specific transporters (NR and NMN) (Grozio et al. 2013; Camacho-Pereira et al. 2016).

Within the cell, NAM is recycled to NMN by iNAMPT (Rongvaux et al. 2002; Ratajczak et al. 2016; Liu et al. 2018), followed by the conversion of NMN to NAD$^+$ by NMN adenylyl transferases 1–3 (NMNAT1–3). The NMNATs are involved in all three main NAD$^+$ synthesis routes converting either NMN or NAMN to NAD$^+$ (Salvage, Kynurenine, Preiss–Handler) (Fig. 1). They have different subcellular localizations, and the expression of NMNAT1 is tissue specific (Berger et al. 2005). NMNAT1 locates to the nucleus and is highly expressed in skeletal muscle, heart, kidney, liver, and pancreas (Emanuelli et al. 2001; Yalowitz et al. 2004). NMNAT2 is localized on the outer membrane of the Golgi apparatus and in the cytosol. NMNAT3 resides mainly in the mitochondria, although the activity responsible for converting NMN to NAD$^+$ within the mitochondria is still debated (Yalowitz et al. 2004; Berger et al. 2005; Yamamoto et al. 2016). Moreover, the expression and activity of NAMPT within the mitochondria may depend on many factors including cell types. In rat liver cells, NAMPT has been detected within the mitochondria (Yang et al. 2007), whereas experiments using immortalized cells show a lack of NAMPT inside the mitochondria (Pittelli et al. 2010). More studies are needed to understand the tissue- and cell-specific expression pattern of NAMPT and related enzymes.

Recently, the hydrogenated form of NR, NRH, was demonstrated to increase NAD$^+$ levels in cells in a more efficient way than using NR/NMN/NAM (Yang et al. 2019). The conversion of NRH to NAD$^+$ provides a potential novel entry point for boosting cellular NAD$^+$ (Fig. 1D; Yang et al. 2020). Adenosine kinase (AK), not NRK1 or NRK2, was demonstrated to convert NRH to the intermediate NMNH (Yang et al. 2020). It was demonstrated in vitro that the adenylation of NMNH to NADH by NNMATs followed by oxidation to NAD$^+$ is a likely route of action, but in vivo studies are needed to establish the mechanism of action and the physiological relevance (Yang et al. 2020; Ziegler and Nikiforov 2020). While the major advantage of using NRH is the

Figure 1. (*Continued*) (*B*) The kynurenine pathway produces NAD$^+$ from the amino acid tryptophan (Trp). Trp is converted to formylkynurenine (FK), which is then catalyzed into kynurenine, which is converted to either quinaldic acid or 3-hydroxykynurenine (3-HK), which by a four-step process is converted to nicotinic acid mononucleotide (NAMN), then following the remaining steps described in the (*C*) Preiss–Handler pathway. Some of the metabolites of the kynurenine pathway are neuroprotective (marked with #), and some are neurotoxic (marked with *). (*C*) The Preiss–Handler pathway describes the conversion of nicotinic acid (NA) to NAD$^+$ via a three-step process. NAMN is an intermediate both in the kynurenine pathway (*B*) and the Preiss–Handler pathway (*C*), and the enzymatic conversion of NAMN to NA adenine dinucleotide (NAAD) is by the NMNATs. Finally, NAD$^+$ synthase (NADS) synthesizes NAAD to NAD$^+$. (*D*) The recently demonstrated NRH salvage pathway uses dihydronicotinamide riboside (NRH), the reduced form of NR, to produce NAD$^+$. The pathway is still relatively unclarified, but the initial step is likely catalyzed by adenosine kinase (AK), providing NMNH from NRH. NMNH is suggested to be converted to NADH through NMNATs, finally being oxidized to NAD$^+$. (*E*) Mitochondrial NAD$^+$ homeostasis. NAD$^+$ is subcellular localized and regulated. SLC25A51, and in specific organs and likely specific cell types SLC25A52, are mammalian mitochondrial transporters for NAD$^+$. The cytosolic and mitochondrial NADH pools communicate indirectly through the transportation of reducing equivalents across the mitochondrial membranes by the glyceraldehyde 3-phosphate and malate-aspartate shuttles. NMNAT3 has been suggested to be an essential participant of the salvage pathway in mitochondria, but recent studies do not support the existence of an active mitochondrial NMNAT3 to synthesize NMN to NAD$^+$ within the mitochondria (Kory et al. 2020; Luongo et al. 2020). Within the mitochondrial matrix, NAD$^+$ is consumed by SIRT3-5, with NAM as a byproduct. NAM is potentially further converted to NMN through NAMPT, although the presence of NAMPT within the mitochondria is not fully understood (Yang et al. 2007; Pittelli et al. 2010). The existence of a mitochondrial NMN transporter is unknown. (*F*) Nuclear NAD$^+$ homeostasis. The nuclear transport of NAD$^+$ remains inconclusive, but nuclear pore-mediated NAD$^+$ diffusion has been speculated. Within the nucleus, the NAD$^+$ pathway involves iNAMPT, converting NAM, produced during the consumption of NAD$^+$, to NMN, and NMNAT1 synthesizing NAD$^+$ from NMN. (Figure is based on data in Reiten et al. 2021, and was created using BioRender.)

efficient increase of cellular NAD$^+$, a major disadvantage is its low stability, which limits broad translational applications.

Kynurenine Pathway

The amino acid tryptophan (Trp) is metabolized to NAD$^+$ de novo via the kynurenine pathway (Fig. 1B). Trp is transported into the cell via the transmembrane solute carrier (SLC) transporters SLC7A5 and SLC36A4 (Pillai and Meredith 2011; Scalise et al. 2018), where it is catabolized via a two-step process to kynurenine, which can be converted to NAD$^+$, kynurenic acid, and xanthurenic acid. The relative contribution of the kynurenine pathway to NAD$^+$ levels is still not well understood, and most cells outside the liver/kidney do not express the enzymes necessary to produce NAD$^+$ from Trp (Liu et al. 2018; Covarrubias et al. 2021). However, evidence suggests that the kynurenine pathway plays an essential role in health. For example, the enzyme α-amino-β-carboxymuconate-ε-semialdehyde (ACMS) decarboxylase (ACMSD) inhibits spontaneous cyclization of ACMS in the kynurenine pathway. Pharmacologic or genetic inhibition of ACMSD enhances de novo NAD$^+$ synthesis, leading to improved mitochondrial function and tissue resilience after damage, especially in kidney and liver tissues (Katsyuba et al. 2018). The liver-dominant kynurenine pathway may also contribute to the generation of NAD$^+$ to detoxify ethanol in the liver: alcohol dehydrogenase complex catalyzes the reaction of ethanol and NAD$^+$ to form acetaldehyde, NADH, and H$^+$ (Edenberg 2000).

In addition to protection against exogenous damage to the kidney and liver, the kynurenine pathway is also linked to common neurodegenerative diseases such as Huntington's and Alzheimer's disease with more details in our recent review (Ogawa et al. 1992; Thevandavakkam et al. 2010; Campesan et al. 2011; Giil et al. 2017; Lautrup et al. 2019; González-Sánchez et al. 2020). The kynurenine pathway is involved in the generation of the neurotransmitters glutamate and acetylcholine, and it regulates N-methyl-D-aspartate receptor activity (Vécsei et al. 2013; Lautrup et al. 2019). Additionally, the intermediates of this pathway include both neurotoxic (3-hydroxykynurenine (3-HK), 3-hydroxyanthranilic acid (3-HAA), quinolinic acid, and free radicals) and neuroprotective metabolites (Trp, kynurenic acid, and picolinic acid) (Vécsei et al. 2013). These findings outline the importance of this de novo NAD$^+$ synthetic pathway in promoting tissue resilience and neuroprotection, among other defensive functions.

Preiss–Handler Pathway

The Preiss–Handler pathway, also called the deamidated biosynthesis pathway, synthesizes NAD$^+$ from the precursor NA via three steps (Fig. 1C). NA is transported into the cell via SLC5A8 and SLC22A13 (Gopal et al. 2005; Bahn et al. 2008). Within the cell, NA is converted to nicotinic acid mononucleotide (NAMN) by nicotinic acid phosphoribosyltransferase (NaPRT) (Houtkooper et al. 2010). Converging with the kynurenine pathway, NAMN is processed to nicotinic acid adenine dinucleotide (NAAD) by NMNAT1–3, and finally NAAD is metabolized to NAD$^+$ by NAD$^+$ synthase (NADS) (Zhang et al. 2003; Houtkooper et al. 2010). NR supplementation can increase the intracellular level of NAAD (Trammell et al. 2016a), connecting the Salvage and Preiss–Handler pathways, although the mechanism is yet to be understood.

CHANGES IN NAD$^+$ DURING AGING

Changes in NAD$^+$ during Normal Aging

During aging, the level of NAD$^+$ declines, and proteins involved in the biosynthesis and consumption of NAD$^+$ are altered (McReynolds et al. 2020). Multiple studies on mice have shown that NAD$^+$ levels decline in various tissues such as pancreas (Yoshino et al. 2011), kidney (McReynolds et al. 2021), white adipose tissue (Yoshino et al. 2011; Camacho-Pereira et al. 2016; McReynolds et al. 2021), spleen (Camacho-Pereira et al. 2016), skeletal muscle and muscle stem (Yoshino et al. 2011; Gomes et al. 2013; Camacho-Pereira et al. 2016; Zhang et al. 2016; Zou et al. 2020; McReynolds et al. 2021), urine-derived stem cells (Zou et al. 2020), liver (Mouchiroud et al. 2013; Camacho-Pereira et al. 2016; McReynolds et al.

2021), skin (Massudi et al. 2012; Zou et al. 2020), and brain (Stein et al. 2014; Zhu et al. 2015), and an age-dependent decline of NAD$^+$ has also been reported in humans (Zhu et al. 2015; Chaleckis et al. 2016; Janssens et al. 2022) and nematodes (Mouchiroud et al. 2013; Fang et al. 2014, 2016a, b). Due to the low stability of NAD$^+$, noninvasive and in vivo methods to detect NAD$^+$ and its related metabolites are needed. An array of fluorescent NAD$^+$ or NAD$^+$/NADH sensors have been developed and used for detection of NAD during aging in zebrafish, mice, and human cells, with all showing an age-dependent decline in levels of NAD$^+$ (Zhao et al. 2011, 2015, 2016, 2018; Zou et al. 2020). Using a magnetic resonance (MR)-based in vivo NAD assay, the level of NAD$^+$, total NAD, and the NAD$^+$/NADH ratio were shown to decline and NADH to increase with age in the human brain (Zhu et al. 2015). Other studies on human tissue samples rely on enzymatic cycling assays or liquid chromatography mass spectrometry (LC-MS)-based analysis of NAD$^+$ and NAD(H) detection (Bernofsky and Swan 1973; Chaleckis et al. 2016; Clement et al. 2019; Sanchez-Roman et al. 2022). Since blood is easily accessible compared to other human tissues, researchers have sought to use blood to examine the age-related changes in NAD$^+$ as a biomarker of aging and disease (Fig. 2). Through use of LC-MS, it has been shown that the level of NAD$^+$ in both whole blood and plasma declines with age (Chaleckis et al. 2016; Clement et al. 2019). Additionally, a positive correlation has been observed between cognitive capacity and plasma levels of NAD$^+$/NADH in centenarians, which might be because NAD$^+$/NADH-consuming enzyme activities are working to decrease the oxidative DNA damage load (Sanchez-Roman et al. 2022). NAD$^+$ is a key regulator of DNA repair mechanisms, including base excision repair and homologous recombination. Reduced NAD$^+$ levels have been shown to impair DNA repair and increase DNA damage, which can contribute to an accumulation of the mutations and cellular dysfunctions generally associated with aging (Fang et al. 2017). Aging is also related to a significant decrease in NAD$^+$ levels in human skeletal muscle; the level of NAD$^+$ correlates with healthy aging (Janssens et al. 2022). Increased physical activity is associ-

ated with increased levels of NAD$^+$ in the skeletal muscle, whereas physical impairments in older people are associated with decreased NAD$^+$ levels when compared with normally active older individuals (Janssens et al. 2022).

Understanding why NAD$^+$ decreases with age remains incomplete, but studies on animal models have provided insight into the important players in age-dependent NAD$^+$ decline; age-related decreases are likely due to reduced production and increased consumption of NAD$^+$. Age-related NAD$^+$ depletion has been linked to increased nuclear DNA damage, which leads to increased activation of PARP1 (Mouchiroud et al. 2013; Fang et al. 2014, 2016a,b; Ryu et al. 2016; Zhang et al. 2016). High PARP1 activity will deplete the cell of NAD$^+$, thereby decreasing the activity of SIRT1 (and other SIRTs). This in turn results in increased acetylation of the transcription factor peroxisome proliferator-activated receptor-γ coactivator 1α (PGC1α) and mitochondrial dysfunction (Mouchiroud et al. 2013; Fang et al. 2014, 2016a,b; Ryu et al. 2016; Zhang et al. 2016). In addition, compromised mitophagy and mitochondrial unfolded protein response (UPR^{mt}), and mitochondrial dysfunction are consequences of NAD$^+$ depletion during aging and age-predisposed diseases (Fang et al. 2014, 2016a,b, 2019a,b; Ryu et al. 2016; Zhang et al. 2016). Depleted NAD$^+$ disrupts cellular metabolism, again leading to decreased cellular functions as shown in both neurons and glial cells, as wells as in stem cells (Ryu et al. 2016; Zhang et al. 2016; Fang et al. 2019b).

Depletion of NAD$^+$ has also been linked to age- and disease-related telomere shortening and dysfunction. In the telomere disorder dyskeratosis congenita, a rare genetic form of bone marrow failure where the marrow is unable to produce sufficient blood cells, decreased NAD$^+$ and imbalance of the NAD$^+$ metabolome was shown to be related to both telomere damage and cellular senescence (Sun et al. 2020). Moreover, NAD$^+$ was found to be reduced both due to the activity of PARP1, SIRT1 while the NAD$^+$ consumer CD38 (Sun et al. 2020), which is increased during aging in mice (Camacho-Pereira et al. 2016). CD38 is required for the age-associated decline in NAD$^+$ levels and age-related

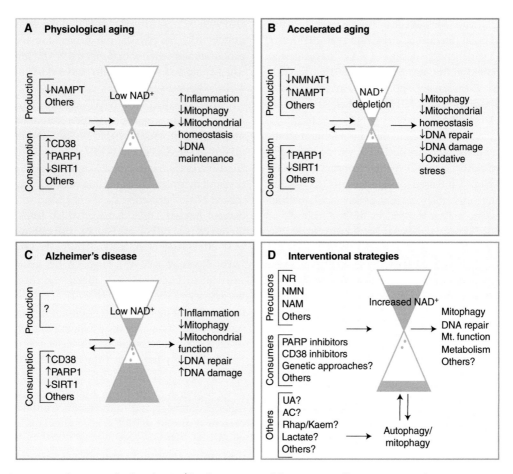

Figure 2. Mechanisms of reduced NAD$^+$ levels in aging and diseases, as well as interventional strategies. During aging and disease, the balance of the production and consumption of NAD$^+$ is altered, resulting in decreased levels of NAD$^+$. (*A–C*) The players involved during (*A*) normal aging, (*B*) accelerated aging, and (*C*) brain diseases such as Alzheimer's disease. (*D*) The known NAD$^+$ up-regulation strategies and outcomes. (UA) Urolithin A, (AC) actinonin, (Rhap) Rhapontigenin, (Kaem) Kaempferol.

mitochondrial dysfunction via a pathway that at least partially depends on the activity of the mitochondrial SIRT3 (Camacho-Pereira et al. 2016). A central role for CD38 in age-dependent NAD$^+$ depletion was also confirmed in activated macrophages from old mice, showing a hyper-activation of CD38, which resulted in lower levels of NAD$^+$ (Covarrubias et al. 2021).

Age-related decrease of NAD$^+$ levels may also be related to a decline in levels or activity of NAD$^+$-producing proteins (Yoshino et al. 2011; Fang et al. 2017). The level of NAMPT, which converts NAM to NMN and is referred to as the rate-limiting enzyme in the salvage path-

way, decreases with age in mice (Yoshino et al. 2011; Stein and Imai 2014), and its expression has been linked to core circadian clock proteins and inflammation (Yaku et al. 2018). On the other hand, it was recently shown through iso-tope tracer experiments that the synthesis of NAD$^+$ across multiple tissues in mice was not altered, pointing at increased consumption as the primary driver for age-related decline of NAD$^+$ availability (McReynolds et al. 2021). Further studies are needed in animal models and in human tissues to further understand the mechanisms that deplete the aging cells and tissues of NAD$^+$.

Changes of NAD$^+$ Levels in Pathological Aging

In addition to normal aging, decreased NAD$^+$ levels have been observed in a number of accelerated aging disorders including Ataxia telangiectasia (A-T), Cockayne syndrome (CS), Werner syndrome (WS), and xeroderma pigmentosum group A (XPA) (Fang et al. 2014, 2016a,b, 2019a; Scheibye-Knudsen et al. 2014). A shared etiological feature of these conditions is the mutation of genes involved in DNA repair and genomic stability. Additionally, patients suffering from these diseases, except for WS, show severe neurodegeneration; lower levels of NAD$^+$ have been observed in *Caenorhabditis elegans* models and mouse brain samples of A-T, CS, WS, and XPA (Fang et al. 2014, 2016a,b; Scheibye-Knudsen et al. 2014). CS is caused by mutations in either the CS complementation group A (*CSA*) or group B (*CSB*) genes. Interestingly, the CS mouse models, *Csb$^{m/m}$* and *Csa$^{m/m}$*, also showed reduced levels of NAD$^+$ and NAD$^+$/NADH ratio in the cochlea associated with reduced hearing in both CS mouse models due to disrupted ribbon synapses and outer hair cell loss (Okur et al. 2020a). These findings suggest that age-related hearing loss in normal aging might also be a consequence of a decline in NAD$^+$. In WS, the main characteristics of the patients include cancer, short stature, dyslipidemia, premature arthrosclerosis, and insulin-resistant diabetes (Takemoto et al. 2013; Oshima et al. 2017). In line with many of the features of WS being related to dysfunctional metabolism, primary fibroblasts, and blood samples from human WS patients showed a decreased level of NAD$^+$ and related metabolites compared to healthy control subjects (Fang et al. 2019a). Additionally, WS *C. elegans* models show a decrease in NAD$^+$ levels throughout the body, which likely contributes to compromised mitophagy, leading to disrupted fat metabolism, mitochondrial dysfunction, and decreased health span and life span (Fang et al. 2019a). As with normal aging, the explanation for the decline in NAD$^+$ levels might be found in an increased consumption, mainly by the DNA damage-activated PARP1, as well as decreased production of NAD$^+$.

In the above-mentioned premature aging diseases an increased activity of PARP1 and decreased activity of SIRT1 has been shown, and in A-T, XPA, and CS (Fang et al. 2014, 2016a,b, 2019a; Scheibye-Knudsen et al. 2014). These studies showed that reduction in NAD$^+$ led to mitochondrial dysfunction and compromised mitophagy, excessive PINK1 cleavage, and increased mitochondrial membrane potential, which in turn resulted in the accumulation of dysfunctional mitochondria, further contributing to oxidative stress and NAD$^+$ depletion, which contributes to a shortened life span, health span, and neurodegeneration (except for WS) (Fang et al. 2014, 2016a,b; Scheibye-Knudsen et al. 2014).

In WS, it was also shown that NMNAT1, responsible for the last step of the salvage pathway, was significantly reduced, while NAMPT was increased (Fang et al. 2019a). The latter might suggest a cellular compensatory feedback mechanism to increase NAD$^+$ (Fang et al. 2019a). To clarify the impact of the altered levels of NAD$^+$ biosynthesis-related proteins, and the direct consequences of NAD$^+$ depletion, more studies are required for both normal and pathological aging in different organisms, tissues, and cell types.

Changes in NAD$^+$ Levels in Age-Associated Diseases with a Focus on AD

NAD$^+$ reduction is evident not only in normal and pathological aging, but also in age-related diseases, including diabetes (Yoshino et al. 2011; Mills et al. 2016), cardiovascular diseases (Diguet et al. 2018), kidney failure (Tran et al. 2016; Poyan Mehr et al. 2018; Morevati et al. 2021), and neurodegenerative diseases (Hou et al. 2019; Yulug et al. 2021a, 2023) with AD being the focus of this review. AD is one of the most common neurodegenerative diseases, and the prevalence of AD increases as the life expectancy of the global population increases. AD is a major global public health problem that needs to be addressed urgently (Livingston et al. 2020). The main clinical features of AD are cognitive deficits, mood swings, and behavioral problems. AD likely results from a combination of genetic and environmental risk factors, plus aging, with common pathological (and also possibly etiological) features being Aβ plaques, Tau aggregation and phosphorylation, inflammation, DNA damage, mitochondrial dysfunction, and compromised autophagy/mitophagy (Goedert 2015; Canter et al. 2016; Fang et al. 2019b; Kobro-Flatmoen et al. 2021).

Recent studies support impairment of the NAD^+-mitophagy axis as a risk factor for, if not an independent cause of AD (Fang et al. 2019b; Xie et al. 2022). Accumulating evidence from rodent AD models suggests that NAD^+ deprivation and defects in NAD^+-dependent pathways are critical for AD pathogenesis (Hou et al. 2019). In mouse models of familial AD, decreased NAD^+ levels, and metabolic abnormalities in the brain have been described (Chambon et al. 1963; Dong and Brewer 2019; Hou et al. 2019). Additionally, rat cortical neurons stimulated with accumulating Aβ showed decreased NAD^+ levels (Liu et al. 2013). Transcriptomic analysis of postmortem brain tissues from AD patients and healthy controls revealed that mitochondrial dysfunction is involved in the underlying mechanism associated with AD (Yulug et al. 2021a), supporting the hypothesis of a compromised NAD^+-mitophagy axis in the development of AD (Kerr et al. 2017).

Moreover, it has previously been shown that reduced levels of NAD^+ resulted in disrupted cellular metabolism and mitochondrial dysfunction as well as compromised mitophagy in AD (Fang et al. 2019b; Hou et al. 2021). Also, heavily increased inflammation seen in the brain of AD patients and animal models has been linked to decreased NAD^+ (Hou et al. 2021). Preclinical studies of NAD^+ precursor-treated AD animal models have given insights into the consequences of NAD^+ and how NAD^+ might be a promising therapeutic target as discussed in the following section for both aging and age-associated diseases.

THE BENEFITS OF NAD^+ AUGMENTATION

NAD^+ Augmentation

Multiple approaches are effective at increasing cellular NAD^+ levels, such as caloric restriction, exercise, inhibiting NAD^+-consuming enzymes, overexpressing NAD^+ synthetic enzymes, or treating with NAD^+ precursors (Cheng et al.

2016; Fang et al. 2019b; Liu et al. 2019). Pharmacological up-regulation of cellular NAD^+ via NAD^+ precursors, such as the use of NR, NMN, or NAM, are in the current scientific spotlight. NR can increase NAD^+ levels in various model organisms as well as humans (Trammell et al. 2016a; Mitchell et al. 2018; Fang et al. 2019a; Hou et al. 2021). In humans, it has been shown that oral NR supplementation (1000 mg/d for 7 d) up-regulated NAD^+ levels up to 2.7-fold, and intermediate NAAD levels increased 45-fold in human blood (Trammell et al. 2016a). NMN supplementation can also increase intracellular NAD^+ levels in animal models (Blacher et al. 2015), and with the results of human clinical trials awaiting (see the section on Clinical Trials with NAD^+ Supplementation).

In mice, short-term (500 mg/kg/d for 14 d) (Fang et al. 2014) or long-term NR treatment (400 mg/kg/d in drinking water for 6 wk, or 570–590 mg/kg/d over 10 mo) had no detectable toxicity (Fang et al. 2016a,b; Frederick et al. 2016). Based on body weight, a dose of 570–590 mg/kg/d in mice is equivalent to 3.19–3.30 g/d for a human (Fang et al. 2016a,b). In rats, a study reported no adverse reactions at 300 mg/kg/d and the lowest NR dose that caused an observable adverse effect was 1000 mg/kg/d (Conze et al. 2016). NMN administration in wild-type C57BL/6N mice in either the short- (500 mg/kg/d, 7 d, IP) (Gomes et al. 2013) or long-term (100 mg/kg/d or 300 mg/kg/d, continuously for 12 mo), produced no signs of toxicity (Mills et al. 2016). Therefore, the low toxicity of NAD^+ precursors in mammals may make these good candidates for clinical intervention, and several studies examining the safety and toxicity of both NR and NMN are now ongoing (see the section on Clinical Trials with NAD^+ Supplementation). A detailed summary of both animal and clinical evidence of increased NAD^+ via NAD^+ precursors is available in Reiten et al. (2021).

Benefits of NAD^+ Augmentation to Normal Aging

How NAD^+ augmentation benefits normally aged individuals is still not clear, although several preclinical studies on age-predisposed diseases

Cite this article as *Cold Spring Harb Perspect Med* doi: 10.1101/cshperspect.a041193

seem optimistic and have been providing ideas for the initial clinical studies on NAD$^+$ precursors (see the section Clinical Trials with NAD$^+$ Supplementation). In wild-type *C. elegans*, NR or NMN treatment increased the organismal level of NAD$^+$ and activated mitophagy resulting in an ~10% increase in life span (Mouchiroud et al. 2013; Li et al. 2014; Fang et al. 2016a,b, 2019a,b). Also, in wild-type mice, supplementation with NMN, NR, and NAM have shown beneficial effects (de Picciotto et al. 2016; Mills et al. 2016; Mitchell et al. 2018). In wild-type C57BL/6N mice, 12 mo of oral treatment with NMN ameliorated age-associated physiological decline including body weight gain, age-associated gene expression changes in key metabolic organs, and improvements in energy and lipid metabolism, insulin sensitivity, and physical activity (Mills et al. 2016). Furthermore, NMN treatment of old mice reversed vascular dysfunction and oxidative stress, likely via a pathway involving SIRT1 activation (de Picciotto et al. 2016; Tarantini et al. 2019). NAM treatment of wild-type mice has been shown to improve health span measures but not life span (Mitchell et al. 2018). NR treatment of wild-type C57BL/6N mice increased skeletal muscle NAD$^+$, thereby inducing anti-inflammatory pathways (Elhassan et al. 2019), the UPR^{mt} and synthesis of prohibitin 1 and 2, which rejuvenated muscle stem cells and improved muscle function in aged mice and in a muscular dystrophy mouse model (Ryu et al. 2016; Zhang et al. 2016). Additionally, NR treatment delayed senescence of neural and melanocytic stem cells and increased the life span of wild-type mice (Zhang et al. 2016). It has also been demonstrated that NAD$^+$ levels were increased after lactate treatment, which restored the mitochondrial function to that of young mice in a SIRT1-dependent manner (Gomes et al. 2013).

Aging is one of the major risk factors for multiple diseases, including obesity, diabetes, acute kidney failure, heart failure, and dementia (see below). In mice, NAM, NMN, or NR treatment has been shown to mitigate age- and high-fat diet-induced diabetes, obesity, and fatty liver disease by increasing the level of NAD$^+$ (Yoshino et al. 2011; Lee et al. 2015; Gariani et al. 2016; Trammell et al. 2016b; Uddin et al. 2016; Mitchell et al.

2018). After NAM or NMN treatment, the diabetic mice showed improved glucose tolerance, insulin sensitivity, and lipid profiles, and gene expression related to oxidative stress and inflammatory responses was restored (Yoshino et al. 2011; Mitchell et al. 2018). Furthermore, both murine heart failure models and cardiac biopsies from human patients with heart failure showed decreased levels of NAD$^+$, in addition to decreased protein levels of NAMPT (Diguet et al. 2018; Breton et al. 2020). Treating mice or isolated cardiomyocytes with NR attenuated heart failure and increased the level of NAD$^+$, NAAD, and related metabolites (Diguet et al. 2018). In mice, age-associated susceptibility to acute kidney injury in has also been shown to be rescued by NMN treatment via a pathway involving SIRT1 and its target PGC1α (Tran et al. 2016; Guan et al. 2017). Moreover, NR or NMN improved kidney function and prevented mitochondrial RNA/RIG-I-dependent inflammation during kidney injury (Doke et al. 2023). Combined, this preclinical data, in both in vitro and animal models, suggests that age-associated diseases might be improved by NAD$^+$ augmentation (Fig. 3A).

Benefits of NAD$^+$ Augmentation to Pathological Aging

In addition to biological aging, supplementation with the NAD$^+$ precursors NR and NMN have shown several benefits in accelerated aging diseases. Human XPA-deficient cells show compromised mitophagy, excessive PINK1 cleavage, and increased mitochondrial membrane potential. The mitochondrial abnormalities are likely due to hyperactive PARP-1 mediated decline of the NAD$^+$-SIRT1-PGC1α axis (Fang et al. 2014). Moreover, *C. elegans* models of XPA (*xpa*-1) also show mitochondrial dysfunction and compromised mitophagy, which at least partially contribute to the shortened life span and reduced health span of the worms. Confirming a central role of PARP1 hyperactivity in NAD$^+$ depletion in XPA, both PARP1 inhibition, NR, or NMN supplementation restored mitochondrial function and mitophagy, and in addition rescued life span defects in the XPA *C. elegans* model (Fang et al. 2014). Mitochondrial dysfunction, compro-

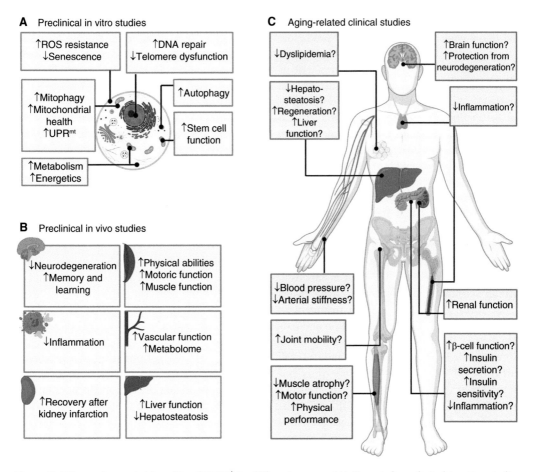

Figure 3. Effects of reported benefits of NAD$^+$ in different organs. (*A*) Reported preclinical in vitro studies showing the effects of treatment with nicotinamide (NAM), nicotinamide riboside (NR), or nicotinamide mononucleotide (NMN). (*B*) Reported preclinical in vivo studies showing the effects of treatment with NAM, NR, or NMN. (*C*) Aging-related features being analyzed in the completed, ongoing, and recruiting clinical trials for NAM, NR, or NMN. "?" represents the unknown effects of supplementation in humans due to lack of published data/results from clinical trials. (This figure was created using BioRender.)

mised mitophagy, and life span defects are also seen in CS and A-T *C. elegans* models and can be at least partially rescued by PARP inhibition (Olaparib) or NAD$^+$ precursor treatment (NR or NMN) in low (micromolar) concentrations via mitophagy induction (Scheibye-Knudsen et al. 2014, 2016; Fang et al. 2016a,b). In *Atm$^{-/-}$* mice and *atm-1* worms treatment with either NR, PARP1 inhibitor, or SIRT1 activator (SRT1720), shortened life span and health span was ameliorated through induction of mitophagy either through activation of the NAD$^+$-SIRTs axis, improved DCT-1 mediated mitophagy (thereby

improving mitochondrial quality), and/or stimulation of DNA repair through activation of the nonhomologous end-joining repair (Ku70 and DNA-PKcs) (Fang et al. 2016a,b). In CS, NR supplementation or high-fat diet extended the life span and improved the health span of *C. elegans* (Fang et al. 2014; Okur et al. 2020a, b) and mouse models of CS (Scheibye-Knudsen et al. 2014; Okur et al. 2020a). *Csa$^{m/m}$* and *Csb$^{m/m}$* mice exhibit hearing deficiencies, which greatly resemble age-associated hearing loss, and short-term supplementation with NR (10 d) rescued this age-associated hearing deficiency (Okur et al.

2020a). Since the mechanism of hearing loss is similar in CS and age-related hearing loss, this provides ideas for therapeutic targets to ameliorate human age-related hearing loss.

Despite WS not being a neurodegeneration-related disease like the above-mentioned, studies suggest that impairment of the NAD⁺-mitophagy-mitochondrial quality axis plays a role in disease etiology. Supplementation with NR or NMN extended life span and health span in *C. elegans* and *Drosophila melanogaster* models of WS (Fang et al. 2019a). In human WS cells and a *C. elegans* WS model (*wrn-1(gk99)*), NR supplementation increased BCL2/adenovirus E1B 19-kDa protein-interacting protein 3-like (NIX) and serine/threonine-protein kinase ULK1 (ULK-1)-dependent mitophagy, improved mitochondrial quality and fat metabolism, and decreased DNA damage and increased DNA repair (homologous recombination) in *C. elegans* (Fang et al. 2019a).

The above studies on premature aging diseases add to our current understanding of the communication between subcellular compartments and how the nuclear–mitochondrial cross talk affects both cellular and organismal health and aging (Fang et al. 2016a,b).

Benefits of NAD⁺ Augmentation to AD

There is increasing evidence that NAD⁺ supplementation is beneficial for the alleviation of cognitive impairment and pathological features of AD in animal models. NAD⁺ augmentation inhibited AD pathogenesis and cognitive impairment in different AD animal models, including NAM-treated triple transgenic (3xTg) AD mice (Liu et al. 2013), NR-treated 3xTgAD/Polβ⁺/⁻ mice, and APP/PS1 mice (Hou et al. 2018; Hou et al. 2021), and NMN-treated transgenic AD *C. elegans* models expressing neuronal $A\beta_{1-42}$ and neuronal Tau (Fang et al. 2019b). Additionally, treatment with combined metabolic activators (CMAs) consisting of NAD⁺ precursors and glutathione precursors improved AD-associated pathology in an AD rat model (Yulug et al. 2021a). Moreover, it has been suggested that Aβ, p-Tau, neuroinflammation, and compromised mitophagy are the pathological occurrences or at least contributors to the development and progression

of AD, and that NAD⁺ supplementation can ameliorate AD (Fang et al. 2019b; Hou et al. 2021).

Two of the main pathological hallmarks of AD are accumulation and formation of extracellular Aβ plaques and intracellular formation of neurofibrillary tangles (NFTs) consisting of hyperphosphorylated Tau protein. Whether NAD⁺ supplementation reduces Aβ pathology seems to be dependent on the animal model used (Gong et al. 2013; Liu et al. 2013). The reduced accumulation of Aβ in NAM- or NR-treated AD mice (APP/PS1 [Fang et al. 2019b] and Tg2576 [Gong et al. 2013]) may be due to reduced production of the pathological $A\beta_{1-42}$, possibly through activation of PGC-1α-regulated BACE1 (β-secretase) degradation; or it may be through enhancing microglia/astrocytes-based phagocytosis of Aβ plaques (Gong et al. 2013; Fang et al. 2019b). However, in 3xTgAD and 3xTg/Polβ⁺/⁻ mice, no detectable effect was observed upon eliminating Aβ pathology (Hou et al. 2018; Fang et al. 2019b). NAD⁺ augmentation has also been reported to reduce Tau pathology in AD models. NAD⁺ supplementation has been demonstrated to inhibit Tau phosphorylation at different sites (Thr181, Ser202, Thr205, and Thr231), possibly by inhibiting the cyclin-dependent kinase 5 (Cdk5)-p25 complex activity (Green et al. 2008; Hou et al. 2018; Fang et al. 2019b).

Increasing NAD⁺ has been shown to affect additional central cellular processes in AD animal models, such as mitochondrial function, mitophagy, DNA repair, inflammation, and senescence. Supplementation of AD mouse models with either NR or NMN improved mitochondrial function and induced mitophagic activity, leading to improvements in brain pathologies, neuronal function and survival, and inflammation (Hou et al. 2018; Fang et al. 2019b; Hou et al. 2021). Interestingly, specific mitophagy inducers, such as urolithin A and the antibiotic actinonin, have also been shown to ameliorate several AD features in both *C. elegans* and mouse models of AD (Fang et al. 2019b), indicating the benefits of stimulating the NAD⁺-mitophagy axis in the treatment of AD. Additionally, through the use of artificial intelligence, we were able to identify novel mitophagy inducers: treatment with these restored memory and improved cognitive deficits in AD *C. elegans* and mouse models (Ai et al. 2022; Xie et al. 2022). NAD$^+$ may ameliorate AD pathology by regulating lysosome and the ubiquitin-proteasome system (UPS) functions via improvement of mitophagic functions. NAD$^+$ augmentation via NR supplementation induced the UPS in the hippocampus and cortex of Tg2576 mice (Gong et al. 2013), and restored UPR^{mt} in APP/PS1 mice. More evidence supporting the function of the lysosome and the UPS in maintaining a healthy brain comes from studies showing that the toxic protein aggregates of Aβ and Tau inhibit the proteasome and autophagy or mitophagy, resulting in protein and mitochondrial accumulation primarily in the hippocampus and prefrontal cortex. Moreover NAD$^+$ supplementation reduces the pathological phenotypes of Aβ and p-Tau (Tseng et al. 2008; Fang et al. 2019b).

As we age, the levels of NAD$^+$ in our bodies gradually decline, and this has been linked to cellular senescence and aging. Cellular senescence is a state in which cells stop dividing and become irreversibly arrested, leading to tissue dysfunction and age-related diseases (López-Otín et al. 2023). Previously, it has been hypothesized that DNA damage is responsible for, or contributes to, the neuronal damage observed in AD, and oxidative stress may be the predominant type of DNA damage primarily repaired by base excision repair. In a base excision repair-deficient AD mouse model (3xTgAD/Polβ$^{+/-}$), and in the APP/PS1 model, NR supplementation reduced the amount of DNA damage as manifested by decreased staining of γH2AX (marking double-strand breaks [DSBs]) in the hippocampus (Hou et al. 2018, 2021). Studies have shown that boosting NAD$^+$ levels can delay the onset of cellular senescence and extend life span in various model organisms. NR supplementation also inhibited neuroinflammation and cellular senescence in AD mice, as well as in the accelerated aging $Atm^{-/-}$ mouse model, which shows severe cerebellar ataxia (Hou et al. 2018, 2021; Yang et al. 2021). The molecular mechanism behind this improvement is likely to include NAD$^+$-dependent induction of mitophagy, which cleans the cells of damaged mitochondria (Hou et al. 2021; Yang et al. 2021). Simultaneously, a NAD$^+$-dependent immune response, activated by NAD$^+$ augmentation, can lead to improved resolution of inflammation and phagocytic activity (Gong et al. 2013; Minhas et al. 2019) as well as inhibition of mitochondrial dysfunction–associated senescence (MiDAS) (Wiley et al. 2016). NAD$^+$ repletion inhibited the NLRP3 inflammasome and the key inflammatory response of cGAS-STING signaling (Fang et al. 2019b; Lautrup et al. 2019; Hou et al. 2021; Yang et al. 2021), providing a mechanism for the inhibitory effect of NAD$^+$ on inflammation and senescence. Senolytics are a type of drug that selectively target and kill senescent cells (Hou et al. 2019; López-Otín et al. 2023), and they could be combined with NAD supplementation to further reduce senescence.

NAD$^+$ augmentation can additionally restore neurogenesis in 3xTgAD and 3xTg/Polβ$^{+/-}$ mice by promoting the proliferation of neural precursor cells (Hou et al. 2018). NR and an allosteric activator of NAMPT, P7C3, have been reported to have neuroprotective abilities in mouse models of AD and PD, respectively (Pieper et al. 2005; De Jesús-Cortés et al. 2012; Hou et al. 2018). Consistent with this, studies of large-scale human brain samples demonstrated that hippocampal neurogenesis gradually decreases with the progression of AD (Moreno-Jiménez et al. 2019). The stem cell regenerative activity of NR and NMN likely also contributes to reducing hippocampus-dependent cognitive deficits seen in AD.

CLINICAL TRIALS WITH NAD$^+$ SUPPLEMENTATION

The preclinical trials presented above have led to numerous clinical trials aiming foremost at establishing the pharmacokinetics and toxicology of the NAD$^+$ precursors focusing on NR, NMN, and NAM, and next to test the effect on aging-related features, age-related diseases, and other diseases. Due to the recent extensive reviews on the clinical trials (Connell et al. 2019; Lautrup et al. 2019; Gilmour et al. 2020; Reiten et al. 2021), we will only present a short summary of the published data from the completed clinical trials related to aging and age-related diseases. Table 1 provides an overview of the clinical trials on NAD$^+$ precursors related to aging and disease. NR is orally bioavailable and tolerated, and supplementation with NR increased NAD$^+$ in

Table 1. A summary of clinical trials related to aging, pathological aging, and age-related diseases

NAD$^+$ precursors	Disease/condition	Dose administration	Duration of treatment	Demographics	Primary outcome and results	Status	NCT/UMIN/jRCT/PMID
NAM	AD	1500 mg BID	12 mo	Age: 50+ Sex: all	Change in p-Tau 231	Recruiting	NCT03061474
		1500 mg BID	6 mo	Age: 50–95 Sex: all	AD symptoms	Completed, results N/A	NCT00580931
	PD	100 mg BID	18 mo	Age: 35+ Sex: all	Inflammation and severity of PD symptoms	Recruiting	NCT03808961
NR	Aging and lipemia	250 mg BID	7 d	Age: 18–35 vs. 60–75 Sex: all	NAD$^+$ in blood / Vasodilatory responsiveness / Lipidemia / Oxidative stress and inflammation	Completed, results N/A	NCT03501433
	AD	1000 mg/d	12 wk	Age: 55–89 Sex: all	Brain NAD$^+$ levels / Brain redox state	Recruiting	NCT04430517
	PD	1000 mg/d	52 wk	Age: 18+ Sex: all	MDS-UPDRS / NAD$^+$ metabolites in blood	Recruiting	NCT03568968
		500 mg BID	30 d	Age: 18+ Sex: all	PD-related patterns, neuronal metabolism, motor function	Completed, results N/A	NCT03816020
	A-T	25 mg/kg/d	4 mo	Age: 2+ Sex: all	Ataxia dysarthria, quality of life, laboratory parameters, intelligibility, and fatigue status	Enrolling, results N/A	NCT03962114
		300 mg/d	2 yr	Age: 3+ Sex: all	NAD$^+$ metabolome / Patient well-being / A-T characteristics and metabolism	Active, results N/A	NCT04870866
	WS	1000 mg/d	52 wk	Age: 20+ Sex: all	Safety / WS characteristics and metabolism	Recruiting	jRCTs031190141
	Mild cognitive impairment	500 mg BID	12 wk	Age: 60–90 Sex: all	Cognitive scores from baseline	Recruiting	NCT03482167
		Dose escalation: 250 mg/d up to 1 g/d, then 1 g/d	4 wk + 6 wk (1 g/d)	Age: 65+ Sex: all	MoCA from baseline at 10 wk	Active, results N/A	NCT02942888
	Cognitive function, mood, and sleep	Crossover study with 300 mg/d and 1000 mg/d	8 wk	Age: 55+ Sex: all	Cognitive function, mood, and sleep	Completed, results N/A	NCT03562468

Continued

Table 1. *Continued*

NAD⁺ precursors	Disease/condition	Dose administration	Duration of treatment	Demographics	Primary outcome and results	Status	NCT/UMIN/jRCT/PMID
	Aging daily function and recovery	1200 mg/d	8 wk	Age: 60+ Sex: all	Cognitive function, mood, and daily activity	Not yet recruiting	NCT04078178
		1000 mg/d	3 wk	Age: 70–80 Sex: male	Skeletal muscle tissue NAD⁺ levels and mitochondrial function	N/A	NCT02950441
		500 mg BID	6 wk	Age: 55–79 Sex: all	Results: NR is well tolerated in healthy middle-aged and older adults	Completed, published	NCT02921659 PMC29599478
		250 or 500 mg/d Basis (NR + PT)	8 wk	Age: 60–80 Sex: all	Safety and efficacy with regard to NAD⁺ sustainability in elderly people	Completed, results submitted	NCT02678611
	Healthy elderly volunteers	500 mg BID	6 mo	Age: 65–80 Sex: female	Maximum oxygen uptake / Muscle function, genes, and mitochondria / Short Physical Performance Battery / Muscle biopsy samples: respiration rate, immunoblot, and polymerase chain reaction (PCR) / Bone metabolism	Recruiting	NCT03818802
	Frailty and sarcopenia	2x 250 mg BID	12 wk	Age: 65–85 Sex: all	Maximal oxygen uptake / Muscle strength / Gait speed	Not yet recruiting	NCT04469186
		500 mg NR/100 mg PT BID	45 d	Age: 55–80 Sex: all	Muscle regeneration in elderly	Completed, results N/A	NCT03754842
		500 mg NR/100 mg PT BID	90 d	Age: 65+	Safety and tolerance / Posttraumatic fall/injury	Unknown	NCT03635411
	Hypertension in elderly	1000 mg/d	6 wk	Age: 65–105 Sex: all	Systolic blood pressure	Recruiting	NCT04112043
		500 mg BID	3 mo	Age: 50–79 Sex: all	Systolic blood pressure and arterial stiffness	Recruiting	NCT03821623
		1000 mg/d	3 mo	Age: 35–80 Sex: all	Arterial stiffness and elevated systolic blood pressure in patients with moderate-to-severe chronic kidney disease (CKD)	Recruiting	NCT04040959

Cite this article as *Cold Spring Harb Perspect Med* doi: 10.1101/cshperspect.a041193

Compound	Condition	Dose	Duration	Age/Sex	Outcome	Status	Identifier
		Dose escalation: 500–2000 mg/d	14 d	Age: 18+ Sex: all	Whole blood NAD$^+$ levels	Recruiting	NCT04528004
	ALS	1500 mg NR/300 mg PT or 1000 mg NR/200 mg PT	?	Age: 35+ Sex: all	Heart failure; Adverse effects; Disease progression; Overall survival	Recruiting	NCT04562831
		1500 mg NR/300 mg PT	?			Recruiting	NCT05095571
	Menopause	500 mg NR/100 mg PT/d	7 d	Age: 35+ Sex: female	Production of estradiol; Change undesirable effects of menopause	Completed, results N/A	NCT04841499
NMN	Glucose metabolism disorders	500 mg/d	8 wk	Age: 55–75 Sex: female	Insulin sensitivity in skeletal muscle	Active	NCT03151239
		300 mg/d	16 wk	Age: 45–75 Sex: all	Muscle insulin sensitivity	Recruiting	NCT04571008
	Aging	300 mg/d	60 d	Age: 40–65 Sex: all	Cellular NAD$^+$ concentration in blood serum, physical performance, blood pressure	Completed, published	NCT04228640
		250 mg/d	12 wk	Age: 65+ Sex: male	Body composition in aging	Completed, published	UMIN000036321
		2% NMN, BID, crème	55 d	Age: 40–65 Sex: females	Wrinkles, fatigue, puffiness around eyes	Completed, results N/A	NCT04685096
	Safety in middle-aged and older individuals	300 mg or 600 or 900 mg/d	60 d	Age: 40–65 Sex: all		Completed, results N/A	NCT04823260
	Safety in middle-aged and older adults	250 mg/d	12 wk	Age: 40–65 Sex: all	Blood vessel conditions	Completed, published	UMIN000045205

(AD) Alzheimer's disease, (A–T) ataxia telangiectasia, (BID) twice a day, (NAM) nicotinamide, (NMN) nicotinamide mononucleotide, (NR) nicotinamide riboside, (PD) Parkinson's disease, (WS) Werner syndrome.

healthy middle-aged and older adults (Trammell et al. 2016a; Martens et al. 2018). Some clinical studies showed NMN safely and effectively elevated NAD^+ metabolism in healthy middle-aged and older-aged adults (Huang 2022; Katayoshi et al. 2023). Currently, multiple studies of the safety, tolerance, and long-term effects of NMN have been completed; results are pending (jRCTs041200034, UMIN000039 527, jRCTs041190080, UMIN000025739, UMIN 000030609, UMIN000021309). NR, in combination with the polyphenol pterostilbene (PT), has been shown to increase NAD^+ levels by 90% in whole blood with no serious adverse events (Dellinger et al. 2017). Currently, the ongoing clinical trials related to aging focus on the effects of NR on cognitive function, daily activity and muscle function, mitochondrial function, hypertension, glucose, and fat metabolism. Several clinical trials are investigating the effects of NAD^+ precursor supplementation on age-related diseases such as heart failure, obesity and diabetes, and neurodegenerative diseases. Two clinical trials with obese and diabetic men have confirmed the bioavailability and safety of NR supplementation, but without seeing effects on weight, glucose intolerance, or insulin sensitivity (Trammell et al. 2016a; Dollerup et al. 2018). One recent clinical study showed that body weight, diastolic blood pressure, total cholesterol, low-density lipoprotein (LDL) cholesterol, and non-high-density lipoprotein cholesterol decreased significantly in the MIB-626 (NMN) group when compared to placebo (Pencina et al. 2023). Chronic NMN supplementation was well tolerated, caused no significant deleterious effect, and showed small but significant improvements in gait speed and performance in a grip test, suggesting alteration to muscle function in healthy older men (Igarashi et al. 2022) (UMIN000036321). One short-term therapeutic study using NR for up to 30 d showed no deleterious impact on methylation homeostasis (Gaare et al. 2023). CMA treatment has been shown to improve the cognitive function of PD patients (Yulug et al. 2021b) and of AD patients after 84 d of treatment compared to placebo (Yulug et al. 2021a). CMA treatment of AD patients resulted in increased plasma levels of NAM

and related metabolites, among others, whereas tryptophan-related metabolites such as kynurenate, kynurenine, and tryptophan betaine decreased after CMA treatment (Yulug et al. 2023). Increased levels of tryptophan-related metabolites have previously been associated with increased neurodegeneration and impaired cognitive function (Guillemin et al. 2003; Ting et al. 2007; O'Farrell and Harkin 2017). Several clinical trials have started or are recruiting (Table 1) and looking at the potential of NAM or NR as preventative therapies for AD or PD, and the next years should reveal whether the effects on human patients are as promising as the preclinical data have been. Last, two clinical trials are ongoing examining the effects of NR on A-T patients (NCT04870866 and NCT03962114), and one on the effects of NR supplementation on WS patients in Japan (jRCTs031190141).

CONCLUSIONS AND FUTURE PERSPECTIVES

The hallmarks of aging include genomic instability, epigenetic alterations, telomere attrition, loss of proteostasis, mitochondrial dysfunction, cellular senescence, deregulated nutrient sensing, altered intercellular communication, stem cell exhaustion (Hou et al. 2019), disabled macroautophagy (Fang et al. 2017), chronic inflammation, and dysbiosis (López-Otín et al. 2023). Most of these pathways are strongly associated with decreased NAD^+ (Lautrup et al. 2019), and NAD^+ supplementation has been demonstrated to have beneficial effects on age-related diseases. However, there are still many challenges and shortcomings in the mechanistic insight. The detection methods are challenging due to the low stability of NAD^+ and some of its precursors and intermediates both physically and while crossing the gut system, and the detection of NAD^+, especially in the brain of human individuals remains a challenge. In vivo MIR scanning is now available (Zhu et al. 2015) and may provide insight into how NAD^+ levels change during aging and disease progression in live human patients. In line with the requirement for better detection methods comes a question on where the metabolites go and what they become. Iso-tope labeling or other tracing experiments would help to determine what actually happens to the supplements during and after uptake, how the NAD$^+$ and its precursors are transferred and to which tissues and/or cell types, and how they are being processed, among other questions.

Even though several studies have contributed to the knowledge we have today of the mechanisms underlying the effects seen after increasing NAD$^+$ with various precursors, more insight into the mechanisms is warranted. It would be interesting to continue the studies on the mechanisms downstream of NAD$^+$, and also to examine upstream pathways to better understand age- and disease-related declines.

Currently, both the preclinical and clinical studies with NAD$^+$ precursors (majorly NR and NMN) have shown a safe and nontoxic profile. However, the long-term effects are yet to be reported. It has been suggested that NAD$^+$ supplementation plays a role in the immune responses, and in cancer research it has been suggested that NAD$^+$ might increase the expression of inflammatory factors (Nacarelli et al. 2019). On the other hand, NAD$^+$ supplementation has been demonstrated to reduce inflammatory responses and the expression of inflammatory factors (Fang et al. 2019b; Hou et al. 2021). There is a continual need to further understand the impact of NAD$^+$ supplementation and its long-term effects. Ongoing clinical trials use short-term treatment, and it would be of interest and importance to evaluate long-term treatment with NAD$^+$ supplementation. It is also important to have larger studies involving more participants than the current ones. There are certain conditions where NAD$^+$ supplementation may want to be avoided, such as certain cancers (Demarest et al. 2019). The results from ongoing clinical trials will hopefully shed light on some of the missing knowledge regarding disease treatment, and hopefully the next decade of research will fill in some of the knowledge gaps in terms of both technical challenges and mechanisms.

COMPETING INTEREST STATEMENT

E.F.F. has an MTA with LMITO Therapeutics, Inc. (South Korea), a CRADA arrangement with ChromaDex (USA), and a commercialization agreement with Molecule AG/VITADAO, and is a consultant to Aladdin Healthcare Technologies (UK and Germany), the Vancouver Dementia Prevention Centre (Canada), Intellectual Labs (Norway), MindRank AI (China), and NYo3 (China).

ACKNOWLEDGMENTS

The authors acknowledge the valuable work of the many investigators whose published articles they were unable to cite owing to space limitations. E.F.F. is supported by Cure Alzheimer's Fund (#282952), HELSE SØR-ØST (#2020001, #2021021, #2023093), the Research Council of Norway (#262175, #334361), Molecule AG/VITADAO (#282942), NordForsk Foundation (#119986), the National Natural Science Foundation of China (#81971327), Akershus University Hospital (#269901, #261973, #262960), the Civitan Norges Forskningsfond for Alzheimers sykdom (#281931), the Czech Republic-Norway KAPPA programme (with Martin Vyhnálek, #TO01000215), and the Rosa Sløyfe/Norwegian Cancer Society & Norwegian Breast Cancer Society (#207819). S.L. has received funding from the European Union's Horizon 2020 research and innovation programme under the Marie Skłodowska-Curie grant agreement No. 801133. Y.H. was supported by the National Natural Science Foundation of China (#82171405), and the Lingang Laboratory (#LG-QS-202205-10). The figures were generated using the subscribed software BioRender. V.A.B. is supported by the intramural program of the National Institute on Aging, National Institutes of Health (NIH), USA.

REFERENCES

Ai R, Zhuang XX, Anisimov A, Lu JH, Fang EF. 2022. A synergized machine learning plus cross-species wet-lab validation approach identifies neuronal mitophagy inducers inhibiting Alzheimer disease. *Autophagy* **18**: 939–941. doi:10.1080/15548627.2022.2031382

Bahn A, Hagos Y, Reuter S, Balen D, Brzica H, Krick W, Burckhardt BC, Sabolić I, Burckhardt G. 2008. Identification of a new urate and high affinity nicotinate transporter, hOAT10 (SLC22A13). *J Biol Chem* **283**: 16332–16341. doi:10.1074/jbc.M800737200

Berger F, Lau C, Dahlmann M, Ziegler M. 2005. Subcellular compartmentation and differential catalytic properties of the three human nicotinamide mononucleotide adenylyltransferase isoforms. *J Biol Chem* **280**: 36334–36341. doi:10.1074/jbc.M508660200

Bernofsky C, Swan M. 1973. An improved cycling assay for nicotinamide adenine dinucleotide. *Anal Biochem* **53**: 452–458. doi:10.1016/0003-2697(73)90094-8

Bieganowski P, Brenner C. 2004. Discoveries of nicotinamide riboside as a nutrient and conserved NRK genes establish a Preiss–Handler independent route to NAD$^+$ in fungi and humans. *Cell* **117**: 495–502. doi:10.1016/s0092-8674(04)00416-7

Billington RA, Travelli C, Ercolano E, Galli U, Roman CB, Grolla AA, Canonico PL, Condorelli F, Genazzani AA. 2008. Characterization of NAD uptake in mammalian cells. *J Biol Chem* **283**: 6367–6374. doi:10.1074/jbc.M706204200

Blacher E, Dadali T, Bespalko A, Haupenthal VJ, Grimm MO, Hartmann T, Lund FE, Stein R, Levy A. 2015. Alzheimer's disease pathology is attenuated in a CD38-deficient mouse model. *Ann Neurol* **78**: 88–103. doi:10.1002/ana.24425

Breton M, Costemale-Lacoste JF, Li Z, Lafuente-Lafuente C, Belmin J, Mericskay M. 2020. Blood NAD levels are reduced in very old patients hospitalized for heart failure. *Exp Gerontol* **139**: 111051. doi:10.1016/j.exger.2020.111051

Canter RG, Penney J, Tsai LH. 2016. The road to restoring neural circuits for the treatment of Alzheimer's disease. *Nature* **539**: 187–196. doi:10.1038/nature20412

Camacho-Pereira J, Tarragó MG, Chini CCS, Nin V, Escande C, Warner GM, Puranik AS, Schoon RA, Reid JM, Galina A, et al. 2016. CD38 dictates age-related NAD decline and mitochondrial dysfunction through an SIRT3-dependent mechanism. *Cell Metab* **23**: 1127–1139. doi:10.1016/j.cmet.2016.05.006

Campesan S, Green EW, Breda C, Sathyasaikumar KV, Muchowski PJ, Schwarcz R, Kyriacou CP, Giorgini F. 2011. The kynurenine pathway modulates neurodegeneration in a *Drosophila* model of Huntington's disease. *Curr Biol* **21**: 961–966. doi:10.1016/j.cub.2011.04.028

Chaleckis R, Murakami I, Takada J, Kondoh H, Yanagida M. 2016. Individual variability in human blood metabolites identifies age-related differences. *Proc Natl Acad Sci* **113**: 4252–4259. doi:10.1073/pnas.1603023113

Chalkiadaki A, Guarente L. 2015. The multifaceted functions of sirtuins in cancer. *Nat Rev Cancer* **15**: 608–624. doi:10.1038/nrc3985

Chambon P, Weill JD, Mandel P. 1963. Nicotinamide mononucleotide activation of a new DNA-dependent polyadenylic acid synthesizing nuclear enzyme. *Biochem Biophys Res Commun* **11**: 39–43. doi:10.1016/0006-291x(63)90024-x

Cheng A, Yang Y, Zhou Y, Maharana C, Lu D, Peng W, Liu Y, Wan R, Marosi K, Misiak M, et al. 2016. Mitochondrial SIRT3 mediates adaptive responses of neurons to exercise and metabolic and excitatory challenges. *Cell Metab* **23**: 128–142. doi:10.1016/j.cmet.2015.10.013

Chi Y, Sauve AA. 2013. Nicotinamide riboside, a trace nutrient in foods, is a vitamin B3 with effects on energy metabolism and neuroprotection. *Curr Opin Clin Nutr Metab Care* **16**: 657–661. doi:10.1097/MCO.0b013e32836510c0

Clement J, Wong M, Poljak A, Sachdev P, Braidy N. 2019. The plasma NAD$^+$ metabolome is dysregulated in "normal" aging. *Rejuvenation Res* **22**: 121–130. doi:10.1089/rej.2018.2077

Connell NJ, Houtkooper RH, Schrauwen P. 2019. NAD$^+$ metabolism as a target for metabolic health: have we found the silver bullet? *Diabetologia* **62**: 888–899. doi:10.1007/s00125-019-4831-3

Conze DB, Crespo-Barreto J, Kruger CL. 2016. Safety assessment of nicotinamide riboside, a form of vitamin B$_3$. *Hum Exp Toxicol* **35**: 1149–1160. doi:10.1177/0960327115626254

Covarrubias AJ, Perrone R, Grozio A, Verdin E. 2021. NAD$^+$ metabolism and its roles in cellular processes during ageing. *Nat Rev Mol Cell Biol* **22**: 119–141. doi:10.1038/s41580-020-00313-x

De Jesús-Cortés H, Xu P, Drawbridge J, Estill SJ, Huntington P, Tran S, Britt J, Tesla R, Morlock L, Naidoo J, et al. 2012. Neuroprotective efficacy of aminopropyl carbazoles in a mouse model of Parkinson disease. *Proc Natl Acad Sci* **109**: 17010–17015. doi:10.1073/pnas.1213956109

Dellinger RW, Santos SR, Morris M, Evans M, Alminana D, Guarente L, Marcotulli E. 2017. Repeat dose NRPT (nicotinamide riboside and pterostilbene) increases NAD$^+$ levels in humans safely and sustainably: a randomized, double-blind, placebo-controlled study. *NPJ Aging Mech Dis* **3**: 17. doi:10.1038/s41514-017-0016-9

Demarest TG, Babbar M, Okur MN, Dan X, Croteau DL, Fakouri NM, Mattson MP, Bohr VA. 2019. NAD$^+$ metabolism in aging and cancer. *Ann Rev Cancer Biol* **3**: 2015–2130. doi:10.1146/annurev-cancerbio-030518-055905

de Picciotto NE, Gano LB, Johnson LC, Martens CR, Sindler AL, Mills KF, Imai S, Seals DR. 2016. Nicotinamide mononucleotide supplementation reverses vascular dysfunction and oxidative stress with aging in mice. *Aging Cell* **15**: 522–530. doi:10.1111/acel.12461

Diguet N, Trammell SAJ, Tannous C, Deloux R, Piquereau J, Mougenot N, Gouge A, Gressette M, Manoury B, Blanc J, et al. 2018. Nicotinamide riboside preserves cardiac function in a mouse model of dilated cardiomyopathy. *Circulation* **137**: 2256–2273. doi:10.1161/CIRCULATIONAHA.116.026099

Doke T, Mukherjee S, Mukhi D, Dhillon P, Abedini A, Davis JG, Chellappa K, Chen B, Baur JA, Susztak K. 2023. NAD$^+$ precursor supplementation prevents mtRNA/RIG-I-dependent inflammation during kidney injury. *Nat Metab* **5**: 414–430. doi:10.1038/s42255-023-00761-7

Dölle C, Niere M, Lohndal E, Ziegler M. 2010. Visualization of subcellular NAD pools and intra-organellar protein localization by poly-ADP-ribose formation. *Cell Mol Life Sci* **67**: 433–443. doi:10.1007/s00018-009-0190-4

Dollerup OL, Christensen B, Svart M, Schmidt MS, Sulek K, Ringgaard S, Stødkilde-Jørgensen H, Møller N, Brenner C, Treebak JT, et al. 2018. A randomized placebo-controlled clinical trial of nicotinamide riboside in obese men: safety, insulin-sensitivity, and lipid-mobilizing effects. *Am J Clin Nutr* **108**: 343–353. doi:10.1093/ajcn/nqy132

Dong Y, Brewer GJ. 2019. Global metabolic shifts in age and Alzheimer's disease mouse brains pivot at NAD$^+$/NADH redox sites. *J Alzheimers Dis* **71:** 119–140. doi:10.3233/JAD-190408

Edenberg HJ. 2000. Regulation of the mammalian alcohol dehydrogenase genes. *Prog Nucleic Acid Res Mol Biol* **64:** 295–341. doi:10.1016/s0079-6603(00)64008-4

Elhassan YS, Kluckova K, Fletcher RS, Schmidt MS, Garten A, Doig CL, Cartwright DM, Oakey L, Burley CV, Jenkinson N, et al. 2019. Nicotinamide riboside augments the aged human skeletal muscle NAD⁺ metabolome and induces transcriptomic and anti-inflammatory signatures. *Cell Rep* **28:** 1717–1728.e6. doi:10.1016/j.celrep.2019.07.043

Elvehjem CA, Madden RJ, Strong FM, Woolley DW. 1974. The isolation and identification of the anti-black tongue factor. *Nutr Rev* **32:** 48–50. doi:10.1111/j.1753-4887.1974.tb06263.x

Emanuelli M, Carnevali F, Saccucci F, Pierella F, Amici A, Raffaelli N, Magni G. 2001. Molecular cloning, chromosomal localization, tissue mRNA levels, bacterial expression, and enzymatic properties of human NMN adenylyltransferase. *J Biol Chem* **276:** 406–412. doi:10.1074/jbc.M008700200

Essuman K, Summers DW, Sasaki Y, Mao X, DiAntonio A, Milbrandt J. 2017. The SARM1 toll/interleukin-1 receptor domain possesses intrinsic NAD⁺ cleavage activity that promotes pathological axonal degeneration. *Neuron* **93:** 1334–1343.e5. doi:10.1016/j.neuron.2017.02.022

Euler HV. 1930. Fermentation of sugars and fermentative enzymes. Nobel Lecture. https://www.nobelprize.org/prizes/chemistry/1929/euler-chelpin/lecture

Fang EF, Scheibye-Knudsen M, Brace LE, Kassahun H, SenGupta T, Nilsen H, Mitchell JR, Croteau DL, Bohr VA. 2014. Defective mitophagy in XPA via PARP-1 hyperactivation and NAD⁺/SIRT1 reduction. *Cell* **157:** 882–896. doi:10.1016/j.cell.2014.03.026

Fang EF, Scheibye-Knudsen M, Chua KF, Mattson MP, Croteau DL, Bohr VA. 2016a. Nuclear DNA damage signalling to mitochondria in ageing. *Nat Rev Mol Cell Biol* **17:** 308–321. doi:10.1038/nrm.2016.14

Fang EF, Kassahun H, Croteau DL, Scheibye-Knudsen M, Marosi K, Lu H, Shamanna RA, Kalyanasundaram S, Bollineni RC, Wilson MA, et al. 2016b. NAD⁺ replenishment improves lifespan and healthspan in ataxia telangiectasia models via mitophagy and DNA repair. *Cell Metab* **24:** 566–581. doi:10.1016/j.cmet.2016.09.004

Fang EF, Lautrup S, Hou Y, Demarest TG, Croteau DL, Mattson MP, Bohr VA. 2017. NAD⁺ in aging: molecular mechanisms and translational implications. *Trends Mol Med* **23:** 899–916. doi:10.1016/j.molmed.2017.08.001

Fang EF, Hou Y, Lautrup S, Jensen MB, Yang B, SenGupta T, Caponio D, Khezri R, Demarest TG, Aman Y, et al. 2019a. NAD⁺ augmentation restores mitophagy and limits accelerated aging in werner syndrome. *Nat Commun* **10:** 5284. doi:10.1038/s41467-019-13172-8

Fang EF, Hou Y, Palikaras K, Adriaanse BA, Kerr JS, Yang B, Lautrup S, Hasan-Olive MM, Caponio D, Dan X, et al. 2019b. Mitophagy inhibits amyloid-β and tau pathology and reverses cognitive deficits in models of Alzheimer's disease. *Nat Neurosci* **22:** 401–412. doi:10.1038/s41593-018-0332-9

Figley MD, DiAntonio A. 2020. The SARM1 axon degeneration pathway: control of the NAD⁺ metabolome regu-lates axon survival in health and disease. *Curr Opin Neurobiol* **63:** 59–66. doi:10.1016/j.conb.2020.02.012

Figley MD, Gu W, Nanson JD, Shi Y, Sasaki Y, Cunnea K, Malde AK, Jia X, Luo Z, Saikot FK, et al. 2021. SARM1 is a metabolic sensor activated by an increased NMN/NAD⁺ ratio to trigger axon degeneration. *Neuron* **109:** 1118–1136.e11. doi:10.1016/j.neuron.2021.02.009

Frederick DW, Loro E, Liu L, Davila A Jr, Chellappa K, Silverman IM, Quinn WJ III, Gosai SJ, Tichy ED, Davis JG, et al. 2016. Loss of NAD homeostasis leads to progressive and reversible degeneration of skeletal muscle. *Cell Metab* **24:** 269–282. doi:10.1016/j.cmet.2016.07.005

Gaare JJ, Dölle C, Brakedal B, Brügger K, Haugarvoll K, Nido GS, Tzoulis C. 2023. Nicotinamide riboside supplementation is not associated with altered methylation homeostasis in Parkinson's disease. *iScience* **26:** 106278. doi:10.1016/j.isci.2023.106278

Gariani K, Menzies KJ, Ryu D, Wegner CJ, Wang X, Ropelle ER, Moullan N, Zhang H, Perino A, Lemos V, et al. 2016. Eliciting the mitochondrial unfolded protein response by nicotinamide adenine dinucleotide repletion reverses fatty liver disease in mice. *Hepatology* **63:** 1190–1204. doi:10.1002/hep.28245

Gerdts J, Brace EJ, Sasaki Y, DiAntonio A, Milbrandt J. 2015. SARM1 activation triggers axon degeneration locally via NAD⁺ destruction. *Science* **348:** 453–457. doi:10.1126/science.1258366

Giil LM, Midttun Ø, Refsum H, Ulvik A, Advani R, Smith AD, Ueland PM. 2017. Kynurenine pathway metabolites in Alzheimer's disease. *J Alzheimers Dis* **60:** 495–504. doi:10.3233/JAD-170485

Gilley J, Coleman MP. 2010. Endogenous Nmnat2 is an essential survival factor for maintenance of healthy axons. *PLoS Biol* **8:** e1000300. doi:10.1371/journal.pbio.1000300

Gilmour BC, Gudmundsrud R, Frank J, Hov A, Lautrup S, Aman Y, Røsjø H, Brenner C, Ziegler M, Tysnes OB, et al. 2020. Targeting NAD⁺ in translational research to relieve diseases and conditions of metabolic stress and ageing. *Mech Ageing Dev* **186:** 111208. doi:10.1016/j.mad.2020.111208

Goedert M. 2015. Neurodegeneration. Alzheimer's and Parkinson's diseases: the prion concept in relation to assembled Aβ, tau, and α-synuclein. *Science* **349:** 1255555. doi:10.1126/science.1255555

Gomes AP, Price NL, Ling AJ, Moslehi JJ, Montgomery MK, Rajman L, White JP, Teodoro JS, Wrann CD, Hubbard BP, et al. 2013. Declining NAD⁺ induces a pseudohypoxic state disrupting nuclear-mitochondrial communication during aging. *Cell* **155:** 1624–1638. doi:10.1016/j.cell.2013.11.037

Gong B, Pan Y, Vempati P, Zhao W, Knable L, Ho L, Wang J, Sastre M, Ono K, Sauve AA, et al. 2013. Nicotinamide riboside restores cognition through an upregulation of proliferator-activated receptor-γ coactivator 1α regulated β-secretase 1 degradation and mitochondrial gene expression in Alzheimer's mouse models. *Neurobiol Aging* **34:** 1581–1588. doi:10.1016/j.neurobiolaging.2012.12.005

González-Sánchez M, Jiménez J, Narváez A, Antequera D, Llamas-Velasco S, Martín AH, Arjona JAM, Munain AL, Bisa AL, Marco MP, et al. 2020. Kynurenic acid levels are increased in the CSF of Alzheimer's disease patients. *Biomolecules* **10:** 571. doi:10.3390/biom10040571

Gopal E, Fei YJ, Miyauchi S, Zhuang L, Prasad PD, Ganapathy V. 2005. Sodium-coupled and electrogenic transport of B-complex vitamin nicotinic acid by slc5a8, a member of the Na/glucose co-transporter gene family. *Biochem J* 388: 309–316. doi:10.1042/BJ20041916

Green KN, Steffan JS, Martinez-Coria H, Sun X, Schreiber SS, Thompson LM, LaFerla FM. 2008. Nicotinamide restores cognition in Alzheimer's disease transgenic mice via a mechanism involving sirtuin inhibition and selective reduction of Thr231-phosphotau. *J Neurosci* 28: 11500–11510. doi:10.1523/JNEUROSCI.3203-08.2008

Grozio A, Sociali G, Sturla L, Caffa I, Soncini D, Salis A, Raffaelli N, De Flora A, Nencioni A, Bruzzone S. 2013. CD73 protein as a source of extracellular precursors for sustained NAD$^+$ biosynthesis in FK866-treated tumor cells. *J Biol Chem* 288: 25938–25949. doi:10.1074/jbc.M113.470435

Guan Y, Wang SR, Huang XZ, Xie QH, Xu YY, Shang D, Hao CM. 2017. Nicotinamide mononucleotide, an NAD$^+$ precursor, rescues age-associated susceptibility to AKI in a sirtuin 1-dependent manner. *J Am Soc Nephrol* 28: 2337–2352. doi:10.1681/ASN.2016040385

Guillemin GJ, Smythe GA, Veas LA, Takikawa O, Brew BJ. 2003. Aβ1-42 induces production of quinolinic acid by human macrophages and microglia. *Neuroreport* 14: 2311–2315. doi:10.1097/00001756-200312190-00005

Gürtler C, Carty M, Kearney J, Schattgen SA, Ding A, Fitzgerald KA, Bowie AG. 2014. SARM regulates CCL5 production in macrophages by promoting the recruitment of transcription factors and RNA polymerase II to the *Ccl5* promoter. *J Immunol* 192: 4821–4832. doi:10.4049/jimmunol.1302980

Harden A, Young WJ. 1906. The alcoholic ferment of yeast-juice. Part II—the coferment of yeast-juice. *Proc R Soc Lond* 78: 369–375. doi:10.1098/rspb.1906.0070

Hou Y, Lautrup S, Cordonnier S, Wang Y, Croteau DL, Zavala E, Zhang Y, Moritoh K, O'Connell JF, Baptiste BA, et al. 2018. NAD$^+$ supplementation normalizes key Alzheimer's features and DNA damage responses in a new AD mouse model with introduced DNA repair deficiency. *Proc Natl Acad Sci* 115: E1876–E1885. doi:10.1073/pnas.1718819115

Hou Y, Dan X, Babbar M, Wei Y, Hasselbalch SG, Croteau DL, Bohr VA. 2019. Ageing as a risk factor for neurodegenerative disease. *Nat Rev Neurol* 15: 565–581. doi:10.1038/s41582-019-0244-7

Hou Y, Wei Y, Lautrup S, Yang B, Wang Y, Cordonnier S, Mattson MP, Croteau DL, Bohr VA. 2021. NAD$^+$ supplementation reduces neuroinflammation and cell senescence in a transgenic mouse model of Alzheimer's disease via cGAS-STING. *Proc Natl Acad Sci* 118: e2011226118. doi:10.1073/pnas.2011226118

Houtkooper RH, Cantó C, Wanders RJ, Auwerx J. 2010. The secret life of NAD$^+$: an old metabolite controlling new metabolic signaling pathways. *Endocr Rev* 31: 194–223. doi:10.1210/er.2009-0026

Huang H. 2022. A multicentre, randomised, double blind, parallel design, placebo controlled study to evaluate the efficacy and safety of uthever (NMN supplement), an orally administered supplementation in middle aged and older adults. *Front Aging* 3: 851698. doi:10.3389/fragi.2022.851698

Igarashi M, Nakagawa-Nagahama Y, Miura M, Kashiwabara K, Yaku K, Sawada M, Sekine R, Fukamizu Y, Sato T, Sakurai T, et al. 2022. Chronic nicotinamide mononucleotide supplementation elevates blood nicotinamide adenine dinucleotide levels and alters muscle function in healthy older men. *NPJ Aging* 8: 5. doi:10.1038/s41514-022-00084-z

Imai S, Armstrong CM, Kaeberlein M, Guarente L. 2000. Transcriptional silencing and longevity protein Sir2 is an NAD-dependent histone deacetylase. *Nature* 403: 795–800. doi:10.1038/35001622

Janssens GE, Grevendonk L, Perez RZ, Schomakers BV, de Vogel-van den Bosch J, Geurts JMW, van Weeghel M, Schrauwen P, Houtkooper RH, Hoeks J. 2022. Healthy aging and muscle function are positively associated with NAD$^+$ abundance in humans. *Nat Aging* 2: 254–263. doi:10.1038/s43587-022-00174-3

Jin D, Liu HX, Hirai H, Torashima T, Nagai T, Lopatina O, Shnayder NA, Yamada K, Noda M, Seike T, et al. 2007. CD38 is critical for social behaviour by regulating oxytocin secretion. *Nature* 446: 41–45. doi:10.1038/nature05526

Kataura T, Sedlackova L, Otten EG, Kumari R, Shapira D, Scialo F, Stefanatos R, Ishikawa KI, Kelly G, Seranova E, et al. 2022. Autophagy promotes cell survival by maintaining NAD levels. *Dev Cell* 57: 2584–2598.e11. doi:10.1016/j.devcel.2022.10.008

Katayoshi T, Uehata S, Nakashima N, Nakajo T, Kitajima N, Kageyama M, Tsuji-Naito K. 2023. Nicotinamide adenine dinucleotide metabolism and arterial stiffness after long-term nicotinamide mononucleotide supplementation: a randomized, double-blind, placebo-controlled trial. *Sci Rep* 13: 2786. doi:10.1038/s41598-023-29787-3

Katsyuba E, Mottis A, Zietak M, De Franco F, van der Velpen V, Gariani K, Ryu D, Cialabrini L, Matilainen O, Liscio P, et al. 2018. De novo NAD$^+$ synthesis enhances mitochondrial function and improves health. *Nature* 563: 354–359. doi:10.1038/s41586-018-0645-6

Kerr JS, Adriaanse BA, Greig NH, Mattson MP, Cader MZ, Bohr VA, Fang EF. 2017. Mitophagy and Alzheimer's disease: cellular and molecular mechanisms. *Trends Neurosci* 40: 151–166. doi:10.1016/j.tins.2017.01.002

Kobro-Flatmoen A, Lagartos-Donate MJ, Aman Y, Edison P, Witter MP, Fang EF. 2021. Re-emphasizing early Alzheimer's disease pathology starting in select entorhinal neurons, with a special focus on mitophagy. *Ageing Res Rev* 67: 101307. doi:10.1016/j.arr.2021.101307

Kornberg A. 1948. The participation of inorganic pyrophosphate in the reversible enzymatic synthesis of diphosphopyridine nucleotide. *J Biol Chem* 176: 1475–1476. doi:10.1016/S0021-9258(18)57167-2

Kory N, Uit de Bos J, van der Rijt S, Jankovic N, Güra M, Arp N, Pena IA, Prakash G, Chan SH, Kunchok T, et al. 2020. MCART1/SLC25A51 is required for mitochondrial NAD transport. *Sci Adv* 6: eabe5310. doi:10.1126/sciadv.abe5310

Lautrup S, Sinclair DA, Mattson MP, Fang EF. 2019. NAD$^+$ in brain aging and neurodegenerative disorders. *Cell Metab* 30: 630–655. doi:10.1016/j.cmet.2019.09.001

Lee HJ, Hong YS, Jun W, Yang SJ. 2015. Nicotinamide riboside ameliorates hepatic metaflammation by modulating NLRP3 inflammasome in a rodent model of type 2 diabetes. *J Med Food* **18**: 1207–1213. doi:10.1089/jmf.2015 .3439

Li X, Fang EF, Scheibye-Knudsen M, Cui H, Qiu L, Li J, He Y, Huang J, Bohr VA, Ng TB, et al. 2014. Di-(2-ethylhexyl) phthalate inhibits DNA replication leading to hyperPAR-ylation, SIRT1 attenuation, and mitochondrial dysfunc-tion in the testis. *Sci Rep* **4**: 6434. doi:10.1038/srep06434

Liu Q, Graeff R, Kriksunov IA, Lam CM, Lee HC, Hao Q. 2008. Conformational closure of the catalytic site of hu-man CD38 induced by calcium. *Biochemistry* **47**: 13966–13973. doi:10.1021/bi801642q

Liu D, Pitta M, Jiang H, Lee JH, Zhang G, Chen X, Kawa-moto EM, Mattson MP. 2013. Nicotinamide forestalls pathology and cognitive decline in Alzheimer mice: evi-dence for improved neuronal bioenergetics and autoph-agy procession. *Neurobiol Aging* **34**: 1564–1580. doi:10 .1016/j.neurobiolaging.2012.11.020

Liu J, Zhao YJ, Li WH, Hou YN, Li T, Zhao ZY, Fang C, Li SL, Lee HC. 2017. Cytosolic interaction of type III human CD38 with CIB1 modulates cellular cyclic ADP-ribose levels. *Proc Natl Acad Sci* **114**: 8283–8288. doi:10.1073/ pnas.1703718114

Liu L, Su X, Quinn WJ, Hui S, Krukenberg K, Frederick DW, Redpath P, Zhan L, Chellappa K, White E, et al. 2018. Quantitative analysis of NAD synthesis-breakdown flux-es. *Cell Metab* **27**: 1067–1080.e5. doi:10.1016/j.cmet.2018 .03.018

Liu Y, Cheng A, Li YJ, Yang Y, Kishimoto Y, Zhang S, Wang Y, Wan R, Raefsky SM, Lu D, et al. 2019. SIRT3 mediates hippocampal synaptic adaptations to intermittent fasting and ameliorates deficits in APP mutant mice. *Nat Com-mun* **10**: 1886. doi:10.1038/s41467-019-09897-1

Livingston G, Huntley J, Sommerlad A, Ames D, Ballard C, Banerjee S, Brayne C, Burns A, Cohen-Mansfield J, Cooper C, et al. 2020. Dementia prevention, intervention, and care: 2020 report of the lancet commission. *Lancet* **396**: 413–446. doi:10.1016/S0140-6736(20)30367-6

López-Otín C, Blasco MA, Partridge L, Serrano M, Kroemer G. 2023. Hallmarks of aging: an expanding universe. *Cell* **186**: 243–278. doi:10.1016/j.cell.2022.11.001

Luongo TS, Eller JM, Lu MJ, Niere M, Raith F, Perry C, Bornstein MR, Oliphint P, Wang L, McReynolds MR, et al. 2020. SLC25A51 is a mammalian mitochondrial NAD$^+$ transporter. *Nature* **588**: 174–179. doi:10.1038/ s41586-020-2741-7

Martens CR, Denman BA, Mazzo MR, Armstrong ML, Reisdorph N, McQueen MB, Chonchol M, Seals DR. 2018. Chronic nicotinamide riboside supplementation is well-tolerated and elevates NAD$^+$ in healthy middle-aged and older adults. *Nat Commun* **9**: 1286. doi:10.1038/ s41467-018-03421-7

Massudi H, Grant R, Braidy N, Guest J, Farnsworth B, Guillemin GJ. 2012. Age-associated changes in oxidative stress and NAD$^+$ metabolism in human tissue. *PLoS ONE* **7**: e42357. doi:10.1371/journal.pone.0042357

Mayer PR, Huang N, Dewey CM, Dries DR, Zhang H, Yu G. 2010. Expression, localization, and biochemical charac-terization of nicotinamide mononucleotide adenylyl-transferase 2. *J Biol Chem* **285**: 40387–40396. doi:10 .1074/jbc.M110.178913

McReynolds MR, Chellappa K, Baur JA. 2020. Age-related NAD$^+$ decline. *Exp Gerontol* **134**: 110888. doi:10.1016/j .exger.2020.110888

McReynolds MR, Chellappa K, Chiles E, Jankowski C, Shen Y, Chen L, Descamps HC, Mukherjee S, Bhat YR, Lingala SR, et al. 2021. NAD$^+$ flux is maintained in aged mice despite lower tissue concentrations. *Cell Syst* **12**: 1160–1172.e4. doi:10.1016/j.cels.2021.09.001

Mills KF, Yoshida S, Stein LR, Grozio A, Kubota S, Sasaki Y, Redpath P, Migaud ME, Apte RS, Uchida K, et al. 2016. Long-term administration of nicotinamide mononucleo-tide mitigates age-associated physiological decline in mice. *Cell Metab* **24**: 795–806. doi:10.1016/j.cmet.2016 .09.013

Minhas PS, Liu L, Moon PK, Joshi AU, Dove C, Mhatre S, Contrepois K, Wang Q, Lee BA, Coronado M, et al. 2019. Macrophage de novo NAD$^+$ synthesis specifies immune function in aging and inflammation. *Nat Immunol* **20**: 50–63. doi:10.1038/s41590-018-0255-3

Mitchell SJ, Bernier M, Aon MA, Cortassa S, Kim EY, Fang EF, Palacios HH, Ali A, Navas-Enamorado I, Di Fran-cesco A, et al. 2018. Nicotinamide improves aspects of healthspan, but not lifespan, in mice. *Cell Metab* **27**: 667–676.e4. doi:10.1016/j.cmet.2018.02.001

Moreno-Jiménez EP, Flor-García M, Terreros-Roncal J, Rá-bano A, Cafini F, Pallas-Bazarra N, Ávila J, Llorens-Mar-tín M. 2019. Adult hippocampal neurogenesis is abun-dant in neurologically healthy subjects and drops sharply in patients with Alzheimer's disease. *Nat Med* **25**: 554–560. doi:10.1038/s41591-019-0375-9

Morevati M, Egstrand S, Nordholm A, Mace ML, Andersen CB, Salmani R, Olgaard K, Lewin E. 2021. Effect of NAD$^+$ boosting on kidney ischemia-reperfusion injury. *PLoS ONE* **16**: e0252554. doi:10.1371/journal.pone.0252554

Mouchiroud L, Houtkooper RH, Moullan N, Katsyuba E, Ryu D, Cantó C, Mottis A, Jo YS, Viswanathan M, Schoonjans K, et al. 2013. The NAD$^+$/sirtuin pathway modulates longevity through activation of mitochondrial UPR and FOXO signaling. *Cell* **154**: 430–441. doi:10 .1016/j.cell.2013.06.016

Murata H, Khine CC, Nishikawa A, Yamamoto KI, Kino-shita R, Sakaguchi M. 2018. c-Jun N-terminal kinase (JNK)-mediated phosphorylation of SARM1 regulates NAD$^+$ cleavage activity to inhibit mitochondrial respira-tion. *J Biol Chem* **293**: 18933–18943. doi:10.1074/jbc .RA118.004578

Nacarelli T, Lau L, Fukumoto T, Zundell J, Fatkhutdinov N, Wu S, Aird KM, Iwasaki O, Kossenkov AV, Schultz D, et al. 2019. NAD$^+$ metabolism governs the proinflammatory senescence-associated secretome. *Nat Cell Biol* **21**: 397–407. doi:10.1038/s41556-019-0287-4

Nikiforov A, Dölle C, Niere M, Ziegler M. 2011. Pathways and subcellular compartment of NAD biosynthesis in human cells: from entry of extracellular precursors to mitochondrial NAD generation. *J Biol Chem* **286**: 21767–21778. doi:10.1074/jbc.M110.213298

O'Farrell K, Harkin A. 2017. Stress-related regulation of the kynurenine pathway: relevance to neuropsychiatric and degenerative disorders. *Neuropharmacology* **112**: 307–323. doi:10.1016/j.neuropharm.2015.12.004

Ogawa T, Matson WR, Beal MF, Myers RH, Bird ED, Mil-bury P, Saso S. 1992. Kynurenine pathway abnormalities

in Parkinson's disease. *Neurology* **42**: 1702–1706. doi:10
.1212/wnl.42.9.1702

Okur MN, Mao B, Kimura R, Haraczy S, Fitzgerald T, Ed-
wards-Hollingsworth K, Tian J, Osmani W, Croteau DL,
Kelley MW, et al. 2020a. Short-term NAD⁺ supplementation prevents hearing loss in mouse models of Cockayne
syndrome. *NPJ Aging Mech Dis* **6**: 1. doi:10.1038/s41514-
019-0040-z

Okur MN, Fang EF, Fivenson EM, Tiwari V, Croteau DL,
Bohr VA. 2020b. Cockayne syndrome proteins CSA and
CSB maintain mitochondrial homeostasis through NAD⁺
signaling. *Aging Cell* **19**: e13268. doi:10.1111/acel.13268

Oshima J, Sidorova JM, Monnat RJ Jr. 2017. Werner syndrome: clinical features, pathogenesis and potential therapeutic interventions. *Ageing Res Rev* **33**: 105–114. doi:10
.1016/j.arr.2016.03.002

Panneerselvam P, Singh LP, Selvarajan V, Chng WJ, Ng SB,
Tan NS, Ho B, Chen J, Ding JL. 2013. T-cell death following immune activation is mediated by mitochondria-
localized SARM. *Cell Death Differ* **20**: 478–489. doi:10
.1038/cdd.2012.144

Pencina KM, Valderrabano R, Wipper B, Orkaby AR, Reid
KF, Storer T, Lin AP, Merugumala S, Wilson L, Latham N,
et al. 2023. Nicotinamide adenine dinucleotide augmentation in overweight or obese middle-aged and older
adults: a physiologic study. *J Clin Endocrinol Metab*
108: 1968–1980. doi:10.1210/clinem/dgad027

Pieper AA, Wu X, Han TW, Estill SJ, Dang Q, Wu LC, Reece-
Fincanon S, Dudley CA, Richardson JA, Brat DJ, et al.
2005. The neuronal PAS domain protein 3 transcription
factor controls FGF-mediated adult hippocampal neurogenesis in mice. *Proc Natl Acad Sci* **102**: 14052–14057.
doi:10.1073/pnas.0506713102

Pillai SM, Meredith D. 2011. SLC36A4 (hPAT4) is a high
affinity amino acid transporter when expressed in *Xeno-
pus laevis* oocytes. *J Biol Chem* **286**: 2455–2460. doi:10
.1074/jbc.M110.172403

Pittelli M, Formentini L, Faraco G, Lapucci A, Rapizzi E,
Cialdai F, Romano G, Moneti G, Moroni F, Chiarugi A.
2010. Inhibition of nicotinamide phosphoribosyltransferase: cellular bioenergetics reveals a mitochondrial insensitive NAD pool. *J Biol Chem* **285**: 34106–34114. doi:10
.1074/jbc.M110.136739

Poyan Mehr A, Tran MT, Ralto KM, Leaf DE, Washco V,
Messmer J, Lerner A, Kher A, Kim SH, Khoury CC, et al.
2018. De novo NAD⁺ biosynthetic impairment in acute
kidney injury in humans. *Nat Med* **24**: 1351–1359. doi:10
.1038/s41591-018-0138-z

Priess J, Handler P. 1958a. Biosynthesis of diphosphopyridine nucleotide. II: Enzymatic aspects. *J Biol Chem* **233**:
493–500.

Priess J, Handler P. 1958b. Biosynthesis of diphosphopyridine nucleotide. I: Identification of intermediates. *J Biol
Chem* **233**: 488–492.

Ratajczak J, Joffraud M, Trammell SA, Ras R, Canela N,
Boutant M, Kulkarni SS, Rodrigues M, Redpath P, Migaud ME, et al. 2016. NRK1 controls nicotinamide mononucleotide and nicotinamide riboside metabolism in
mammalian cells. *Nat Commun* **7**: 13103. doi:10.1038/
ncomms13103

Ray Chaudhuri A, Nussenzweig A. 2017. The multifaceted
roles of PARP1 in DNA repair and chromatin remodel-

ling. *Nat Rev Mol Cell Biol* **18**: 610–621. doi:10.1038/nrm
.2017.53

Reiten OK, Wilvang MA, Mitchell SJ, Hu Z, Fang EF. 2021.
Preclinical and clinical evidence of NAD⁺ precursors in
health, disease, and ageing. *Mech Ageing Dev* **199**:
111567. doi:10.1016/j.mad.2021.111567

Rongvaux A, Shea RJ, Mulks MH, Gigot D, Urbain J, Leo O,
Andris F. 2002. Pre-B-cell colony-enhancing factor,
whose expression is up-regulated in activated lymphocytes, is a nicotinamide phosphoribosyltransferase, a cytosolic enzyme involved in NAD biosynthesis. *Eur J Immunol* **32**: 3225–3234. doi:10.1002/1521-4141(200211)
32:11<3225::AID-IMMU3225>3.0.CO;2-L

Rouleau M, Patel A, Hendzel MJ, Kaufmann SH, Poirier GG.
2010. PARP inhibition: PARP1 and beyond. *Nat Rev Cancer* **10**: 293–301. doi:10.1038/nrc2812

Ryu D, Zhang H, Ropelle ER, Sorrentino V, Mázala DA,
Mouchiroud L, Marshall PL, Campbell MD, Ali AS,
Knowels GM, et al. 2016. NAD⁺ repletion improves mus-
cle function in muscular dystrophy and counters global
PARylation. *Sci Transl Med* **8**: 361ra139. doi:10.1126/sci
translmed.aaf5504

Sanchez-Roman I, Ferrando B, Holst CM, Mengel-From J,
Rasmussen SH, Thinggaard M, Bohr VA, Christensen K,
Stevnsner T. 2022. Molecular markers of DNA repair and
brain metabolism correlate with cognition in centenarians. *Geroscience* **44**: 103–125. doi:10.1007/s11357-021-
00502-2

Scalise M, Galluccio M, Console L, Pochini L, Indiveri C.
2018. The human SLC7A5 (LAT1): the intriguing histi-
dine/large neutral amino acid transporter and its relevance to human health. *Front Chem* **6**: 243. doi:10
.3389/fchem.2018.00243

Scheibye-Knudsen M, Mitchell SJ, Fang EF, Iyama T, Ward
T, Wang J, Dunn CA, Singh N, Veith S, Hasan-Olive MM,
et al. 2014. A high-fat diet and NAD⁺ activate Sirt1 to
rescue premature aging in Cockayne syndrome. *Cell
Metab* **20**: 840–855. doi:10.1016/j.cmet.2014.10.005

Scheibye-Knudsen M, Tseng A, Borch Jensen M, Scheibye-
Alsing K, Fang EF, Iyama T, Bharti SK, Marosi K,
Froetscher L, Kassahun H, et al. 2016. Cockayne syn-
drome group A and B proteins converge on transcrip-
tion-linked resolution of non-B DNA. *Proc Natl Acad
Sci* **113**: 12502–12507. doi:10.1073/pnas.1610198113

Stein LR, Imai S. 2014. Specific ablation of Nampt in adult
neural stem cells recapitulates their functional defects
during aging. *EMBO J* **33**: 1321–1340. doi:10.1002/embj
.201386917

Stein LR, Wozniak DF, Dearborn JT, Kubota S, Apte RS,
Izumi Y, Zorumski CF, Imai S. 2014. Expression of Nampt
in hippocampal and cortical excitatory neurons is critical
for cognitive function. *J Neurosci* **34**: 5800–5815. doi:10
.1523/JNEUROSCI.4730-13.2014

Sun C, Wang K, Stock AJ, Gong Y, Demarest TG, Yang B,
Giri N, Harrington L, Alter BP, Savage SA, et al. 2020. Re-
equilibration of imbalanced NAD metabolism ameliorates the impact of telomere dysfunction. *EMBO J* **39**:
e103420. doi:10.15252/embj.2019103420

Takemoto M, Mori S, Kuzuya M, Yoshimoto S, Shimamoto
A, Igarashi M, Tanaka Y, Miki T, Yokote K. 2013. Diagnostic criteria for Werner syndrome based on Japanese

nationwide epidemiological survey. *Geriatr Gerontol Int* **13:** 475–481. doi:10.1111/j.1447-0594.2012.00913.x

Tarantini S, Valcarcel-Ares MN, Toth P, Yabluchanskiy A, Tucsek Z, Kiss T, Hertelendy P, Kinter M, Ballabh P, Süle Z, et al. 2019. Nicotinamide mononucleotide (NMN) supplementation rescues cerebromicrovascular endothelial function and neurovascular coupling responses and improves cognitive function in aged mice. *Redox Biol* **24:** 101192. doi:10.1016/j.redox.2019.101192

Thevandavakkam MA, Schwarcz R, Muchowski PJ, Giorgini F. 2010. targeting kynurenine 3-monooxygenase (KMO): implications for therapy in Huntington's disease. *CNS Neurol Disord Drug Targets* **9:** 791–800. doi:10.2174/187152710793237430

Ting KK, Brew B, Guillemin G. 2007. The involvement of astrocytes and kynurenine pathway in Alzheimer's disease. *Neurotox Res* **12:** 247–262. doi:10.1007/BF03033908

Trammell SA, Schmidt MS, Weidemann BJ, Redpath P, Jaksch F, Dellinger RW, Li Z, Abel ED, Migaud ME, Brenner C. 2016a. Nicotinamide riboside is uniquely and orally bioavailable in mice and humans. *Nat Commun* **7:** 12948. doi:10.1038/ncomms12948

Trammell SA, Weidemann BJ, Chadda A, Yorek MS, Holmes A, Coppey LJ, Obrosov A, Kardon RH, Yorek MA, Brenner C. 2016b. Nicotinamide riboside opposes type 2 diabetes and neuropathy in mice. *Sci Rep* **6:** 26933. doi:10.1038/srep26933

Tran MT, Zsengeller ZK, Berg AH, Khankin EV, Bhasin MK, Kim W, Clish CB, Stillman IE, Karumanchi SA, Rhee EP, et al. 2016. PGC1α drives NAD biosynthesis linking oxidative metabolism to renal protection. *Nature* **531:** 528–532. doi:10.1038/nature17184

Tseng BP, Green KN, Chan JL, Blurton-Jones M, LaFerla FM. 2008. Aβ inhibits the proteasome and enhances amyloid and tau accumulation. *Neurobiol Aging* **29:** 1607–1618. doi:10.1016/j.neurobiolaging.2007.04.014

Uddin GM, Youngson NA, Sinclair DA, Morris MJ. 2016. Head-to-head comparison of short-term treatment with the NAD$^+$ precursor nicotinamide mononucleotide (NMN) and 6 weeks of exercise in obese female mice. *Front Pharmacol* **7:** 258. doi:10.3389/fphar.2016.00258

Vécsei L, Szalárdy L, Fülöp F, Toldi J. 2013. Kynurenines in the CNS: recent advances and new questions. *Nat Rev Drug Discov* **12:** 64–82. doi:10.1038/nrd3793

Verdin E. 2015. NAD$^+$ in aging, metabolism, and neurodegeneration. *Science* **350:** 1208–1213. doi:10.1126/science.aac4854

Warburg O, Christian W. 1936. Pyridin, der wasserstoffübertragende Bestandteil von Gärungsfermenten [Pyridin, the hydrogen-transferring component of the fermentation enzymes]. *Helvetica* **19:** E79–E88. doi:10.1002/hlca.193601901199

Wiley CD, Velarde MC, Lecot P, Liu S, Sarnoski EA, Freund A, Shirakawa K, Lim HW, Davis SS, Ramanathan A, et al. 2016. Mitochondrial dysfunction induces senescence with a distinct secretory phenotype. *Cell Metab* **23:** 303–314. doi:10.1016/j.cmet.2015.11.011

Wilson DM III, Cookson MR, Van Den Bosch L, Zetterberg H, Holtzman DM, Dewachter I. 2023a. Hallmarks of neurodegenerative diseases. *Cell* **186:** 693–714. doi:10.1016/j.cell.2022.12.032

Wilson N, Kataura T, Korsgen ME, Sun C, Sarkar S, Korolchuk VI. 2023b. The autophagy-NAD axis in longevity and disease. *Trends Cell Biol* S0962-8924(23)00023-5.

Xie C, Zhuang XX, Niu Z, Ai R, Lautrup S, Zheng S, Jiang Y, Han R, Gupta TS, Cao S, et al. 2022. Amelioration of Alzheimer's disease pathology by mitophagy inducers identified via machine learning and a cross-species workflow. *Nat Biomed Eng* **6:** 76–93. doi:10.1038/s41551-021-00819-5

Yaku K, Okabe K, Nakagawa T. 2018. NAD metabolism: implications in aging and longevity. *Ageing Res Rev* **47:** 1–17. doi:10.1016/j.arr.2018.05.006

Yalowitz JA, Xiao S, Biju MP, Antony AC, Cummings OW, Deeg MA, Jayaram HN. 2004. Characterization of human brain nicotinamide 5′-mononucleotide adenylyltransferase-2 and expression in human pancreas. *Biochem J* **377:** 317–326. doi:10.1042/BJ20030518

Yamamoto M, Hikosaka K, Mahmood A, Tobe K, Shojaku H, Inohara H, Nakagawa T. 2016. Nmnat3 is dispensable in mitochondrial NAD level maintenance in vivo. *PLoS ONE* **11:** e0147037. doi:10.1371/journal.pone.0147037

Yang H, Yang T, Baur JA, Perez E, Matsui T, Carmona JJ, Lamming DW, Souza-Pinto NC, Bohr VA, Rosenzweig A, et al. 2007. Nutrient-sensitive mitochondrial NAD$^+$ levels dictate cell survival. *Cell* **130:** 1095–1107. doi:10.1016/j.cell.2007.07.035

Yang Y, Mohammed FS, Zhang N, Sauve AA. 2019. Dihydronicotinamide riboside is a potent NAD$^+$ concentration enhancer in vitro and in vivo. *J Biol Chem* **294:** 9295–9307. doi:10.1074/jbc.RA118.005772

Yang Y, Zhang N, Zhang G, Sauve AA. 2020. NRH salvage and conversion to NAD$^+$ requires NRH kinase activity by adenosine kinase. *Nat Metab* **2:** 364–379. doi:10.1038/s42255-020-0194-9

Yang B, Dan X, Hou Y, Lee JH, Wechter N, Krishnamurthy S, Kimura R, Babbar M, Demarest T, McDevitt R, et al. 2021. NAD$^+$ supplementation prevents STING-induced senescence in ataxia telangiectasia by improving mitophagy. *Aging Cell* **20:** e13329. doi:10.1111/acel.13329

Yoshino J, Mills KF, Yoon MJ, Imai S. 2011. Nicotinamide mononucleotide, a key NAD$^+$ intermediate, treats the pathophysiology of diet- and age-induced diabetes in mice. *Cell Metab* **14:** 528–536. doi:10.1016/j.cmet.2011.08.014

Yulug B, Altay O, Li X, Hanoglu L, Cankaya S, Lam S, Yang H, Coskun E, Idil E, Nogaylar R, et al. 2021a. Combined metabolic activators improves cognitive functions in Alzheimer's disease. medRxiv doi:10.1101/2021.07.14.21260511

Yulug B, Altay O, Li X, Hanoglu L, Cankaya S, Lam S, Yang H, Coskun E, Idil E, Nogaylar N, et al. 2021b. Combined metabolic activators improve cognitive functions without altering motor scores in Parkinson's disease. medRxiv doi:10.1101/2021.07.28.21261293

Yulug B, Altay O, Li X, Hanoglu L, Cankaya S, Lam S, Velioglu HA, Yang H, Coskun E, Idil E, et al. 2023. Combined metabolic activators improve cognitive functions in Alzheimer's disease patients: a randomised, double-blinded, placebo-controlled phase-II trial. *Transl Neurodegener* **12:** 4. doi:10.1186/s40035-023-00336-2

Zhang X, Kurnasov OV, Karthikeyan S, Grishin NV, Osterman AL, Zhang H. 2003. Structural characterization of a human cytosolic NMN/NaMN adenylyltransferase and implication in human NAD biosynthesis. *J Biol Chem* **278:** 13503–13511. doi:10.1074/jbc.M300073200

Zhang H, Ryu D, Wu Y, Gariani K, Wang X, Luan P, D'Amico D, Ropelle ER, Lutolf MP, Aebersold R, et al. 2016. NAD$^+$ repletion improves mitochondrial and stem cell function and enhances life span in mice. *Science* **352:** 1436–1443. doi:10.1126/science.aaf2693

Zhao Y, Jin J, Hu Q, Zhou HM, Yi J, Yu Z, Xu L, Wang X, Yang Y, Loscalzo J. 2011. Genetically encoded fluorescent sensors for intracellular NADH detection. *Cell Metab* **14:** 555–566. doi:10.1016/j.cmet.2011.09.004

Zhao Y, Hu Q, Cheng F, Su N, Wang A, Zou Y, Hu H, Chen X, Zhou HM, Huang X, et al. 2015. Sonar, a highly responsive NAD+/NADH sensor, allows high-throughput metabolic screening of anti-tumor agents. *Cell Metab* **21:** 777–789. doi:10.1016/j.cmet.2015.04.009

Zhao Y, Wang A, Zou Y, Su N, Loscalzo J, Yang Y. 2016. In vivo monitoring of cellular energy metabolism using SoNar, a highly responsive sensor for NAD$^+$/NADH redox state. *Nat Protoc* **11:** 1345–1359. doi:10.1038/nprot.2016.074

Zhao Y, Zhang Z, Zou Y, Yang Y. 2018. Visualization of nicotine adenine dinucleotide redox homeostasis with genetically encoded fluorescent sensors. *Antioxid Redox Signal* **28:** 213–229. doi:10.1089/ars.2017.7226

Zhao ZY, Xie XJ, Li WH, Liu J, Chen Z, Zhang B, Li T, Li SL, Lu JG, Zhang L, et al. 2019. A cell-permeant mimetic of NMN activates SARM1 to produce cyclic ADP-ribose and induce non-apoptotic cell death. *iScience* **15:** 452–466. doi:10.1016/j.isci.2019.05.001

Zhu XH, Lu M, Lee BY, Ugurbil K, Chen W. 2015. In vivo NAD assay reveals the intracellular NAD contents and redox state in healthy human brain and their age dependences. *Proc Natl Acad Sci* **112:** 2876–2881. doi:10.1073/pnas.1417921112

Ziegler M, Nikiforov AA. 2020. NAD on the rise again. *Nat Metab* **2:** 291–292. doi:10.1038/s42255-020-0197-6

Zou Y, Wang A, Huang L, Zhu X, Hu Q, Zhang Y, Chen X, Li F, Wang Q, Wang H, et al. 2020. Illuminating NAD$^+$ metabolism in live cells and in vivo using a genetically encoded fluorescent sensor. *Dev Cell* **53:** 240–252.e7. doi:10.1016/j.devcel.2020.02.017

Evolutionary Approaches in Aging Research

Melissa Emery Thompson

Department of Anthropology, University of New Mexico, Albuquerque, New Mexico 87131, USA
Correspondence: memery@unm.edu

While evolutionary explanations for aging have been widely acknowledged, the application of evolutionary principles to the practice of aging research has, until recently, been limited. Aging research has been dominated by studies of populations in evolutionarily novel industrialized environments and by use of short-lived animal models that are distantly related to humans. In this review, I address several emerging areas of "evolutionarily relevant" aging research, which provide a valuable complement to conventional biomedical research on aging. Nonhuman primates offer particular value as both translational and comparative models due to their long life spans, shared evolutionary history with humans, and social complexity. Additionally, because the human organism evolved in a radically different environment than that in which most humans live today, studying populations living in diverse ecologies has redefined our understanding of healthy aging by revealing the contribution of industrialized human environments to age-related pathologies.

EVOLUTIONARY THEORY OF AGING

Evolutionary theory has long been at the heart of aging science as a way to explain *why* we age. Purely mechanical views of aging propose that like any machine, biological systems inevitably deteriorate over time. In contrast, evolutionary biologists have rooted their inquiry into how and why the negative effects of aging have been maintained in the face of natural selection, a process that is expected to eliminate detrimental traits. Early evolutionary theories of aging attempted to address why natural selection may simply be unable to counteract the aging process. For example, the Mutation Accumulation Theory explains that natural selection has a diminished capacity to eliminate genetic mutations that cause disease or dysfunction late in the life span, as these traits will be passed on through reproduction before their negative effects begin to manifest (Haldane 1941; Medawar 1946, 1952). Subsequent theories embraced this core idea but proposed that the imbalance between the force of selection early versus late in life may not just fail to remove harmful late-acting genes but may actively promote them. Williams originally formalized the concept of "antagonistic pleiotropy," demonstrating that genes that have positive effects on reproductive success early in life will be favored even if they produce negative effects on survival (Williams 1957). Williams' observation was central to the development of life history theory, which poses that when organisms spend energy on reproduction, they have less energy available to invest in somatic maintenance (Williams 1966; Stearns 1989).

These core ideas have evolved as the understanding of aging biology has increased. One of the most prominent contemporary evolutionary theories of aging, the Disposable Soma theory, proposes a mechanistic extension of antagonistic pleiotropy: damage accumulates over the life span because it is less advantageous to spend energy on damage repair and prevention than it is to spend the same energy on reproductive effort (Kirkwood 1977; Kirkwood and Rose 1991). Although Kirkwood's original formulation of this theory focused on the accumulation of errors during cell divisions, this essential trade-off can affect diverse aging mechanisms. The Disposable Soma theory is frequently applied to proximate trade-offs within species, whereby individuals with higher reproductive investment are expected to experience accelerated aging. However, persistence of these trade-offs over evolutionary time is predicted to set a rate of somatic repair that promotes senescence even in the absence of reproduction.

The Developmental Theory of Aging interprets the principle of antagonistic pleiotropy in a different way, by positing that aging results as a side effect of mechanisms that have been optimized by natural selection to promote successful development (de Magalhães and Church 2005). Some physiological processes calibrated for healthy development appear to exert damaging effects when maintained over time, while other types of age-related deterioration occur because processes important in development become less active over time. Together, these theories contribute to a growing explanatory framework, which, while still incomplete, can be used to generate new lines of research.

Whereas evolutionary influences on aging are widely acknowledged, evolutionarily minded approaches to aging are uncommon. The perspective that aging is a natural biological process is often juxtaposed with the medical view of aging as a "disease" that could be cured to extend human life spans (de Magalhães 2014; Bulterijs et al. 2015; Blagosklonny 2018). The emerging field of geroscience shifts this perspective in that it embraces aging as an inevitable part of our biology, but targets the extension of disease-free life, or "health span" (Burch et al. 2014; Kennedy et al.

2014). Nevertheless, research effort remains largely focused on the diseases of aging rather than on the biology of aging itself (Hayflick 2000, 2004). To a certain extent, this is necessary to target interventions at the leading causes of death and disability. Yet, by asking how the biology of aging has been shaped by natural selection, evolutionary approaches can generate unique perspectives on the origins of disease and the potential success (or harm) of interventions. Embedded in this way of thinking is that biological traits evolve in response to challenges posed by the environment across the life course. Exposure to different environments affects health directly but may also alter the salience of particular risk factors or the effects of interventions.

The evolutionary approach to aging has undergone a recent revolution, guided by the principles of evolutionary medicine, which uses knowledge about how human biology evolved to better understand the factors influencing health (Grunspan et al. 2018). Here, I highlight "evolutionarily relevant" approaches that are being used alongside conventional biomedical approaches to develop a holistic science of aging. These involve comparative biodemography to identify evolutionary trends in aging, the selection of model species with longer life spans and closer genetic relationships to humans, and the study of aging across a broader range of ecological contexts.

EVOLUTIONARY BIODEMOGRAPHY OF AGING

Evolutionary biodemographers have made important contributions toward understanding aging in the context of broader life history evolution. With this approach, the effects of aging are identified at the species or population level via the expected increase in mortality rates across adulthood (Jones et al. 2014). Broad cross-species comparisons identify patterns of evolutionary change, such as in similarities in life span or patterns of mortality shared by species with a common ancestry. However, in revealing the diversity of life history patterns possible, these studies have also challenged assumptions and identified

Cite this article as *Cold Spring Harb Perspect Med* doi: 10.1101/cshperspect.a041195

limitations to existing evolutionary theories of aging (Baudisch 2012).

Among the most surprising revelations from evolutionary biodemographic approaches is that aging is not a universal characteristic of living things, or even of animals. Whereas mammals share a pattern of accelerated mortality with age, mortality rates of some animals remain relatively constant throughout adulthood, and some even exhibit "negative aging," whereby mortality risks are reduced at later ages (Jones et al. 2014). Within this variation are clear phylogenetic effects, supporting the hypothesis that some attributes of aging in a given species are likely to be inherited from deep in the evolutionary past and may be subject to selective constraints. Mammals show more evidence of these constraints than do other broad taxa, such as birds. However, important variation in mortality patterns exists even among closely related taxa. Following the logic of evolutionary trade-offs, it is hypothesized that much of this variation may be linked to the effects of widely varying growth and reproductive patterns across species (Jones et al. 2014). This hypothesis is supported by the considerable sex differences observed in many species where reproductive effort of males and females differs in timing or intensity. Surprisingly, the shape of mortality profiles does not appear to be intrinsically related to life span.

Accordingly, biodemographers have found it useful to distinguish the "shape" of aging, defined as above by the relative rate at which mortality changes across the adult life span, from the "pace" of aging defined by measures like longevity or life expectancy (Baudisch 2011). Humans' long life spans would suggest a slow rate of senescence, but when standardized for differences in life span, humans experience a steeper increase in mortality than many shorter-lived species. This pace-standardized approach also provides a way to examine "life span equality," or how evenly ages of death are distributed across the life span (Wrycza et al. 2015).

Primates are long-lived compared to other mammals of equivalent body size (Charnov and Berrigan 1993). Within the Primate Order, human mortality patterns are not distinct, but fall along a continuum with other primates species

(Bronikowski et al. 2011) Whereas life span and life span equality vary independently across mammals, they are positively correlated across primate species (Colchero et al. 2016) and are very tightly correlated across populations in any particular primate species or genus (Colchero et al. 2021). For example, variation in life expectancy across human populations experiencing diverse environments is overwhelmingly explained by differences in life span equality (Edwards and Tuljapurkar 2005; Colchero et al. 2016; Németh 2017). In other words, populations that experience higher life expectancy do so because fewer individuals die at young ages and not because they exhibit slower aging. By contrast, selection on the rate of aging explains differences in longevity observed between primate species (Colchero et al. 2021). An important implication is that although life expectancy has rapidly increased in industrialized populations, as life span equality plateaus, we may be reaching the natural limits of human life spans.

EVOLUTIONARY-RELEVANT ANIMAL MODELS

Laboratory animal models have been a critical resource for investigating the mechanisms of aging (Conn 2011). Selected species are typically small and short-lived, making it feasible to study the effects of experimental interventions across entire life spans and large samples. Many model organisms are selected because they exhibit extraordinary anti-aging mechanisms, or alternatively because they experience close analogs to human age-related diseases. However, significant physiological differences result from the great evolutionary distance that separates humans from these species (Chiou et al. 2020), yielding a high rate of translation failures from simple animal models (McGonigle and Ruggeri 2014). Indeed, even the relatively small differences between rats and mice or among different strains of these species can influence the outcomes of experiments, and the effects of artificial laboratory breeding and environments may confound the generalizability of results (Mitchell et al. 2015). Aside from the problems of taxonomic divergence, it may also be unrealistic to generalize findings from short-lived species when the evolution of longer life spans likely involved fundamental changes to the aging process.

Nonhuman primate models present an attractive middle ground (Fig. 1). Their close evolutionary relationship to humans is associated with increased genetic and physiological similarities, yet life spans are often short enough to be feasible for study (Lavery 2000; Shively and Clarkson 2009; Colman 2018; Emery Thompson et al. 2020d). Where similarities to humans can be identified, they are likely to be a result of common descent, increasing the probability that these are true functional similarities. Whereas studying nonhuman primates involves stricter ethical considerations, many species can be practicably housed and managed in captivity. Most captive nonhuman primate populations also offer greater genetic diversity than is typical of other model organisms.

Two primate models, mouse lemurs and callitrichids (a neotropical group including marmosets and tamarins), offer several of the advantages of conventional animal models in that they are small, short-lived, and easy to maintain in captivity. However, as primates, they live considerably longer than other mammals of the same size. For example, the gray mouse lemur, a prosimian primate, is rodent-sized but can live 12 years (Languille et al. 2012). Rather than being used explicitly as genetic or disease models, mouse lemurs have been used primarily to study natural aging processes, including changes in physiological regulation, motor function, and cognition (Languille et al. 2012), although they also show promise as models for Alzheimer's disease and related pathologies (Bons et al. 2006). Marmosets, the smallest and shortest lived of the anthropoid primates, develop many human-like aging diseases in captivity, distinguishing them from rodent models (Tardif et al. 2011; Ross 2019).

The most abundant and commonly used nonhuman primate models in captivity are macaques, which take a significant step closer to humans in terms of body size, life span, and genetic relatedness (Chiou et al. 2020). They are attractive models not because of any specific shared aging mechanisms, but because they exhibit many similarities in aging across domains,

offering enhanced potential to model complex aging phenotypes. Additionally, they are particularly prone to obesity when fed processed captive diets, and develop associated metabolic diseases (Simmons 2016). Thus, macaques were instrumental in developing the paradigm that caloric restriction is associated with healthier aging (Masoro 2000; Lane et al. 2001; Mattison et al. 2017). Captive macaques have also been useful for studying interactions of diets with other risk factors in the development of atherosclerosis (Shively and Clarkson 1994; Shively et al. 2009). Whereas rhesus macaques have scarcely been studied in the wild, a large research colony of free-ranging rhesus macaques are maintained on the island of Cayo Santiago in Puerto Rico (Rawlins and Kessler 1986). Here, animals can be studied in a relatively naturalistic social and ecological context, yet it is still possible to perform some procedures that could not be done routinely in a fully wild setting, such as blood draws, veterinary examinations, and histopathology. This setting is emerging as a natural laboratory for aging research (Chiou et al. 2020).

PRIMATES AS ESSENTIAL MODELS FOR SOCIAL DETERMINANTS OF AGING

Nonhuman primates are of special significance for the study of social aging and the social determinants of health. Whereas research in human populations has established clear and compelling interactions between social relationships and health (Sapolsky 2004; Uchino 2009; Holt-Lunstad et al. 2010), progress in this area is hampered by the difficulty of deriving tractable social experience variables, particularly when influential environments may have occurred decades prior to enrollment in a research study. Many nonhuman primate species live in large, stable social groups with status hierarchies and complex differentiation of social relationships, but social networks can be more easily defined than in many human populations. Nonhuman primate social behavior can also be freely observed and objectively quantified. Several long-term research studies of free-ranging and wild primates have recorded social behavior of the same cohorts of animals on a

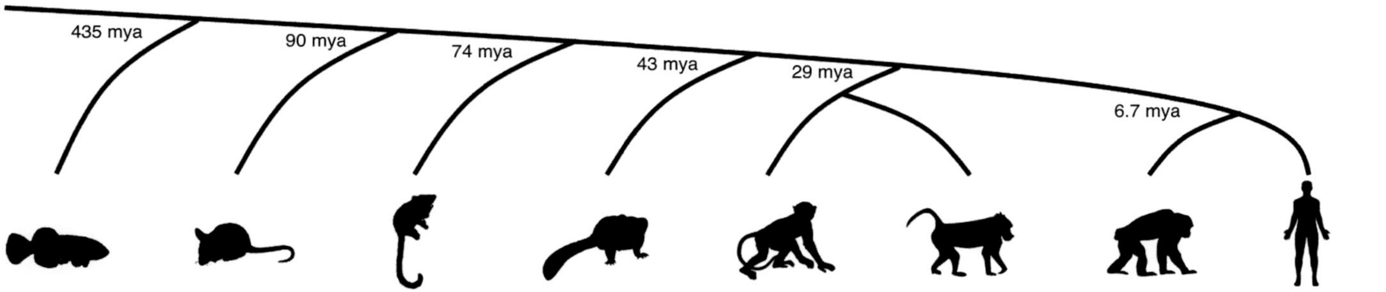

	African turquoise killifish (*Nothobranchius fruzeri*)	House mouse (*Mus musculus*)	Gray mouse lemur (*Microcebus murinus*)	Common marmoset (*Callithrix jacchus*)	Rhesus macaque (*Macaca mulatta*)	Baboon (*Papio cynocephalus*)	Chimpanzee (*Pan troglodytes*)	Human (*Homo sapiens*)
Life expectancy	3–7 mo	2–3 yr	5–6 yr	5–7 yr	10–30 yr	10–20 yr	15–40 yr	50–80 yr
Max life span	<1 yr	5 yr	12 yr	16 yr	40 yr	30 yr	60+ yr	100+ yr
Typical body mass	<5 g	18–35 g	60–120 g	350–400 g	7–15 kg	10–30 kg	30–60 kg	40–100 kg

Figure 1. Common vertebrate aging models: life history comparison and relatedness to humans (see Dyban et al. 1991; Altmann et al. 1993; Colman et al. 1998; Altmann and Alberts 2003; Tardif et al. 2011; Languille et al. 2012; Reuter et al. 2018; Chiou et al. 2020; Emery Thompson and Sabbi 2022). Estimated divergence time from humans in millions of years ago (mya): Timetree.org (Kumar et al. 2017).

near-daily basis for decades, and these studies have generated rigorous metrics of social relationship quality and social status.

Like humans, nonhuman primates experience significant and independent influences of social integration and social status on survival (Silk et al. 2003, 2010; McFarland and Majolo 2013; Archie et al. 2014; Brent et al. 2017; Thompson and Cords 2018; Ellis et al. 2019; Campos et al. 2020), indicating that they are not only a convenient model but an appropriate one for investigating the mechanisms by which social environments impact human aging. Studies of primates allow for investigation of social influences on health without many of the confounding factors affecting human studies, such as variable access to medical care and health information, smoking, and substance use.

Status (or dominance) hierarchies are near-universal features of primate societies and, as in humans, are associated with unequal access to resources. The complexity of social competition in many primates is also thought to lead to a relatively unique association between status and chronic psychosocial stress, compounding the direct effects of resource inequality (Sapolsky 2021). Like in humans, low social status in primates is typically associated with elevated glucocorticoids and increased mortality (Cavigelli and Caruso 2015; Shively and Day 2015; Snyder-Mackler et al. 2020), supporting the hypothesis that stress may be a common pathway by which social factors influence multiple dimensions of health (Sapolsky et al. 1987; Sapolsky 2005). Primate affiliative bonds are hypothesized to influence health through similar pathways, such as by increasing access to resources, reducing exposure to stressful events, or by buffering the stress response (Ostner and Schülke 2018; Thompson 2019). The form and function of social relationships vary considerably within and between primate species, offering excellent potential for modeling different feature of social environments.

Researchers studying the interaction of primate social environments and health have increasingly favored naturalistic studies where individuals have greater freedom of association and experience the full range of environmental selection pressures that are likely to have shaped the evolution of both social behavior and of aging. However, there are ethical and logistical impediments to obtain detailed biomedical data. The Amboseli Baboon Research Project has conducted a continuous, longitudinal study of individually recognized wild baboons (*Papio cynocephalus*) in Kenya for five decades, amassing extensive ecological, behavioral, and demographic data sets (Alberts and Altmann 2012). Routine, noninvasive fecal sampling is conducted, allowing for the quantification of glucocorticoids, parasites, and genetic relatedness. Because baboons are primarily terrestrial, it is also possible to safely immobilize the baboons with tranquilizer darts, allowing for occasional sampling of skin and blood for high-quality DNA and RNA. In this wild system, females acquire rank through maternal inheritance and subsequent alliances with kin, while male ranks are continually renegotiated via aggressive competition. Whereas high status is associated with lower glucocorticoid activity in females (Levy et al. 2020), it is associated with higher glucocorticoid activity in males (Gesquiere et al. 2011). Accordingly, social status is associated with inverse effects on immune cell gene regulation in males and females (Anderson et al. 2022). While status does not directly predict longevity in females (Campos et al. 2020), the high glucocorticoid exposure typical of low rank reduces adult female survival (Campos et al. 2021), while high rank is associated with reduced survival and accelerated epigenetic aging in males (Campos et al. 2020; Anderson et al. 2021). In contrast, social bonds yield survival advantages in both sexes (Archie et al. 2014; Campos et al. 2020). While both social status and social integration affect gene expression and regulation, the specific targets of these effects are distinct (Runcie et al. 2013; Anderson et al. 2022).

An inherent limitation of wild studies is inferring causality if the relationship between social environment and health is bidirectional. However, many of the above results are supported by captive experiments on rhesus macaques, where social status can be reliably manipulated by removing females from established groups and introducing them sequentially to a newly created group. Both in baseline and post-manipulation groups, status is associated with widespread effects on the immune system, where the effects of low status closely resemble those of senescence (Tung et al. 2012; Snyder-Mackler et al. 2014). Status affects glucocorticoid regulation, proliferation of immune cells, gene expression and regulation, and chromatin accessibility (Kohn et al. 2016; Snyder-Mackler et al. 2016, 2019; Debray et al. 2019; Sanchez-Rosado et al. 2021). These differences reflect a more proinflammatory phenotype and greater glucocorticoid resistance in low-ranking individuals and a stronger antiviral phenotype in high-status individuals. The effects of status on health are mediated by differential rates of harassment and degree of social integration (Snyder-Mackler et al. 2016), although as in baboons, social integration appears to have independent positive effects on health, such as improved mtDNA regulation in immune cells (Debray et al. 2019).

COMPARATIVE PRIMATE AGING MODELS

While nonhuman primates offer significant promise as experimental and translational models of aging, evolutionary approaches to aging also emphasize the value of primates as comparative models to trace how recent evolutionary history has shaped human aging biology. By identifying shared ancestry of particular facets of aging biology, we are better equipped to evaluate how unique features of human aging are linked to other recently evolved features of our species, as well as to our unusual longevity and changes in vulnerability to age-related diseases.

While many aging processes are broadly shared across primates, even relatively small evolutionary distances between species are associated with significant differences. For example, aging humans experience physiological dysregulation, an emergent aging phenomenon marked by more frequent or extreme departures from homeostasis and increased risk of disease and mortality (Arbeev et al. 2019). This phenomenon is detectable in multivariate biomarker data sets from other primates, but more distantly related species show increasingly divergent patterns (Dansereau et al. 2019). Only chimpanzees, the species most closely related to humans, exhibit a

pattern that strongly correlates with that of humans. Similar findings are beginning to emerge for CpG methylation, a highly conserved aging feature across primates (Horvath et al. 2020). While it is possible to construct a broadly applicable primate "molecular clock," species differ markedly in the specific sites and rates of methylation (Horvath et al. 2020). A human-derived reference, adjusted for differences in longevity, can predict rhesus macaque ages ($R^2\sim0.5$), but with considerable error (Chiou et al. 2020), while performing substantially better when predicting chimpanzee ages ($R^2\sim0.9$) (Guevara et al. 2020).

Humans are a part of the hominid family (the "great apes"), which also includes seven extant species of orangutans, gorillas, chimpanzees, and bonobos. As a group, the hominids are characterized by extended life histories compared with other primates (Emery Thompson and Sabbi 2022). All great apes can live over 40 years in the wild, and chimpanzees can survive into their 60s. Comparative data on the great apes is of unique value for understanding the evolution of human aging because this can allow us to reconstruct the probable features of a last common ancestor at the origins of the human lineage (Muller et al. 2017). Yet, remarkably little is known about the aging biology of these species.

Until recently, most of the aging information available for great apes derived from veterinary screening of captive chimpanzees in biomedical research laboratories. For example, aging captive chimpanzees exhibit declining liver and kidney function and increased risk of hypertension and anemia (Videan et al. 2008; Ely et al. 2013). Compared with healthy humans, captive chimpanzees maintain markedly higher levels of biomarkers typically associated with cardiovascular risk and accelerated aging, including blood pressure, cholesterol, fibrinogen, and insulin (Videan et al. 2009; Ely et al. 2013; Cole et al. 2020). Despite this, chimpanzees and other captive great apes are at relatively low risk of most age-related pathologies that plague industrialized human populations, including coronary artery disease, cancers, osteoporosis, degenerative joint disease, and Alzheimer's-related pathologies, although strokes are not uncommon (Lowenstine et al. 2015; Edler et al. 2020). Like humans, heart disease is the most common cause of death for captive chimpanzees, yet the nature of the pathology differs. Great apes develop myocardial fibrosis and aortic dissections, rare conditions for humans, while they rarely develop advanced atherosclerosis (Kenny et al. 1994; Schulman et al. 1995; Seiler et al. 2009; Varki et al. 2009). This contrast has led to novel consideration of how human endurance activities may have shaped the evolution of the cardiovascular system and vulnerability to disease (Shave et al. 2019). Additionally, comparative genetic study reveals that apolipoprotein E4 (apoE4), an allele that increases risk of cardiovascular disease in humans, is the ancestral allele found in chimpanzees and bonobos (Hanlon and Rubinsztein 1995; McIntosh et al. 2012), whereas novel polymorphisms associated with reduced risk have evolved more recently in humans.

Other apparent differences between humans and chimpanzees may be side effects of captivity. Studies of free-living chimpanzees in sanctuaries observe significantly lower levels of blood pressure, glucose, cholesterol, and triglycerides than in zoos or laboratories (Ely et al. 2013; Ronke et al. 2015; Cole et al. 2020). In contrast to most captive laboratory chimpanzees, which are relatively sedentary and are fed processed animal chows, most wild-born sanctuary chimpanzees consume fresh fruits and vegetables and free range over large, forested areas. They are accordingly less likely to be obese, a factor that raises the levels of unhealthy biomarkers in both species (Nehete et al. 2014; Obanda et al. 2014).

Valid comparisons of aging physiology between humans and closely related species thus depend on evaluating how they age in in their natural environments. One such model system has been developed in the Kibale National Park, Uganda, where wild chimpanzees have been under continuous observation for more than 30 years (Emery Thompson et al. 2020c). Because chimpanzees are endangered in the wild, this research is limited to noninvasive measures; yet a wide range of informative data are possible from urine and fecal samples in addition to observational health and activity surveys. Aging in these wild chimpanzees is associated with increased parasite loads, greater diversity of viral infection,

and increased morbidity and mortality from respiratory disease, implicating immunosenescence as a driver of declining health (Emery Thompson et al. 2018; Negrey et al. 2019, 2022; Phillips et al. 2020). Chimpanzees also exhibit age-related dysregulation of the hypothalamic-pituitary-adrenal (HPA) axis, characterized by increases in glucocorticoid production and a human-like blunting of the circadian rhythm (Emery Thompson et al. 2020a). Shared patterns of immunosenescence and physiological dysregulation between humans and chimpanzees indicate dimensions of our natural aging biology that are evolutionarily ancient.

Despite shorter life spans and challenging environments characterized by resource constraints and infectious disease, wild chimpanzees age quite successfully. For example, wild chimpanzees do not show evidence of a physical frailty syndrome, despite maintaining physically demanding foraging strategies that involve climbing high into the forest canopy. They experience only moderate changes in body condition and physical activity with age, and variation in condition does not predict mortality (Emery Thompson et al. 2020b). Similarly, studies of skeletal collections indicate that, despite high rates of healed fractures and moderate bone loss with age, wild chimpanzees and mountain gorillas rarely experience advanced osteoporosis, osteoarthritis, or degenerative joint disease (Jurmain 2000; Morbeck et al. 2002; Ruff et al. 2020). In an analogous fashion, captive chimpanzees exhibit cognitive aging, moderate neuronal loss, and even lesions characteristic of Alzheimer's disease, but they do not exhibit the severity of neurodegeneration associated with dementia in humans (Finch and Austad 2015; Edler et al. 2020; Lacreuse et al. 2020).

The process of senescence for great apes is at once very human-like, with age-related functional losses in the same domains, but it is not commonly associated with the aging pathologies that are leading causes of death for humans. Chronic inflammation has been identified as a key variable distinguishing healthy and pathological aging in humans (Franceschi et al. 2007, 2018; Baylis et al. 2013). The data from free-living chimpanzees in sanctuaries predict that wild populations may resist inflammaging, but noninvasive tools for direct measurement of inflammation in wild chimpanzees are limited. With opportunistic sampling, it can be also be difficult to distinguish the effects of immunosenescence, causing older individuals to experience more frequent acute bouts of inflammation, from the effects of chronic inflammation. For example, urinary neopterin, a proinflammatory marker of cellular immune activation, increased with age in one short-term study of wild chimpanzees (Negrey et al. 2021), but not in a longitudinal study within the same population (Thompson González et al. 2020). The latter study found that increased inflammation was only detectable in the 2–3 years before the death of some older chimpanzees, suggesting the expected association with declining health but not with aging per se. In support of this, aging was not associated with elevation of oxidative stress, a signature of human inflammaging (Zuo et al. 2019), in two independent studies of wild chimpanzees (Thompson González et al. 2020; Costantini et al. 2021).

AGING IN HUMANS IN EVOLUTIONARILY RELEVANT ENVIRONMENTS

Overwhelmingly, human aging research has been conducted in postindustrial populations. It has been only ~10,000 years since the origins of agriculture and only a few generations since the first nations underwent the industrial transition. Prior to these transitions, the vast majority of human existence was spent in a hunting and gathering (i.e., foraging) context. Thus, a major guiding principle of evolutionary medicine is that human biology has been shaped by these environments of the past (Stearns 2012). We have had little time to adapt to the radical lifestyle changes of industrial development, and this environmental mismatch may lead to novel, and even maladaptive, health outcomes (Gurven and Lieberman 2020).

Whereas medical innovations have increased longevity in industrialized populations, all available evidence suggests that the human species is naturally long-lived. For example, modal ages of death for contemporary foraging populations are ~68–78 years when individuals survive to adulthood, closely matching demographics from pre-industrialized Europe (Gurven and Kaplan 2007).

Recent insights from studies of contemporary foragers and other small-scale subsistence populations (e.g., pastoralists, horticulturalists) have fundamentally challenged our understanding of human aging. It is important to note that foraging populations cannot be considered relics of our evolutionary past, nor is their lifestyle untouched by the market-integrated populations that surround them. Rather, the environments and lifestyle of these communities replicate key selection pressures that would have shaped the evolution of the modern human organism: resource limitations, high workload, unprocessed wild diets, small kin-based communities, and fewer barriers to infectious disease and environmental stress.

Small-scale subsistence populations appear to be models of successful aging, resisting many of the age-associated diseases that plague industrialized populations (Pontzer et al. 2018; Gurven et al. 2022). Heart disease and strokes are rare causes of death (Hill and Hurtado 1996; Gurven et al. 2007), and screening of forager and forager-horticulturalist populations find little evidence for underlying atherosclerosis, chronic inflammation, or hypertension (Lindeberg and Lundh 1993; Vasunilashorn et al. 2010; Kaplan et al. 2017; Raichlen et al. 2017). This is remarkable given that forager diets are often heavily meat-based. It is hypothesized that the relatively high balance of protein to carbohydrates, prevalence of "good" fats, low sodium, high fiber, and rich micronutrients in forager diets may counteract atherogenic effects that might typically arise from high fat content (Cordain et al. 2002). Resistance to chronic inflammation is also surprising given that subsistence populations experience relatively high rates of infection, leading to frequent acute bouts of inflammation (Gurven et al. 2008). High prevalence of helminth infections is suspected to help to resist cardiovascular disease and diabetes by increasing anti-inflammatory immune responses, consuming blood lipids, and diverting resources that might otherwise contribute to obesity or arterial plaques (Gurven et al. 2016).

Cross-cultural studies also highlight the importance of gene–environment interactions in moderating Alzheimer's disease (AD) risk. Whereas the apoE4 allele has been widely implicated in increased risk of AD in industrialized populations, and was similarly associated with increased risk of dementia in the Tsimane and Moseten forager-horticulturalists of Bolivia (Gatz et al. 2022), the allele was associated with increased cognitive performance among Tsimane with moderate-to-severe eosinophilia, characteristic of parasitic infection (Trumble et al. 2017). Tsimane with the apoE4 allele do not suffer higher mortality than others (Vasunilashorn et al. 2011).The apoE4 allele has also been implicated in improved child health and cognitive development in a Brazilian population experiencing high rates of early life mortality (Oriá et al. 2010). These findings suggest reasons why this allele, deleterious in industrialized environments, may have been conserved in humans. While the Tsimane exhibit mild cognitive impairment with age, they exhibit very low rates of dementia (~1%) compared with industrialized populations (Gurven et al. 2017; Gatz et al. 2022). It is not yet clear how generalizable this finding is to other subsistence settings. A meta-analysis of 15 "indigenous" populations found widely varying rates of dementia (Warren et al. 2015), but the most affected populations, such as Australian aborigines, are already significantly market-integrated and experience high rates of obesity and sedentism (Radford et al. 2019).

Subsistence workloads involve considerable investment in physical activity. Rather than contributing to accelerated wear and tear, intensive workloads appear to be protective against frailty. Studies of Hadza foragers of Tanzania and Pokot pastoralists of Kenya find that strength and daily duration of physical activity declines by about half across adulthood, but rates of physical performance among the oldest adults remain remarkable remarkably high (Sayre et al. 2019, 2020). For example, the average 60-year-old Hadza or Pokot engages in ~150 min of moderate-to-vigorous physical activity per day, while most Americans fail to meet the recommended 30 min per day. Physical inactivity and obesity are also implicated in the severity of knee osteoarthritis (Berenbaum et al. 2018; Wallace et al. 2022), which may help to explain a doubling in

prevalence in the industrial era (Wallace et al. 2017).

Physical activity is likely to be a key mechanism by which subsistence populations resist chronic inflammation and its damaging consequences for health (Pontzer et al. 2018; Gurven and Lieberman 2020). Indeed, many aspects of human anatomy and physiology are optimized for the long periods of physical activity that would have characterized prehistoric lifeways, setting us apart from our close primate relatives (Bramble and Lieberman 2004; Kraft et al. 2021). These adaptations that increased fitness throughout most of our evolutionary history predispose us to disease when mismatched to sedentary environments (Shave et al. 2019; Lieberman et al. 2021). The recent "active grandparent" hypothesis goes one step further in posing that adaptation to physically active lifestyles were integral to the evolution of extended human life spans (Lieberman et al. 2021). Two mechanisms are proposed. First, activity could promote healthy aging by drawing energy away from excess fat storage and reproduction, thus reducing harmful downstream effects of inflammation, high steroid production, and insulin resistance. In addition, exercise induces mild stress, activating mechanisms of cellular repair and maintenance that combat senescence (Lieberman et al. 2021).

CONCLUDING REMARKS

Evolutionary approaches to aging research aim to move beyond the acknowledgment that aging has evolved toward reconstructing how the mechanisms of aging and disease have been shaped by our evolutionary past. There has been a conspicuous gap in our knowledge of aging biology during our recent evolutionary history that is now being filled in by anthropologists and primatologists studying our closest primate relatives and humans living in preindustrial environments. While this body of work is still new, it has already demonstrated the potential to redefine our understanding of the relationship between aging, health, and disease.

While the findings of the evolutionary aging program demonstrate that human aging biology retains many features from our evolutionary

Cite this article as *Cold Spring Harb Perspect Med* doi: 10.1101/cshperspect.a041195

past, our capacity for healthy aging is dramatically affected by current environments. On the one hand, there is evidence that unique human adaptations may predispose us to severe degenerative disease risks not experienced by our close evolutionary relatives. On the other hand, there is mounting evidence to support the hypothesis that these risks may be limited to novel environments to which humans are not yet adapted. If so, there is even more reason to consider that natural aging and disease emerge from distinct, although interacting, processes. Diversifying the contexts for aging research will provide increased capacity to discriminate these processes and how they respond to complex social and ecological phenomena across the life course.

ACKNOWLEDGMENTS

The author is supported by a grant from the National Institute on Aging R01AG049395.

REFERENCES

Alberts SC, Altmann J. 2012. The Amboseli baboon research project: 40 years of continuity and change. In *Long-term field studies of primates*, pp. 261–287. Springer, Berlin.

Altmann J, Alberts SC. 2003. Variability in reproductive success viewed from a life-history perspective in baboons. *Am J Hum Biol* 15: 401–409. doi:10.1002/ajhb.10157

Altmann J, Schoeller D, Altmann SA, Muruthi P, Sapolsky RM. 1993. Body size and fatness of free-living baboons reflect food availability and activity levels. *Am J Primatol* 30: 149–161. doi:10.1002/ajp.1350300207

Anderson JA, Johnston RA, Lea AJ, Campos FA, Voyles TN, Akinyi MY, Alberts SC, Archie EA, Tung J. 2021. High social status males experience accelerated epigenetic aging in wild baboons. *eLife* 10: e66128. doi:10.7554/eLife.66128

Anderson JA, Lea AJ, Voyles TN, Akinyi MY, Nyakundi R, Ochola L, Omondi M, Nyundo F, Zhang Y, Campos FA, et al. 2022. Distinct gene regulatory signatures of dominance rank and social bond strength in wild baboons. *Philos Trans R Soc Lond B Biol Sci* 377: 20200441. doi:10.1098/rstb.2020.0441

Arbeev KG, Ukraintseva SV, Bagley O, Zhbannikov IY, Cohen AA, Kulminski AM, Yashin AI. 2019. "Physiological dysregulation" as a promising measure of robustness and resilience in studies of aging and a new indicator of preclinical disease. *J Gerontol A* 74: 462–468. doi:10.1093/gerona/gly136

Archie EA, Tung J, Clark M, Altmann J, Alberts SC. 2014. Social affiliation matters: both same-sex and opposite-sex relationships predict survival in wild female baboons. *Proc Biol Sci* 281: 20141261. doi:10.1098/rspb.2014.1261

Baudisch A. 2011. The pace and shape of ageing. *Methods Ecol Evol* 2: 375–382. doi:10.1111/j.2041-210X.2010.00087.x

Baudisch A. 2012. Birds do it, bees do it, we do it: contributions of theoretical modelling to understanding the shape of ageing across the tree of life. *Gerontology* 58: 481–489. doi:10.1159/000341861

Baylis D, Bartlett DB, Patel HP, Roberts HC. 2013. Understanding how we age: insights into inflammaging. *Longev Healthspan* 2: 8. doi:10.1186/2046-2395-2-8

Berenbaum F, Wallace IJ, Lieberman DE, Felson DT. 2018. Modern-day environmental factors in the pathogenesis of osteoarthritis. *Nat Rev Rheumatol* 14: 674–681. doi:10.1038/s41584-018-0073-x

Blagosklonny MV. 2018. Disease or not, aging is easily treatable. *Aging (Albany NY)* 10: 3067–3078. doi:10.18632/aging.101647

Bons N, Rieger F, Prudhomme D, Fisher A, Krause KH. 2006. *Microcebus murinus*: a useful primate model for human cerebral aging and Alzheimer's disease? *Genes Brain Behav* 5: 120–130. doi:10.1111/j.1601-183X.2005.00149.x

Bramble DM, Lieberman DE. 2004. Endurance running and the evolution of Homo. *Nature* 432: 345–352. doi:10.1038/nature03052

Brent LJ, Ruiz-Lambides A, Platt ML. 2017. Family network size and survival across the lifespan of female macaques. *Proc Biol Sci* 284: 20170515.

Bronikowski AM, Altmann J, Brockman DK, Cords M, Fedigan L, Pusey A, Stoinski T, Morris WF, Strier KB, Alberts SC. 2011. Aging in the natural world: comparative data reveal similar mortality patterns across primates. *Science* 331: 1325–1328. doi:10.1126/science.1201571

Bulterijs S, Hull RS, Björk VCE, Roy AG. 2015. It is time to classify biological aging as a disease. *Front Genet* 6: 205. doi:10.3389/fgene.2015.00205

Burch JB, Augustine AD, Frieden LA, Hadley E, Howcroft TK, Johnson R, Khalsa PS, Kohanski RA, Li XL, Macchiarini F, et al. 2014. Advances in geroscience: impact on healthspan and chronic disease. *J Gerontol A* 69: S1–S3. doi:10.1093/gerona/glu041

Campos FA, Villavicencio F, Archie EA, Colchero F, Alberts SC. 2020. Social bonds, social status and survival in wild baboons: a tale of two sexes. *Philos Trans R Soc Lond B Biol Scii* 375: 20190621. doi:10.1098/rstb.2019.0621

Campos FA, Archie EA, Gesquiere LR, Tung J, Altmann J, Alberts SC. 2021. Glucocorticoid exposure predicts survival in female baboons. *Sci Adv* 7: eabf6759. doi:10.1126/sciadv.abf6759

Cavigelli SA, Caruso MJ. 2015. Sex, social status and physiological stress in primates: the importance of social and glucocorticoid dynamics. *Philos Trans R Soc Lond B Biol Sci* 370: 20140103. doi:10.1098/rstb.2014.0103

Charnov EL, Berrigan D. 1993. Why do female primates have such long lifespans and so few babies? Or life in the slow lane. *Evol Anthropol* 1: 191–194. doi:10.1002/evan.1360010604

Chiou KL, Montague MJ, Goldman EA, Watowich MM, Sams SN, Song J, Horvath JE, Sterner KN, Ruiz-Lambides A, Martinez MI, et al. 2020. Rhesus macaques as a tractable physiological model of human ageing. *Philos Trans*

R Soc Lond B Biol Sci **375:** 20190612. doi:10.1098/rstb .2019.0612

Colchero F, Rau R, Jones OR, Barthold JA, Conde DA, Lenart A, Nemeth L, Scheuerlein A, Schoeley J, Torres C, et al. 2016. The emergence of longevous populations. *Proc Natl Acad Sci* **113:** E7681–E7690. doi:10.1073/pnas.1612 191113

Colchero F, Aburto J, Archie EA, Boesch C, Breuer T, Campos F, Collins A, Conde DA, Cords M, Crockford C, et al. 2021. The long lives of primates and the 'invariant rate of ageing' hypothesis. *Nat Commun* **12:** 1–10. doi:10.1038/ s41467-021-23894-3

Cole MF, Cantwell A, Rukundo J, Ajarova L, Fernandez-Navarro S, Atencia R, Rosati AG. 2020. Healthy cardiovascular biomarkers across the lifespan in wild-born chimpanzees (*Pan troglodytes*). *Philos Trans R Soc Lond B Biol Sci* **375:** 20190609. doi:10.1098/rstb.2019.0609

Colman RJ. 2018. Non-human primates as a model for aging. *Biochim Biophys Acta* **1864:** 2733–2741. doi:10.1016/ j.bbadis.2017.07.008

Colman RJ, Roecker EB, Ramsey JJ, Kemnitz JW. 1998. The effect of dietary restriction on body composition in adult male and female rhesus macaques. *Age Clin Exper Res* **10:** 83–92. doi:10.1007/BF03339642

Conn PM. 2011. *Handbook of models for human aging.* Elsevier, Burlington, MA.

Cordain L, Eaton SB, Miller JB, Mann N, Hill K. 2002. The paradoxical nature of hunter-gatherer diets: meat-based, yet non-atherogenic. *Eur J Clin Nutr* **56:** S42–S52. doi:10 .1038/sj.ejcn.1601353

Costantini D, Masi S, Rachid L, Beltrame M, Rohmer M, Krief S. 2021. Mind the food: rapid changes in antioxidant content of diet affect oxidative status of chimpanzees. *Am J Physiol Regul Integr Comp Physiol* **320:** R728–R734. doi:10.1152/ajpregu.00003.2021

Dansereau G, Wey TW, Legault V, Brunet MA, Kemnitz JW, Ferrucci L, Cohen AA. 2019. Conservation of physiological dysregulation signatures of aging across primates. *Aging Cell* **18:** e12925. doi:10.1111/acel.12925

Debray R, Snyder-Mackler N, Kohn JN, Wilson ME, Barreiro LB, Tung J. 2019. Social affiliation predicts mitochondrial DNA copy number in female rhesus macaques. *Biol Lett* **15:** 20180643. doi:10.1098/rsbl.2018.0643

de Magalhães JP. 2014. The scientific quest for lasting youth: prospects for curing aging. *Rejuvenation Res* **17:** 458–467. doi:10.1089/rej.2014.1580

de Magalhães JP, Church GM. 2005. Genomes optimize reproduction: aging as a consequence of the developmental program. *Physiology* **20:** 252–259. doi:10.1152/physiol .00010.2005

Dyban AP, Puchkov VF, Samoshkina NA, Khozhai LI, Chebotar' NA, Baranov VS. 1991. Laboratory mammals: mouse (*Mus musculus*), rat (*Rattus norvegicus*), rabbit (*Oryctolagus cuniculus*), and golden hamster (*Cricetus auratus*). In *Animal species for developmental studies: vertebrates* (ed. Dettlaff TA, Vassetzky SG), pp. 351–443. Springer, Boston, MA.

Edler MK, Munger EL, Meindle RS, Hopkins WD, Ely JJ, Erwin JM, Mufson EJ, Hof PR, Sherwood CC, Raghanti MA. 2020. Neuron loss associated with age but not Alzheimer's disease pathology in the chimpanzee brain.

Philos Trans R Soc Lond B Biol Sci **375:** 20190619. doi:10.1098/rstb.2019.0619

Edwards RD, Tuljapurkar S. 2005. Inequality in life spans and a new perspective on mortality convergence across industrialized countries. *Popul Dev Rev* **31:** 645–674. doi:10.1111/j.1728-4457.2005.00092.x

Ellis S, Snyder-Mackler N, Ruiz-Lambides A, Platt ML, Brent LJ. 2019. Deconstructing sociality: the types of social connections that predict longevity in a group-living primate. *Proc Biol Sci* **286:** 20191991. doi:10.1098/rspb.2019.1991

Ely JJ, Zavaskis T, Lammey ML. 2013. Hypertension increases with aging and obesity in chimpanzees (*Pan troglodytes*). *Zoo Biol* **32:** 79–87. doi:10.1002/zoo.21044

Emery Thompson M, Sabbi KH. 2022. Evolutionary demography of the great apes. In *Human evolutionary demography* (ed. Sear R, Burger O, Lee R). Open Book Publishers, Cambridge, UK.

Emery Thompson M, Machanda ZP, Scully EJ, Enigk DK, Otali E, Muller MN, Goldberg TG, Chapman CA, Wrangham RW. 2018. Risk factors for respiratory illness in a community of wild chimpanzees (*Pan troglodytes schweinfurthii*). *R Soc Open Sci* **5:** 180840. doi:10.1098/ rsos.180840

Emery Thompson M, Fox SA, Berghänel A, Sabbi K, Phillips-Garcia S, Enigk DK, Otali E, Machanda ZP, Wrangham RW, Muller MN. 2020a. Wild chimpanzees exhibit humanlike aging of glucocorticoid regulation. *Proc Natl Acad Sci* **117:** 8424–8430. doi:10.1073/pnas.1920593117

Emery Thompson M, Machanda ZP, Fox SA, Sabbi KH, Otali E, Thompson González N, Muller MN, Wrangham RW. 2020b. Evaluating the impact of physical frailty during ageing in wild chimpanzees (*Pan troglodytes schweinfurthii*). *Philos Trans R Soc Lond B Biol Sci* **375:** 20190607. doi:10.1098/rstb.2019.0607

Emery Thompson M, Muller MN, Machanda ZP, Otali E, Wrangham RW. 2020c. The Kibale Chimpanzee Project: over thirty years of research, conservation, and change. *Biol Conserv* **252:** 108857. doi:10.1016/j.biocon.2020 .108857

Emery Thompson M, Rosati AG, Snyder-Mackler N. 2020d. Insights from evolutionarily relevant models for human ageing. *Philos Trans R Soc Lond B Biol Sci* **375:** 20190605. doi:10.1098/rstb.2019.0605

Finch CE, Austad SN. 2015. Commentary: is Alzheimer's disease uniquely human? *Neurobiol Aging* **36:** 553–555. doi:10.1016/j.neurobiolaging.2014.10.025

Franceschi C, Capri M, Monti D, Giunta S, Olivieri F, Sevini F, Panourgia MP, Invidia L, Celani L, Scurti M, et al. 2007. Inflammaging and anti-inflammaging: a systemic perspective on aging and longevity emerged from studies in humans. *Mech Ageing Dev* **128:** 92–105. doi:10.1016/j .mad.2006.11.016

Franceschi C, Garagnani P, Parini P, Giuliani C, Santoro A. 2018. Inflammaging: a new immune–metabolic viewpoint for age-related diseases. *Nat Rev Endocrinol* **14:** 576–590. doi:10.1038/s41574-018-0059-4

Gatz M, Mack WJ, Chui HC, Law EM, Barisano G, Sutherland ML, Sutherland JD, Eid Rodriguez D, Quispe Gutierrez R, Copajira Adrian J, et al. 2022. Prevalence of dementia and mild cognitive impairment in indigenous Bolivian forager-horticulturalists. *Alzheimers Dement* doi:10.1002/alz.12626

Gesquiere LR, Learn NH, Simao MCM, Onyango PO, Alberts SC, Altmann J. 2011. Life at the top: rank and stress in wild male baboons. *Science* **333:** 357–360. doi:10.1126/science.1207120

Grunspan DZ, Nesse RM, Barnes ME, Brownell SE. 2018. Core principles of evolutionary medicine: a Delphi study. *Evol Med Public Health* **2018:** 13–23. doi:10.1093/emph/eox025

Guevara EE, Lawler RR, Staes N, White CM, Sherwood CC, Ely JJ, Hopkins WD, Bradley BJ. 2020. Age-associated epigenetic change in chimpanzees and humans. *Philos Trans R Soc Lond B Biol Sci* **375:** 20190616. doi:10.1098/rstb.2019.0616

Gurven M, Kaplan H. 2007. Longevity among hunter-gatherers: a cross-cultural examination. *Popul Dev Rev* **33:** 321–365. doi:10.1111/j.1728-4457.2007.00171.x

Gurven MD, Lieberman DE. 2020. WEIRD bodies: mismatch, medicine and missing diversity. *Evol Hum Behav* **41:** 330–340. doi:10.1016/j.evolhumbehav.2020.04.001

Gurven M, Kaplan HS, Zelada Supa A. 2007. Mortality experience of Tsimane Amerindians of Bolivia: regional variation and temporal trends. *Am J Hum Biol* **19:** 379–398. doi:10.1002/ajhb.20600

Gurven M, Kaplan HS, Winking J, Finch C, Crimmins EM. 2008. Aging and inflammation in two epidemiological worlds. *J Gerontol* **63:** 196–199. doi:10.1093/gerona/63.2.196

Gurven MD, Trumble BC, Stieglitz J, Blackwell AD, Michalik DE, Finch CE, Kaplan HS. 2016. Cardiovascular disease and type 2 diabetes in evolutionary perspective: a critical role for helminths? *Evol Med Public Health* **2016:** 338–357. doi:10.1093/emph/eow028

Gurven M, Fuerstenberg E, Trumble B, Stieglitz J, Beheim B, Davis H, Kaplan H. 2017. Cognitive performance across the life course of Bolivian forager-farmers with limited schooling. *Dev Psychol* **53:** 160–176. doi:10.1037/dev0000175

Gurven M, Kaplan H, Trumble B, Stieglitz J. 2022. The biodemography of human health in contemporary non-industrial populations: insights from the Tsimane Health and Life History Project. In *Human evolutionary demography* (ed. Sear R, Burger O, Lee R). Open Book Publishers, Cambridge, UK.

Haldane J. 1941. *New paths in genetics*. Allen & Unwin, London.

Hanlon CS, Rubinsztein DC. 1995. Arginine residues at codons 112 and 158 in the apolipoprotein E gene correspond to the ancestral state in humans. *Atherosclerosis* **112:** 85–90. doi:10.1016/0021-9150(94)05402-5

Hayflick L. 2000. The future of ageing. *Nature* **408:** 267–269. doi:10.1038/35041709

Hayflick L. 2004. Debates: the not-so-close relationship between biological aging and age-associated pathologies in humans. *J Gerontol A* **59:** B547–B550. doi:10.1093/gerona/59.6.B547

Hill KR, Hurtado AM. 1996. *Ache life history: the ecology and demography of a foraging people*. Transaction, Piscataway, NJ.

Holt-Lunstad J, Smith TB, Layton JB. 2010. Social relationships and mortality risk: a meta-analytic review. *PLoS Med* **7:** e1000316. doi:10.1371/journal.pmed.1000316

Horvath S, Haghani A, Zoller J, Lu A, Ernst J, Pellegrini M, Jasinska A, Mattison J, Salmon A, Raj K, et al. 2020. Pan-primate DNA methylation clocks. bioRxiv doi:10.1101/2020.11.29.402891

Jones OR, Scheuerlein A, Salguero-Gómez R, Camarda CG, Schaible R, Casper BB, Dahlgren JP, Ehrlén J, García MB, Menges ES, et al. 2014. Diversity of ageing across the tree of life. *Nature* **505:** 169–173. doi:10.1038/nature12789

Jurmain R. 2000. Degenerative joint disease in African great apes: an evolutionary perspective. *J Hum Evol* **39:** 185–203. doi:10.1006/jhev.2000.0413

Kaplan H, Thompson RC, Trumble BC, Wann LS, Allam AH, Beheim B, Frohlich B, Sutherland ML, Sutherland JD, Stieglitz J, et al. 2017. Coronary atherosclerosis in indigenous south American Tsimane: a cross-sectional cohort study. *Lancet* **389:** 1730–1739. doi:10.1016/S0140-6736(17)30752-3

Kennedy BK, Berger SL, Brunet A, Campisi J, Cuervo AM, Epel ES, Franceschi C, Lithgow GJ, Morimoto RI, Pessin JE, et al. 2014. Geroscience: linking aging to chronic disease. *Cell* **159:** 709–713. doi:10.1016/j.cell.2014.10.039

Kenny DE, Cambre RC, Alvarado TP, Prowten AW, Allchurch AF, Marks SK, Zuba JR. 1994. Aortic dissection: an important cardiovascular disease in captive gorillas (*Gorilla gorilla gorilla*). *J Zoo Wildl Med* **25:** 561–568.

Kirkwood T. 1977. Evolution of ageing. *Nature* **270:** 301–304. doi:10.1038/270301a0

Kirkwood TB, Rose MR. 1991. Evolution of senescence: late survival sacrificed for reproduction. *Philos Trans R Soc Lond B Biol Sci* **332:** 15–24. doi:10.1098/rstb.1991.0028

Kohn JN, Snyder-Mackler N, Barreiro LB, Johnson ZP, Tung J, Wilson ME. 2016. Dominance rank causally affects personality and glucocorticoid regulation in female rhesus macaques. *Psychoneuroendocrinology* **74:** 179–188. doi:10.1016/j.psyneuen.2016.09.005

Kraft TS, Venkataraman VV, Wallace IJ, Crittenden AN, Holowka NB, Stieglitz J, Harris J, Raichlen DA, Wood B, Gurven M, et al. 2021. The energetics of uniquely human subsistence strategies. *Science* **374:** eabf0130. doi:10.1126/science.abf0130

Kumar S, Stecher G, Suleski M, Hedges SB. 2017. Timetree: a resource for timelines, timetrees, and divergence times. *Mol Biol Evol* **34:** 1812–1819. DOI: 10.1093/molbev/msx116

Lacreuse A, Raz N, Schmidtke D, Hopkins WD, Herndon JG. 2020. Age-related decline in executive function as a hallmark of cognitive ageing in primates: an overview of cognitive and neurobiological studies. *Philos Trans R Soc Lond B Biol Sci* **375:** 20190618. doi:10.1098/rstb.2019.0618

Lane MA, Black A, Handy A, Tilmont EM, Ingram DK, Roth GS. 2001. Caloric restriction in primates. *Ann NY Acad Sci* **928:** 287–295. doi:10.1111/j.1749-6632.2001.tb05658.x

Languille S, Blanc S, Blin O, Canale CI, Dal-Pan A, Devau G, Dhenain M, Dorieux O, Epelbaum J, Gomez D, et al. 2012. The grey mouse lemur: a non-human primate model for ageing studies. *Age Res Rev* **11:** 150–162. doi:10.1016/j.arr.2011.07.001

Lavery WL. 2000. How relevant are animal models to human ageing? *J R Soc Med* **93:** 296–298. doi:10.1177/014107680009300605

Levy EJ, Gesquiere LR, McLean E, Franz M, Warutere JK, Sayialel SN, Mututua RS, Wango TL, Oudu VK, Altmann J, et al. 2020. Higher dominance rank is associated with lower glucocorticoids in wild female baboons: a rank metric comparison. *Horm Behav* 125: 104826. doi:10.1016/j.yhbeh.2020.104826

Lieberman DE, Kistner TM, Richard D, Lee IM, Baggish AL. 2021. The active grandparent hypothesis: physical activity and the evolution of extended human healthspans and lifespans. *Proc Natl Acad Sci* 118: e2107621118. doi:10.1073/pnas.2107621118

Lindeberg S, Lundh B. 1993. Apparent absence of stroke and ischaemic heart disease in a traditional Melanesian island: a clinical study in Kitava. *J Intern Med* 233: 269–275. doi:10.1111/j.1365-2796.1993.tb00986.x

Lowenstine LJ, McManamon R, Terio KA. 2016. Comparative pathology of aging great apes. *Vet Pathol* 53: 250–276. doi:10.1177/0300985815612154

Masoro EJ. 2000. Caloric restriction and aging: an update. *Exper Gerontol* 35: 299–305. doi:10.1016/S0531-5565(00)00084-X

Mattison JA, Colman RJ, Beasley TM, Allison DB, Kemnitz JW, Roth GS, Ingram DK, Weindruch R, de Cabo R, Anderson RM. 2017. Caloric restriction improves health and survival of rhesus monkeys. *Nat Commun* 8: 14063. doi:10.1038/ncomms14063

McFarland R, Majolo B. 2013. Coping with the cold: predictors of survival in wild Barbary macaques, *Macaca sylvanus*. *Bio Lett* 9: 20130428. doi:10.1098/rsbl.2013.0428

McGonigle P, Ruggeri B. 2014. Animal models of human disease: challenges in enabling translation. *Biochem Pharmacol* 87: 162–171. doi:10.1016/j.bcp.2013.08.006

McIntosh AM, Bennett C, Dickson D, Anestis SF, Watts DP, Webster TH, Fontenot MB, Bradley BJ. 2012. The apolipoprotein E (APOE) gene appears functionally monomorphic in chimpanzees (*Pan troglodytes*). *PLoS ONE* 7: e47760. doi:10.1371/journal.pone.0047760

Medawar PB. 1946. Old age and natural death. *Modern Quarterly* 1: 30–56.

Medawar PB. 1952. *An unsolved problem of biology*. HK Lewis, London.

Mitchell SJ, Scheibye-Knudsen M, Longo DL, Cabo RD. 2015. Animal models of aging research: implications for human aging and age-related diseases. *Annu Rev Anim Biosci* 3: 283–303. doi:10.1146/annurev-animal-022114-110829

Morbeck M, Galloway A, Sumner DR. 2002. Getting old at Gombe: skeletal aging in wild-ranging chimpanzees. *Interdisc Top Gerontol* 31: 48–62. doi:10.1159/000061458

Muller MN, Wrangham RW, Pilbeam DR. 2017. *Chimpanzees and human evolution*. Harvard University Press, Cambridge, MA.

Negrey JD, Reddy RB, Scully EJ, Phillips-Garcia S, Owens L, Langergraber KE, Mitani J, Emery Thompson M, Wrangham RW, Muller MN, et al. 2019. Simultaneous outbreaks of respiratory disease in wild chimpanzees caused by distinct viruses of human origin. *Emerg Microbes Infect* 8: 139–149. doi:10.1080/22221751.2018.1563456

Negrey JD, Behringer V, Langergraber KE, Deschner T. 2021. Urinary neopterin of wild chimpanzees indicates that cell-mediated immune activity varies by age, sex, and female reproductive status. *Sci Rep* 11: 1–11. doi:10.1038/s41598-021-88401-6

Negrey JD, Mitani JC, Wrangham RW, Otali E, Reddy RB, Pappas TE, Grindle KA, Gern JE, Machanda ZP, Muller MN. 2022. Viruses associated with ill health in wild chimpanzees. *Am J Primatol* 84: e23358. doi:10.1002/ajp.23358

Nehete P, Magden ER, Nehete B, Hanley PW, Abee CR. 2014. Obesity related alterations in plasma cytokines and metabolic hormones in chimpanzees. *Int J Inflam* 2014: 856749.

Németh L. 2017. Life expectancy versus lifespan inequality: a smudge or a clear relationship? *PLoS ONE* 12: e0185702. doi:10.1371/journal.pone.0185702

Obanda V, Omondi GP, Chiyo PI. 2014. The influence of body mass index, age and sex on inflammatory disease risk in semi-captive chimpanzees. *PLoS ONE* 9: e104602. doi:10.1371/journal.pone.0104602

Oriá RB, Patrick PD, Oriá MOB, Lorntz B, Thompson MR, Azevedo OGR, Lobo RNB, Pinkerton RF, Guerrant RL, Lima AAM. 2010. Apoe polymorphisms and diarrheal outcomes in Brazilian shanty town children. *Braz J Med Biol Res* 43: 249–256. doi:10.1590/S0100-879X2010007500003

Ostner J, Schülke O. 2018. Linking sociality to fitness in primates: a call for mechanisms. *Adv Study Behav* 50: 127–175. doi:10.1016/bs.asb.2017.12.001

Phillips SR, Goldberg T, Muller M, Machanda Z, Otali E, Friant S, Carag J, Langergraber K, Mitani J, Wroblewski E, et al. 2020. Faecal parasites increase with age but not reproductive effort in wild female chimpanzees. *Philos Trans R Soc Lond B Biol Sci* 375: 20190614. doi:10.1098/rstb.2019.0614

Pontzer H, Wood BM, Raichlen DA. 2018. Hunter-gatherers as models in public health. *Obes Rev* 19: 24–35. doi:10.1111/obr.12785

Radford K, Lavrencic LM, Delbaere K, Draper B, Cumming R, Daylight G, Mack HA, Chalkley S, Bennett H, Garvey G, et al. 2019. Factors associated with the high prevalence of dementia in older aboriginal Australians. *J Alzheimers Dis* 70: S75–S85. doi:10.3233/JAD-180573

Raichlen DA, Pontzer H, Harris JA, Mabulla AZP, Marlowe FW, Josh Snodgrass J, Eick G, Colette Berbesque J, Sancilio A, Wood BM. 2017. Physical activity patterns and biomarkers of cardiovascular disease risk in hunter-gatherers. *Am J Hum Biol* 29: e22919. doi:10.1002/ajhb.22919

Rawlins RG, Kessler MJ. 1986. *The Cayo Santiago macaques: history, behavior, and biology*. SUNY Press, Albany, NY.

Reuter H, Krug J, Singer P, Englert C. 2018. The African turquoise killifish *Nothobranchius furzeri* as a model for aging research. *Drug Discovery Today: Disease Models* 27: 15–22. doi:10.1016/j.ddmod.2018.12.001

Ronke C, Dannemann M, Halbwax M, Fischer A, Helmschrodt C, Brügel M, André C, Atencia R, Mugisha L, Scholz M, et al. 2015. Lineage-specific changes in biomarkers in great apes and humans. *PLoS ONE* 10: e0134548. doi:10.1371/journal.pone.0134548

Ross CN. 2019. Marmosets in aging research. In *The common marmoset in captivity and biomedical research* (ed. Marini R, et al.), pp. 355–376. Academic, Cambridge, MA.

Cite this article as *Cold Spring Harb Perspect Med* doi: 10.1101/cshperspect.a041195

Ruff CB, Junno JA, Eckardt W, Gilardi K, Mudakikwa A, McFarlin SC. 2020. Skeletal ageing in Virunga mountain gorillas. *Philos Trans R Soc Lond B Biol Sci* **375**: 20190606. doi:10.1098/rstb.2019.0606

Runcie DE, Wiedmann RT, Archie EA, Altmann J, Wray GA, Alberts SC, Tung J. 2013. Social environment influences the relationship between genotype and gene expression in wild baboons. *Philos Trans R Soc Lond B Biol Sci* **368**: 20120345. doi:10.1098/rstb.2012.0345

Sanchez-Rosado M, Snyder-Mackler N, Higham J, Brent L, Marzan-Rivera N, Pavez-Fox M, Watowich M, Sariol CA. 2021. Effects of age and social adversity on immune cell populations in a non-human primate model of human aging. *Innov Aging* **5**: 530–530. doi:10.1093/geroni/igab046.2044

Sapolsky RM. 2004. Social status and health in humans and other animals. *Annu Rev Anthropol* **33**: 393–418. doi:10.1146/annurev.anthro.33.070203.144000

Sapolsky RM. 2005. The influence of social hierarchy on primate health. *Science* **308**: 648–652. doi:10.1126/science.1106477

Sapolsky RM. 2021. Glucocorticoids, the evolution of the stress-response, and the primate predicament. *Neurobiol Stress* **14**: 100320. doi:10.1016/j.ynstr.2021.100320

Sapolsky R, Armanini M, Packan D, Tombaugh G. 1987. Stress and glucocorticoids in aging. *Endocrinol Metab Clin North Am* **16**: 965–980. doi:10.1016/S0889-8529(18)30453-5

Sayre MK, Pike IL, Raichlen DA. 2019. High levels of objectively measured physical activity across adolescence and adulthood among the pokot pastoralists of Kenya. *Am J Hum Biol* **31**: e23205. doi:10.1002/ajhb.23205

Sayre MK, Pontzer H, Alexander GE, Wood BM, Pike IL, Mabulla AZ, Raichlen DA. 2020. Ageing and physical function in East African foragers and pastoralists. *Philos Trans R Soc Lond B Biol Sci* **375**: 20190608. doi:10.1098/rstb.2019.0608

Schulman FY, Farb A, Virmani R, Montali RJ. 1995. Fibrosing cardiomyopathy in captive western lowland gorillas (*Gorilla gorilla gorilla*) in the United States: a retrospective study. *J Zoo Wildl Med* **26**: 43–51.

Seiler BM, Dick EJ Jr, Guardado-Mendoza R, VandeBerg JL, Williams JT, Mubiru JN, Hubbard GB. 2009. Spontaneous heart disease in the adult chimpanzee (*Pan troglodytes*). *J Med Primatol* **38**: 51–58. doi:10.1111/j.1600-0684.2008.00307.x

Shave RE, Lieberman DE, Drane AL, Brown MG, Batterham AM, Worthington S, Atencia R, Feltrer Y, Neary J, Weiner RB, et al. 2019. Selection of endurance capabilities and the trade-off between pressure and volume in the evolution of the human heart. *Proc Natl Acad Sci* **116**: 19905–19910. doi:10.1073/pnas.1906902116

Shively CA, Clarkson TB. 1994. Social status and coronary artery atherosclerosis in female monkeys. *Arterioscler Thromb* **14**: 721–726. doi:10.1161/01.ATV.14.5.721

Shively CA, Clarkson TB. 2009. The unique value of primate models in translational research. *Am J Primatol* **71**: 715–721. doi:10.1002/ajp.20720

Shively CA, Day SM. 2015. Social inequalities in health in nonhuman primates. *Neurobiol Stress* **1**: 156–163. doi:10.1016/j.ynstr.2014.11.005

Shively CA, Register TC, Clarkson TB. 2009. Social stress, visceral obesity, and coronary artery atherosclerosis: product of a primate adaptation. *Am J Primatol* **71**: 742–751. doi:10.1002/ajp.20706

Silk JB, Alberts SC, Altmann J. 2003. Social bonds of female baboons enhance infant survival. *Science* **302**: 1231–1234. doi:10.1126/science.1088580

Silk JB, Beehner JC, Bergman TJ, Crockford C, Engh AL, Moscovice LR, Wittig RM, Seyfarth RM, Cheney DL. 2010. Strong and consistent social bonds enhance the longevity of female baboons. *Curr Biol* **20**: 1359–1361. doi:10.1016/j.cub.2010.05.067

Simmons HA. 2016. Age-associated pathology in rhesus macaques (*Macaca mulatta*). *Vet Pathol* **53**: 399–416. doi:10.1177/0300985815620628

Snyder-Mackler N, Somel M, Tung J. 2014. Shared signatures of social stress and aging in peripheral blood mononuclear cell gene expression profiles. *Aging Cell* **13**: 954–957. doi:10.1111/acel.12239

Snyder-Mackler N, Sanz J, Kohn JN, Brinkworth JF, Morrow S, Shaver AO, Grenier JC, Pique-Regi R, Johnson ZP, Wilson ME, et al. 2016. Social status alters immune regulation and response to infection in macaques. *Science* **354**: 1041–1045. doi:10.1126/science.aah3580

Snyder-Mackler N, Sanz J, Kohn JN, Voyles T, Pique-Regi R, Wilson ME, Barreiro LB, Tung J. 2019. Social status alters chromatin accessibility and the gene regulatory response to glucocorticoid stimulation in rhesus macaques. *Proc Natl Acad Sci* **116**: 1219–1228. doi:10.1073/pnas.1811758115

Snyder-Mackler N, Burger JR, Gaydosh L, Belsky DW, Noppert GA, Campos FA, Bartolomucci A, Yang YC, Aiello AE, O'Rand A, et al. 2020. Social determinants of health and survival in humans and other animals. *Science* **368**: eaax9553. doi:10.1126/science.aax9553

Stearns SC. 1989. Trade-offs in life history evolution. *Funct Ecol* **3**: 259–268. doi:10.2307/2389364

Stearns SC. 2012. Evolutionary medicine: its scope, interest and potential. *Proc Biol Sci* **279**: 4305–4321.

Tardif SD, Mansfield KG, Ratnam R, Ross CN, Ziegler TE. 2011. The marmoset as a model of aging and age-related diseases. *ILAR J* **52**: 54–65. doi:10.1093/ilar.52.1.54

Thompson NA. 2019. Understanding the links between social ties and fitness over the life cycle in primates. *Behaviour* **156**: 859–908. doi:10.1163/1568539X-00003552

Thompson NA, Cords M. 2018. Stronger social bonds do not always predict greater longevity in a gregarious primate. *Ecol Evol* **8**: 1604–1614. doi:10.1002/ece3.3781

Thompson González NA, Otali E, Machanda ZP, Muller MN, Wrangham RW, Emery Thompson M. 2020. Urinary markers of oxidative stress respond to infection and late life in wild chimpanzees. *PLoS ONE* **15**: e0238066. doi:10.1371/journal.pone.0238066

Trumble BC, Stieglitz J, Blackwell AD, Allayee H, Beheim B, Finch CE, Gurven M, Kaplan H. 2017. Apolipoprotein E4 is associated with improved cognitive function in Amazonian forager-horticulturalists with a high parasite burden. *FASEB J* **31**: 1508–1515. doi:10.1096/fj.201601084R

Tung J, Barreiro LB, Johnson ZP, Hansen KD, Michopoulos V, Toufexis D, Michelini K, Wilson ME, Gilad Y. 2012. Social environment is associated with gene regulatory variation in the rhesus macaque immune system. *Proc Natl Acad Sci* **109:** 6490–6495. doi:10.1073/pnas.1202 734109

Uchino BN. 2009. Understanding the links between social support and physical health: a life-span perspective with emphasis on the separability of perceived and received support. *Perspect Psychol Sci* **4:** 236–255. doi:10.1111/j .1745-6924.2009.01122.x

Varki N, Anderson D, Herndon JG, Pham T, Gregg CJ, Cheriyan M, Murphy J, Strobert E, Fritz J, Else JG, et al. 2009. Heart disease is common in humans and chimpanzees, but is caused by different pathological processes. *Evol Appl* **2:** 101–112. doi:10.1111/j.1752-4571.2008 .00064.x

Vasunilashorn S, Crimmins EM, Kim JK, Winking J, Gurven M, Kaplan H, Finch CE. 2010. Blood lipids, infection, and inflammatory markers in the Tsimane of Bolivia. *Am J Hum Biol* **22:** 731–740. doi:10.1002/ajhb.21074

Vasunilashorn S, Finch C, Crimmins EM, Vikman SA, Stielitz J, Gurven M, Kaplan HS, Allayee H. 2011. Inflammatory gene variants in the Tsimane, an indigenous Bolivian population with a high infectious load. *Biodemography Soc Biol* **57:** 33–52. doi:10.1080/19485565.2011.564475

Videan EN, Fritz J, Murphy J. 2008. Effects of aging on hematology and serum clinical chemistry in chimpanzees (*Pan troglodytes*). *Am J Primatol* **70:** 327–338. doi:10 .1002/ajp.20494

Videan EN, Heward CB, Chowdhury K, Plummer J, Su Y, Cutler RG. 2009. Comparison of biomarkers of oxidative stress and cardiovascular disease in humans and chimpanzees. *Comp Med* **59:** 287–296.

Wallace IJ, Worthington S, Felson DT, Jurmain RD, Wren KT, Maijanen H, Woods RJ, Lieberman DE. 2017. Knee osteoarthritis has doubled in prevalence since the mid-20th century. *Proc Natl Acad Sci* **114:** 9332–9336. doi:10 .1073/pnas.1703856114

Wallace IJ, Riew GJ, Landau R, Bendele AM, Holowka NB, Hedrick TL, Konow N, Brooks DJ, Lieberman DE. 2022. Experimental evidence that physical activity inhibits osteoarthritis: implications for inferring activity patterns from osteoarthritis in archeological human skeletons. *Am J Biol Anthropol* **177:** 223–231. doi:10.1002/ajpa .24429

Warren LA, Shi Q, Young K, Borenstein A, Martiniuk A. 2015. Prevalence and incidence of dementia among indigenous populations: a systematic review. *Int Psychoger* **27:** 1959–1970. doi:10.1017/S1041610215000861

Williams GC. 1957. Pleiotropy, natural selection and the evolution of senescence. *Evolution* **11:** 398–411. doi:10 .1111/j.1558-5646.1957.tb02911.x

Williams GC. 1966. Natural selection, the costs of reproduction, and a refinement of lack's principle. *Am Nat* **100:** 687–690. doi:10.1086/282461

Wrycza TF, Missov TI, Baudisch A. 2015. Quantifying the shape of aging. *PLoS ONE* **10:** e0119163. doi:10.1371/ journal.pone.0119163

Zuo L, Prather ER, Stetskiv M, Garrison DE, Meade JR, Peace TI, Zhou T. 2019. Inflammaging and oxidative stress in human diseases: from molecular mechanisms to novel treatments. *Int J Mol Sci* **20:** 4472. doi:10.3390/ijms 20184472

Aging and Inflammation

Amit Singh,[1,6] Shepherd H. Schurman,[2,6] Arsun Bektas,[3] Mary Kaileh,[1] Roshni Roy,[1,5] David M. Wilson III,[4] Ranjan Sen,[1] and Luigi Ferrucci[3]

[1]Laboratory of Molecular Biology and Immunology, National Institute on Aging, Baltimore, Maryland 21224, USA

[2]Clinical Research Unit, National Institute on Aging, Baltimore, Maryland 21224, USA

[3]Translational Gerontology Branch, National Institute on Aging, Baltimore, Maryland 21224, USA

[4]Biomedical Research Institute, Hasselt University, Diepenbeek 3500, Belgium

Correspondence: ferruccilu@grc.nia.nih.gov

Aging can be conceptualized as the progressive disequilibrium between stochastic damage accumulation and resilience mechanisms that continuously repair that damage, which eventually cause the development of chronic disease, frailty, and death. The immune system is at the forefront of these resilience mechanisms. Indeed, aging is associated with persistent activation of the immune system, witnessed by a high circulating level of inflammatory markers and activation of immune cells in the circulation and in tissue, a condition called "inflammaging." Like aging, inflammaging is associated with increased risk of many age-related pathologies and disabilities, as well as frailty and death. Herein we discuss recent advances in the understanding of the mechanisms leading to inflammaging and the intrinsic dysregulation of the immune function that occurs with aging. We focus on the underlying mechanisms of chronic inflammation, in particular the role of NF-κB and recent studies targeting proinflammatory mediators. We further explore the dysregulation of the immune response with age and immunosenescence as an important mechanistic immune response to acute stressors. We examine the role of the gastrointestinal microbiome, age-related dysbiosis, and the integrated stress response in modulating the inflammatory "response" to damage accumulation and stress. We conclude by focusing on the seminal question of whether reducing inflammation is useful and the results of related clinical trials. In summary, we propose that inflammation may be viewed both as a clinical biomarker of the failure of resilience mechanisms and as a causal factor in the rising burden of disease and disabilities with aging. The fact that inflammation can be reduced through nonpharmacological interventions such as diet and exercise suggests that a life course approach based on education may be a successful strategy to increase the health span with few adverse consequences.

[5]Present address: Department of Microbiology and Immunology, Emory University School of Medicine, Atlanta, Georgia 30322, USA.

[6]These authors contributed equally to this work.

AGING AND THE RISE OF INFLAMMATION

Aging—the complex array of phenotypic and functional manifestations that eventually lead to the death of the individual—occurs in all living species with only a few rare exceptions. Much has been written about the biological significance of aging and why individual mortality exists, with many theories coming back to the idea that, for the good of the population, there is an evolutionary advantage to "eliminate" aged organisms, particularly when past reproductive prime, because they consume significant resources and present a burden on the community (Cleveland and Jacobs 1999). At the beginning of life, a magnificent, extremely robust, and redundant program encoded by the genome aims to create an organism that is fully functional and in perfect homeostatic equilibrium within its environment. This status of perfect molecular order though cannot escape the second law of thermodynamics. To counteract the trend toward a higher level of entropy and facilitate a longer life span, a cadre of compensatory mechanisms have evolved that continuously surveil the integrity and functionality of molecules, organelles, cells, tissues, and organs, repairing or recycling and replacing severely damaged structures when needed (Alzeer 2022). These mechanisms are initially so effective that the progression of entropy is almost imperceptible. However, over time, the efficiency of these resilience mechanisms declines because their core molecular components become damaged through entropy, and because cumulative internal and external stressors impose an increasing burden beyond the level at which these systems can fully cope. Intrinsic to this model, as organisms age, resilience mechanisms shift from intermittent activation (e.g., during acute infection) to a chronic state of activation that is more typical of chronic disease. The immune system is a prototypical example of a resilience system.

An optimally functioning immune system protects against danger signals. Easily recognizable environmental danger signals include infection by pathogenic viruses or bacteria. The immune system is also a surveillance mechanism that maintains tissue homeostasis by repairing damage induced by extrinsic (UV radiation, oxygen deprivation, etc.) and intrinsic (protein aggregates, mitochondrial respiration, uric acid crystals, etc.) sources. The cardinal components of immunity are the inherent mechanisms that accurately tune the response to the need. Excessive and uncontrolled immunity leads to autoimmunity and hyperinflammatory syndromes (such as rheumatoid arthritis, intestinal bowel disease, and acute phase responses), whereas suboptimal responses result in immune deficiencies. Because the immune system is at the heart of all resilience mechanisms, it is not surprising that activation of the immune system, as indicated by high circulating levels of inflammatory markers and a state of active immune responses in multiple tissues, has been considered as one of the "pillars" of aging, now known as "inflammaging" (Ferrucci and Fabbri 2018).

In this article, after introducing the evidence that supports the concept of inflammaging, we explore some of the mechanisms that may be at the root of this chronic inflammatory state. Figure 1 provides a comprehensive view of the many causes and consequences of inflammaging proposed in the literature. However, rather than going through this long list, we will limit our discussion to a few topics that are receiving considerable attention at present. We describe instances where inflammation is mostly interpreted as a "response" to damage accumulation or stress, focusing on the role of the microbiome and the integrated stress response (ISR). We approach the literature on inflammaging from a mechanistic perspective. Next, we explore the existing evidence that inflammaging is driven by age-related intrinsic dysregulation. Finally, we review the literature on the available evidence that interventions aimed at reducing inflammation prevent or slow down the adverse phenotypic and functional effects of aging.

INFLAMMAGING AND UNDERLYING MECHANISMS

Several articles have described the characteristics of inflammaging, initially from the prospective of circulating biomarkers and more recently as the infiltration and activation of immune cells in

Cite this article as *Cold Spring Harb Perspect Med* doi: 10.1101/cshperspect.a041197

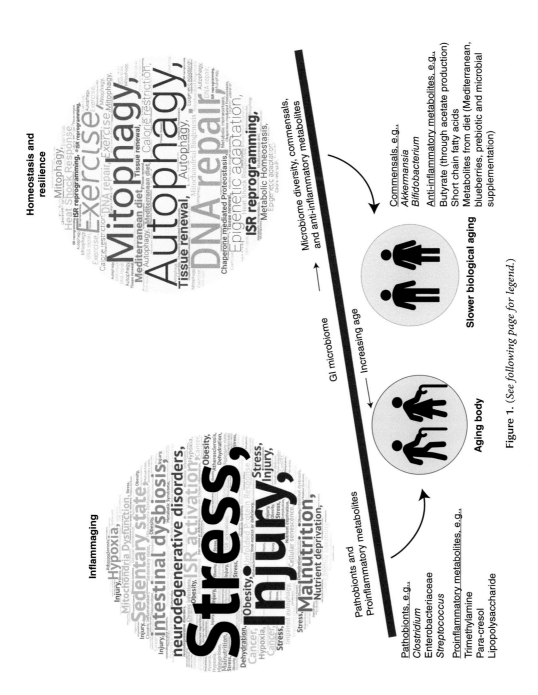

Homeostasis and resilience

Mitophagy, Autophagy, DNA repair

Exercise, Mediterranean diet, Tissue renewal, Calorie restriction, ISR reprogramming,

Microbiome diversity, commensals, and anti-inflammatory metabolites

GI microbiome

Increasing age

Slower biological aging

Commensals, e.g.,
Akkermansia
Bifidobacterium

Anti-inflammatory metabolites, e.g.,
Butyrate (through acetate production)
Short chain fatty acids
Metabolites from diet (Mediterranean, blueberries, prebiotic and microbial supplementation)

Inflammaging

Stress, Injury,

neurodegenerative disorders, intestinal dysbiosis, Sedentary state, ISR activation, Malnutrition, Nutrient deprivation, Hypoxia, Mitochondria Dysfunction, Obesity, Atherosclerosis, Dehydration, Cancer, Cellular senescence

Pathobionts and Proinflammatory metabolites

Aging body

Pathobionts, e.g.,
Clostridium
Enterobacteriaceae
Streptococcus

Proinflammatory metabolites, e.g.,
Trimethylamine
Para-cresol
Lipopolysaccharide

Figure 1. (*See following page for legend.*)

multiple tissues. Studies have found that circulating levels of interleukin 6 (IL)-6, tumor necrosis factor (TNF)-α, IL-1, and other proinflammatory markers increase with aging, even in individuals who are deemed to be extremely healthy (Furman et al. 2019). In addition, high levels of inflammatory markers have been associated with, and in some cases predictive of, a large variety of age-related adverse health outcomes or conditions, including major chronic diseases (e.g., diabetes, atherosclerosis, dementia), viral infections (COVID-19 and flu), disability, frailty, nursing home admission, and death. Although a mechanistic understanding of the connection between inflammaging and adverse outcomes is still lacking, many authors have hypothesized that these pathologies are directly caused by the endocrine and metabolic effects of inflammatory mediators. For example, the shift toward catabolism and insulin resistance induced by inflammation may play a role in sarcopenia and neurodegenerative diseases. Nevertheless, other hypotheses should be considered.

Chronic inflammation that does not resolve, such as seen in inflammaging, could be a normal response to a persistent proinflammatory stimulus and most certainly involves a number of contributory mechanisms. For instance, aging is associated with changes in the gut microbiome due to the leakage of pathogen-associated molecular patterns (PAMPs), which are recognized by pattern-recognition receptors (PRRs) and trigger innate immunity (Conway and Duggal 2021). Moreover, there is evidence that mitochondrial function declines with aging, and it has been recently recognized that mitochondrial stress can trigger an inflammatory response through the release of oxidated mitochondrial DNA (mtDNA) and oxidated cardiolipin (also called damage-associated molecular patterns [DAMPs]), triggering the NLRP3 inflammasome, NF-κB, and the cGAS-STING pathway (Walker et al. 2022). Of note, dysfunctional mitochondria are physiologically removed by mitophagy, and the persistence of damaged mitochondria with age is at least in part explained by defective mitophagy (Kaushik et al. 2021). Finally, aging is associated with the accumulation of senescent cells that assume a senescent-associated inflammatory phenotype (SASP) and produce a large variety of bioactive molecules, including a collection of cytokines and chemokines (Walker et al. 2022). As the integrity and functionality of the immune system itself is progressively challenged by damage accumulation, an important question is whether a primary defect in the immune system contributes to the rise of inflammaging. Despite the strong rationale, the evidence for this hypothesis is still weak and limited to animal models.

Figure 1. Inflammaging, homeostasis, and resilience mechanisms. The rate of aging and progressive systemic entropy can be viewed as a continuing dynamic equilibrium between the forces of inflammaging and its consequences and counteractive mechanisms to maintain homeostasis. Affecting these opposing influences on the human body and the rate of biological aging are members of the gastrointestinal (GI) microbiome, including the positive effects of commensals and anti-inflammatory metabolites on the one hand and pathobionts and proinflammatory metabolites on the other. Many causes of inflammaging have been proposed (large blue circle) and, to name a few, include stress, injury, malnutrition, a sedentary state, intestinal dysbiosis, integrated stress response (ISR) activation, hypoxia, mitochondrial dysfunction, obesity, metabolic syndrome, chronic inflammation, the unfolded protein response, nutrient deprivation, cellular senescence, iron excess or deficiency, impaired autophagy, genomic instability, dysregulated nutrient sensing, protein precipitation, chronic infections, and dehydration. The possible consequences of inflammaging are numerous and are hypothesized to lead to age-related disorders including neurodegenerative disease, cancer, atherosclerosis, and impaired tissue renewal. Countering the effects of inflammaging are many proposed mechanisms and resilience strategies that maintain homeostasis (large pink circle) and include autophagy, mitophagy, DNA repair, exercise, epigenetic adaptation, ISR reprogramming, the heat shock response, diets such as the Mediterranean diet, tissue renewal, calorie restriction, chaperone-mediated proteostasis, mitochondrial bioenergetics, and metabolic homeostasis. Inflammaging, pathobionts, and proinflammatory metabolites will favor increasing age and an aging body (small blue circle), whereas homeostasis and resilience mechanisms and microbiome diversity, commensals, and anti-inflammatory metabolites may favor slower biological aging (small pink circle).

 Cite this article as *Cold Spring Harb Perspect Med* doi: 10.1101/cshperspect.a041197

The above age-related biological phenomena are far from being an exhaustive list of the persistent outcomes that likely drive inflammaging (see Fig. 1) yet highlight the important role of chronic inflammation in aging. The described outcomes also raise two opposite and complex questions of (1) whether inflammaging is contributing to pathology, or (2) whether inflammaging is a resilience mechanism itself and its absence would lead to an even more severe accumulation of damage. Assuming the latter, chronic inflammation would signify the presence of persistent, unresolved pathology and, thus, it is not surprising that inflammaging is associated with adverse health outcomes. From a more general prospective, the emergence of chronic inflammation with aging may designate the time when resilience mechanisms no longer match the rise in entropy and damage accumulation, suggesting that in chronic disease and frailty, inflammaging may be both a biomarker of resilience exhaustion and a causal factor.

One of the most popular theories about the origin of inflammaging is that the up-regulation of inflammation is linked to the effect of aging on endocrine regulation and metabolism. Supporting this concept are observations that chronic inflammation is significantly more prevalent and severe in older individuals with visceral obesity, metabolic syndrome, type 2 diabetes, cardiovascular disease, and neurodegenerative disorders (Furman et al. 2019; Bektas et al. 2020). These conditions are caused by a combination of genetic predisposition and lifestyle or environmental stressors, such as pollution, smoking, sedentary behavior, and an unhealthy diet, as well as social and psychological stress, just to name a few (Bektas et al. 2020). Mechanistically, exogenous compounds, such as bacteria or viral fragments and certain microbiota elements, act as PAMPs, whereas endogenous processes generate DAMPs. PAMPs and DAMPs interact with sensors present on the cell surface or in the cytoplasm that in combination trigger inflammatory responses and proinflammatory cytokine secretion, which are hallmarks of inflammaging (Franceschi et al. 2018). Indeed, studies have underlined the role of immunobiography (the cumulative history of exposure to certain microorganisms (e.g., HIV and CMV) or antigens in causing chronic inflammation via the modulation of inflammatory responses (Franceschi et al. 2017, 2018; Ferrucci and Fabbri 2018; Fulop et al. 2018).

INFLAMMAGING AS A CAUSE OF PATHOLOGY AND ACCELERATED AGING

The prediction of the inflammaging hypothesis would be that suppression of age-associated chronic inflammation will coordinately attenuate multiple aging phenotypes and improve overall health and longevity. The immense implications for extending human health span via this strategy motivates rigorous tests of the hypothesis to identify nodes that can be therapeutically manipulated to meet this goal. Causal connections between two observables can be established by either activating or down-regulating one and assessing the effects on the other. In the case of inflammaging, this means (1) inducing chronic inflammation and assaying the development of aging phenotypes, or (2) attenuating chronic inflammation and exploring the health consequences. Major hurdles in experimentally testing this are (1) molecular characteristics (known as markers) of chronic inflammation, especially those instrumental in causing aging phenotypes, remain unclear, and (2) inducing inflammation for a long period of time is probably harmful. Thus, challenges to the inflammaging hypothesis usually entail studying the effects of increasing inflammation in animal models and reducing inflammation in both animal and human experiments. In this section, we highlight recent studies that exemplify both approaches.

Inducing Inflammation

One consistent theme in inflammation is the essential role of the transcription factor NF-κB (Taniguchi and Karin 2018). NF-κB, a heterodimer comprised of p50 and p65 components, is a well-known universal stress sensor, which when activated by different types of stimuli upregulates the transcription of inflammatory cytokines, chemokines, and adhesion molecules, thereby causing inflammation. Additionally,

NF-κB induces the expression of transcripts that encode for proteins that regulate cell proliferation, apoptosis, morphogenesis, and differentiation. Moreover, NF-κB is activated in response to DNA damage (via ATM/ATR activation), mitochondrial dysfunction (via generation of reactive oxygen species) or proinflammatory cytokines in the milieu. Whether we consider the proinflammatory cytokines associated with human aging (such as IL-1, IL-6 or TNF-α) or the proinflammatory components of the SASP (widely believed to be a major cause of inflammaging), there is the unifying theme that many of the genes involved in these outcomes are regulated by NF-κB. Thus, it is not surprising that NF-κB is implicated in inflammaging and many of the hallmarks of aging (Songkiatisak et al. 2022). However, it is important to note that NF-κB responses are inducer- and cell-specific and have a strong kinetic dimension (Sen and Smale 2010), which makes it difficult to formulate a simple model for its contribution to age-associated chronic inflammation. Two kinds of observations provide causal connections between NF-κB and aging.

First, mice that lack NFKB1, the p50 component of NF-κB, manifest several characteristics of premature aging (Jurk et al. 2014). These include high systemic IL-6 levels and immune cell infiltration in the liver. Regeneration capacity of both liver and gut is also significantly reduced, and telomere-dysfunctional senescent cells accumulate in various tissues. Furthermore, the frequency of senescent cells in the liver or intestinal crypts correlates with mean and maximum life span of *NFKB1* knockout animals. Although accelerated aging in mice that lack an NF-κB component may appear counter to the hypothesis (i.e., that NF-κB supports a major protective response), one plausible explanation is that p50 homodimers have been previously suggested to dampen NF-κB-dependent responses. That is, p50 homodimers act as functional repressors of NF-κB-dependent gene expression in some circumstances (Cartwright et al. 2018). Thus, the absence of p50 may accentuate NF-κB activity resulting in chronic inflammation. A specific role for inflammation in the aging phenotypes of NFKB1-deficient mice is supported by the observation that treatment with the nonsteroidal anti-inflammatory ibuprofen ameliorates cognitive defects in these animals (Fielder et al. 2020). Interestingly, rapamycin treatment also improved aging phenotypes in NFKB1-deficient mice (Correia-Melo et al. 2019). Because low-dose rapamycin has been hailed as one of the most robust anti-aging treatments (Selvarani et al. 2021), the positive effects in NFKB1-deficient mice supports the idea that aging phenotypes in this model recapitulate features of normal aging.

Second, down-modulation of NF-κB activity via genetic deletion of one allele of RelA, the p65 component of NF-κB, has been shown to overcome aging in mouse models (Tilstra et al. 2012; García-García et al. 2021). These observations were extended recently with the use of a selective inhibitor of NF-κB activation. Zhang et al. (2021) showed that treatment of the $Ercc1^{-/\Delta}$ mouse model of accelerated aging (see more below) with SR12343, an agent that blocks IKK/NF-κB activation by disrupting the association between IKKβ and NEMO, two key NF-κB signaling proteins, reduced aging phenotypes such as elevated levels of senescent cells in tissues, expression of p16, and muscle pathologies. Concurrently, NF-κB activation, as measured by phosphorylation of RelA and expression of NF-κB target genes (e.g., *Tnfa*, *Cox2*, and *Mcp1*), was reduced following SR12343 administration. Thus, targeting NF-κB activation has therapeutic potential in ameliorating certain aging phenotypes. However, a caveat that must be considered is that NF-κB activation serves important physiological functions in most tissues via control of cell adhesion, cell viability, and cell cycle, among many others. The challenge will therefore be to find the "sweet spot" whereby effects against persistent activation that lead to sustained expression of inflammatory markers during aging are maximized, while minimally affecting acute activation in response to environmental or pathogenic stress.

Attenuating Chronic Inflammation

The geroscience hypothesis posits that manipulating underlying causes of aging has the potential to simultaneously alleviate multiple physiological characteristics of aging. As discussed, inflammaging has emerged as one of the most robust "underlying causes" of the phenotypes of aging. Several ongoing clinical trials have therefore explored the use of rapamycin and metformin, two compounds with immunosuppressive activity, to alleviate inflammaging and, thereby, age-associated comorbidities. The molecular targets and benefits of these compounds have been previously discussed and will not be further considered here (Selvarani et al. 2021). Instead, we will focus on recent studies in which select proinflammatory mediators were targeted, because specific mediators of inflammaging are less likely to have broad spectrum effects. Selective intervention may prove to be more effective, with fewer side effects, and more in line with the coming era of individualized medicine. Moreover, because inflammaging is a classic example of pleiotropic antagonism, long-term suppression of inflammatory responses may have detrimental consequences that are yet to be fully defined, again pointing to the need for more directed therapies beyond generalized anti-inflammatory treatments.

IL-6 and TNF-α are frequently associated with inflammaging, and biologics against these cytokines have proven to be effective in situations of acute inflammation, such as in psoriatic arthritis (using anti-IL-6 receptor) and rheumatoid arthritis (using therapies directed against TNF-α). Several recent examples indicate that interfering with TNF-α function can also overcome certain aging phenotypes. Davison-Castillo et al. (2019) showed that skewed hematopoiesis during aging results in the generation of hyperactive platelets that may contribute to increased thrombotic risk. Defective platelet generation in old mice was reduced by depleting TNF-α with anti-TNF antibodies, reducing predisposition to thrombosis. Perturbations of hematopoietic stem cells (HSCs) also underlies myeloid-biased hematopoiesis and an increased incidence of myeloid malignancies with age (Pang et al. 2017). This adverse phenotype was partially reversed by suppressing TNF-α signaling (Davizon-Castillo et al. 2019). At the functional level, in a mouse model of pneumococcal infection, the susceptibility of old mice to bacterial colonization was circumvented by pharmacological reduction of

TNF-α or removal of a subset of proinflammatory monocytes (Puchta et al. 2016). Finally, a synthetic derivative of myosmine that suppresses TNF-α production ameliorated several phenotypes in aging mice, including muscle loss and frailty (Sabini et al. 2023). In these examples, neutralizing one inflammatory cytokine appears to have substantial beneficial effects. This may be because, unlike many other age-associated proinflammatory markers, TNF-α is an activator of NF-κB. Thus, its specific inhibition has the potential to mitigate proinflammatory NF-κB-dependent gene expression. One such NF-κB target is the *IL6* gene. Neutralizing IL-6/IL-6R signaling has recently been shown to overcome accelerated aging features in a mouse model of Hutchinson–Gilford progeria syndrome (Squarzoni et al. 2021). IL-6 has also been implicated in HSC dysfunction with age via the micro-RNA, miR146a (Grants et al. 2020). Unlike TNF-α, however, IL-6 cannot perpetuate NF-κB activity, resulting in more restricted outcomes.

A somewhat new player in the inflammaging cytokine milieu is IL-17, which is associated with inflammatory immune diseases such as rheumatoid arthritis, psoriasis, and multiple sclerosis (Mills 2023). Solá et al. (2023) found that IL-17 producing innate lymphoid cells and a subset of T cells increase with age in mouse skin and that neutralizing IL-17 delayed many symptoms of skin aging. Increased IL-17 production was also observed in human CD4$^+$ T cells from older compared to younger individuals. Expression of this inflammatory cytokine was connected to defective autophagy and disrupted the redox balance in old CD4$^+$ T cells, outcomes that were reversed by metformin treatment ex vivo (Bharath et al. 2020). It is possible that IL-17 has not been featured prominently as an inflammaging cytokine so far, because its production and function may be localized in specific tissue environments.

Overall, a review of this literature suggests that the chronic proinflammatory state observed in many older persons is causally linked with age-associated chronic disease and other aging phenotypes and that inflammation is an important target for interventions aimed at improving health span and longevity.

INFLAMMAGING AND IMMUNOSENESCENCE

Dysregulation of immune responses during aging accentuates the deleterious rather than the protective immune responses, a phenomenon termed immunosenescence (Walford 1969; Franceschi et al. 2000). The varied and complex phenotypes associated with immunosenescence, presumably due to the involvement of multiple cell types and their interactions with various tissues (Fig. 2), is distinct from the phenomenon of cellular senescence (Sharma 2021; Lee et al. 2022). Because both inflammaging and immunity have essential inflammatory components, it is sometimes considered paradoxical that functional immunity declines with age as chronic low-grade inflammation increases. The key distinction is that optimal immunity requires regulated control of inflammation, both increased and decreased depending on need, a balance that is upset during aging. Accordingly, elderly people are more susceptible to infectious diseases, more prone to autoimmune diseases and cancer, and less responsive to vaccination (Goronzy and Weyand 2012, 2013). These facts, as well as the negative consequences of rampant and uncontrolled inflammation, have been highlighted during the COVID-19 pandemic (Demaret et al. 2021; Levin et al. 2021).

Immunity is broadly subclassified into innate or adaptive responses. Innate immunity is mediated by many different cell types, including monocytes/macrophages, granulocytes, natural killer (NK) cells, and innate lymphoid cells. These cells are first responders to danger signals and eliminate pathogens by mechanisms such as phagocytosis, NETosis, and the production of toxic reactive oxygen species (Ogawa et al. 2008; Simell et al. 2011; Brubaker et al. 2013; Hazeldine et al. 2014). They are also classic inflammatory cells in that they produce chemokines and cytokines that result in systemic inflammation. Although slower than innate responses, adaptive immunity features the generation of memory in B and T lymphocytes and natural killer T (NKT) cells. These so-called memory cells carry receptors that are selected for during an immune response to target and destroy specific pathogens. Adaptive immune memory permits more rapid and effective responses to reinfection with the same (or closely related) pathogens and is the basis of all vaccinations. CD4$^+$ T cells are required to generate optimal B-cell responses and, along with NKT cells, produce inflammatory cytokines, such as TNF-α, IFN-γ, and IL-17, which have been implicated in rheumatoid arthritis and psoriasis (Chemin et al. 2019; Povoleri et al. 2020; Nussbaum et al. 2021; Hu et al. 2022). Finally, CD8$^+$ T cells kill cells that have been infected with intracellular pathogens such as viruses. Recently a form of memory has been identified in innate cells as well and is referred to as trained immunity (Netea et al. 2011; Brueggeman et al. 2022). This form of memory is relatively short-lived and not pathogen specific.

Virtually all aspects of immunity are affected with age (reviewed recently and comprehensively in Goronzy and Weyand 2013; Nikolich-Žugich 2018; Nikolich-Zugich et al. 2020; Santoro et al. 2021; Shive and Pandiyan 2022; Teissier et al. 2022; Fulop et al. 2023). Key new developments are summarized in Table 1. The complexities of age-associated immunosenescence can be divided into three elements.

First, immune cell populations change with age. For adaptive immune cells, this change entails a decreased proportion of naïve (antigen inexperienced) cells and an increased proportion of memory cells (resulting from prior infections and vaccinations) in both B and T lymphocyte compartments (Listì et al. 2006; Britanova et al. 2014). The impact of trained immunity on age-associated immune dysregulation remains to be determined. Additionally, the aging immune system features the emergence of cells that are barely detectable in early life. Prominent among such cells are the exhausted T cells, marked by the absence of the cell-surface marker CD28. Exhausted T cells do not participate in effective immune responses and may constitute one major cause of reduced immunity with age (Boucher et al. 1998; Weng et al. 2009). These cells exhibit features of classic cellular senescence and may, thus, contribute to inflammaging via proinflammatory cytokine and chemokine expression (Lee and Lee 2016; Coleman et al. 2021). Moreover, recent single-cell RNA sequencing studies identified aging-related increased proportions of cy-

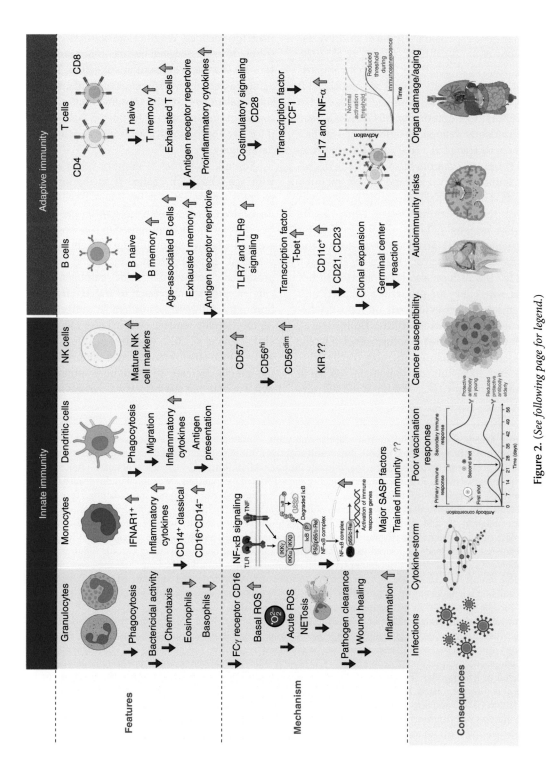

Figure 2. (*See following page for legend.*)

totoxic and regulatory subsets of CD4$^+$ T cells with marked pro- and anti-inflammatory patterns of gene expression (Elyahu et al. 2019; Hashimoto et al. 2019; Cano-Gamez et al. 2020; Mogilenko et al. 2022). In the B-cell compartment, a subset of cells, named age-associated B cells (ABCs), increases with age in mice (Hao et al. 2011; Cortegano et al. 2017). ABCs were independently defined by different cell-surface markers by Hao et al. (2011) and Rubtsov et al. (2011) and are commonly associated with microbial immune responses and B-cell memory (Chang et al. 2017; Knox et al. 2017). These cells express the transcription factor T-bet, require Toll-like receptor (TLR)7 and 9 signaling for their generation (Naradikian et al. 2016), and are metabolically active (Frasca et al. 2021). CD11c$^+$ B cells have also been reported in humans, where they are primarily associated with autoimmune diseases like systemic lupus erythematosus and rheumatoid arthritis (Rubtsov et al. 2011; Wang et al. 2018). Another subset of B cells in old mice are exhausted memory B cells (Ehrhardt et al. 2008; Rubtsova et al. 2015). ABCs and exhausted memory B cells share some cell-surface characteristics, such as low levels of CD21 and CD23 markers, but further relationships remain to be defined. Whether and how ABCs contribute to age-associated decline in humoral responses is an active area of investigation. Thus, aging is associated with the emergence of new cell subpopulations that alter immune homeostasis toward proinflammatory phenotypes that can reduce effective immunity while exaggerating inflammaging.

Second, properties of immune cells change with age. One such change is in the antigen receptor repertoires of naive B and T cells. Reduced diversity of antigen recognition specificities with age has been proposed to contribute to reduced adaptive immunity during aging (Gibson et al. 2009; Tabibian-Keissar et al. 2016), presumably because the "right" pathogen-specific receptor is not present to trigger effective immunity. However, considerable antigen receptor diversity remains even in older individuals (Verma et al. 2012; Joseph et al. 2022), suggesting that other features must contribute to the overall decrease in immune responses as well. For example, age-associated changes in cel-

Figure 2. Effects of aging on innate and adaptive immunity—"multiple shades of immunosenescence." Immunosenescence with age is rooted in both innate and adaptive arms of immunity and its extent dictates the health status of a host. Immunosenescence in major innate immune cells is featured by either loss of normal function or by hyperresponsiveness. Reduction in functionality and associated mechanisms are denoted by downward facing red arrows, whereas up-regulated features are indicated by upward green arrows. Contradicting reports are represented by gradient-filled arrows, whereas still not reported events have "?" symbols. Innate immune cells reduce phagocytotic and chemotactic properties, which can be mediated by reduction in expression of Fcγ receptors or other chemokine receptors, respectively. In granulocytes, reactive oxygen species (ROS) levels are dysregulated, which leads to delayed pathogen clearance and wound healing, fostering chronic inflammation. Monocytes having interferon α-receptor1 (IFNAR1) are markedly increased in the lungs, whereas, systemically, classical monocytes (which are more responsive to lipopolysaccharide [LPS]) are reduced. NF-κB signaling dysregulation is a major culprit in age-related monocyte dysregulation (see text for p50 knockout studies). These cells further participate in generating major senescent-associated inflammatory phenotype (SASP) factors. Meanwhile, the emerging concept of "trained immunity" has not yet been linked with immunosenescence or aging. Adaptive immunity is globally characterized by a reduction in naive lymphocytes and up-regulation of memory and exhausted cells. These, in part, can be explained by selective Toll-like receptor (TLR) signaling in B cells and reduced expression of costimulatory CD28 on T cells. The antigen receptor repertoire is significantly hindered in lymphocytes. Transcription factor T-bet in B cells are overexpressed, whereas the T-cell factor 1 (TCF1) is down-regulated, leading to a loss in their optimal functionality. The inflammatory environment of interleukin (IL)-17 and tumor necrosis factor (TNF)-α reduces the activation threshold of T cells and leads them to be unnecessarily hyperactive with age, which can create an autoimmunity-like situation. Ultimately, interplay of these immunosenescence properties make the host susceptible to infections, cytokine-storm (after uncontrolled infections), poor outcome of vaccinations in the elderly, and increased susceptibility toward cancers and autoimmunity. Furthermore, immunosenescence can cause organ damage and accelerate aging of various organs. (Figure created using BioRender.com.)

 Cite this article as *Cold Spring Harb Perspect Med* doi: 10.1101/cshperspect.a041197

Table 1. Age-associated immunosenescence features in main immune cell populations

Cell type	Effects of immunosenescence/effects with age	References
Adaptive immune cells		
B cells	Loss of naive IgD$^+$ B cells	Listi et al. 2006; Pritz et al. 2015; Cortegano et al. 2017
	Decrease in IgM and IgG increases with age mostly in men	
	Significant IgD$^-$ memory B-cell increase	
	Lack of clonotypic immune response	
	Higher proportion of memory B cells in PBMC than bone marrow (BM)	
	BM has fewer plasma cells in old age	
	Loss of marginal zone B lymphocytes	
	An enhancement of a CD19$^+$CD45R^{lo} innate-like B-cell population (B1REL) and the so-called aged B-cell compartment (ABC, D45R$^+$CD21^{lo}CD23^{lo}CD5$^-$CD11b$^-$) in aged senescence-accelerated (SAMP8) mice but not in aged senescence-resistant (SAMR1) mice	
T cells	Decline in proportion of CD28$^+$ T cells	Boucher et al. 1998; Sakata-Kaneko et al. 2000; Britanova et al. 2014; Elyahu et al. 2019; Pereira et al. 2020; Rodriguez et al. 2021; Yang et al. 2021
	Age-related diminution of T-cell responsiveness to mitogenic signals	
	T-cell receptor (TCR)-β diversity decrease	
	Decrease in naive and increase in memory cells with senescent phenotype	
	Increased CD57$^+$ and KLRG1$^+$ (senescent markers) in terminally differentiated memory T cells	
	The sestrin-driven senescence of CD8$^+$ T cells has recently been reported to lead to loss of TCR	
	Expression together with the acquisition of natural killer (NK) features	
	Increase of proinflammatory cytokines	
	Decrease in telomere length	
	Greater type I interferon (IFN), interleukin (IL)-2, but less IL-4	
	Gene-expression profile of T cells reveal up-regulation of immunosuppressive markers and immune checkpoints; aged CD4 memory T cells exhibited proapoptotic gene signatures, aged CD8 memory T cells expressed antiapoptotic genes	
	Microenvironment in which CD4$^+$ T cells develop in older individuals may cause production of more cells committed to Th1	
	Accumulation of activated Tregs with anti-inflammatory features in mice; proinflammatory phenotype in cytotoxic CD4 cells in mice	

Continued

Table 1. *Continued*

Innate immune cells

Cell type	Effects of immunosenescence/effects with age	References
Monocyte	Alterations of monocyte NF-κB p65/RelA signaling in a cohort of older medical patients, age-matched controls, and healthy young adults	Tavenier et al. 2020; D'Souza et al. 2021
	Novel type-1 IFN signaling-dependent monocyte subset (MO-IFN) that up-regulated IFNAR1 expression identified in the aged lung	
	Higher inflammatory markers	
	Reduced pNF-κB induction in response to lipopolysaccharide (LPS) and tumor necrosis factor α (TNF-α)	
Granulocytes/ neutrophils	Reduced phagocytic activity due to decreased surface expression of FCγ receptor CD16	Wenisch et al. 2000; Ogawa et al. 2008; Simell et al. 2011; Brubaker et al. 2013; Hazeldine et al. 2014; Sauce et al. 2017; Teissier et al. 2022
	Opsonic activities to antibodies against pneumococci impaired	
	Significant reduction in the intracellular reactive oxygen species (ROS) production after stimulation with *Staphylococcus aureus*	
	Acute ROS production decreases but higher basal ROS levels leading to inflammaging	
	Neutrophil bactericidal activity impaired with age	
	Reduced neutrophil phagocytosis and chemotaxis with age	
	NETosis decline	
	Delay in pathogen clearance and wound healing contributing to local inflammation	
	Very few eosinophils and basophils and some contradiction	
Natural killer cells	NK cells in cord blood displayed specific features associated with immaturity, including poor expression of KIR and LIR-1/ILT-2 and high expression of both NKG2A and IFN-γ	Wendt et al. 2006; Le Garff-Tavernier et al. 2010
	NK cells from older subjects, on the other hand, preserved their major phenotypic and functional characteristics, but with their mature features accentuated	
	The expression of CD57, a marker of highly differentiated NK cells, is increased in the elderly	
	Profound decline of CD56^high subset, rise of CD56^dim population	
	Conflicting reports on killer immunoglobulin-like receptor	
Dendritic cells	Diminished functions, impaired migration, and phagocytosis	Agrawal et al. 2009; Kornete and Piccirillo 2012; Teissier et al. 2022
	Increased production of TNF-α and IL-6	
	Reduced IL-10 upon stimulation	
	Reduced phagocytosis leads to decreased antigen presentation, hence less B- and T-cell priming	

Cite this article as *Cold Spring Harb Perspect Med* doi: 10.1101/cshperspect.a041197

lular responses to antigen receptor stimulation may reduce the extent of clonal expansion (by cell division) of antigen-specific cells required for effective immunity or alter qualitatively the patterns of gene expression in activated lymphocytes. The latter mechanism has been recently proposed to contribute to inflammaging via increased expression of inflammatory cytokines by cells in older individuals (Bharath et al. 2020).

Third, the impact of age-associated immune dysregulation on the health span of the elderly must consider interactions between immunity and other physiological changes that occur with age. Studies that investigated relationships between immune characteristics and physiological parameters, such as frailty and multimorbidity, have found limited correlation with classic inflammaging markers (e.g., C-reactive protein, TNF-α, and IL-6) (Marcos-Pérez et al. 2018; Alberro et al. 2021). Instead, more recent investigations have moved toward multiomics approaches to identify biomarker panels that summarize changes in immune function with aging and, independent of chronological age, predict health outcomes. Alpert and colleagues (2019) used multiomic technologies on immune cells of 135 healthy adult individuals of different ages sampled longitudinally over a 9-yr period to generate an immune aging (IMM-AGE) score, which produced a more accurate estimate of one's immune status than chronological age. The same group more recently conducted a comprehensive analysis of 50 circulating immune proteins to develop an inflammatory clock of aging (iAge) that predicts multimorbidity. In this study, the authors quantified serum cytokine, chemokine, and growth factor levels in over a thousand donors between ages 8 and 96 yr. Using a neural network–based deep learning model, the investigators were able to reliably predict age-associated deterioration of immune function (Furman et al. 2017; Sayed et al. 2021). Moreover, iAge, which tracks age-associated frailty and multimorbidity in humans, identified the interferon-induced chemokine CXCL9 as a prominent inflammatory component contributing to cardiovascular aging.

It is important to point out that immune dysfunction and immunosenescence are widely considered as two components of the same age-related phenomenon (i.e., inflammaging) and that some talk about immunosenescence and inflammaging as the same dimension. Because inflammaging was originally defined by high circulating levels of proinflammatory cytokines, in this discussion we will define inflammaging as chronic immune activation, whereas we reserve the term immunosenescence to the cadre of mechanisms that reduce the immune response to acute stressors. From this perspective, clear-cut evidence of a connection between immunosenescence and inflammaging is lacking. It is possible that inflammaging promotes immunosenescence or, in other words, that immune dysregulation and inflammaging are mutually reinforcing forces that drive many aging phenotypes. The best evidence that defective immune cells can lead to an aging-like proinflammatory state comes from the studies of Yousefzadeh et al. (2021). These authors engineered a hematopoietic-specific deletion in mice of the *Ercc1* gene, which encodes a protein involved in DNA repair. Mutant animals exhibited many symptoms of age-associated immune dysfunction, including increased proportions of senescent immune cells, increased levels of SASP markers, and compromised cellular and humoral function, thus resembling normal aged mice. Importantly, prominent aging phenotypes were also evident in tissues where *Ercc1* was intact, such as the liver and kidney, and cytokine levels were elevated in the serum. These observations strongly support the notion that selective and persistent activation of inflammatory responses in immune cells (i.e., immune dysfunction) is sufficient to drive inflammaging and systemic aging features in mice. An important implication of these studies is that reducing immunosenescence, and thereby inflammaging, may have beneficial effects in the elderly beyond immune-specific outcomes, such as improved vaccine efficacy and protection against infectious disease.

The converse issue is equally important, that is, does inflammaging induce immune dysregulation? This is more difficult to address because of the complexity in disentangling inflammaging from immunosenescence. One mechanism by which inflammaging can affect immunity is by changing the milieu in which immune responses take place, the most obvious effects being conferred by cytokines and chemokines that are hallmarks of inflammaging. For example, CD4+ T-cell responses in an IL-6-rich environment skew effector phenotypes toward proinflammatory IL-17-producing cells (Ghoreschi et al. 2010). This mechanism may underlie increased IL-17 production by CD4+ T cells from older humans. Similarly, IL-17 and TNF-α have been shown to lower the threshold for CD4+ T cell activation (Banerjee et al. 2005; Ben-Sasson et al. 2009, 2011) that may predispose the emergence of self-reactive cells and increased autoimmunity during aging. Such cells are constrained in a noninflammatory youthful environment by mechanisms of immune tolerance. The resulting picture is one whereby multiple features of inflammaging and immune senescence establish positive feedback effects that increase steadily with age.

INFLAMMAGING AND THE INTEGRATED STRESS RESPONSE

Several lines of evidence suggest that inflammaging is directly connected to the biological mechanisms of aging and results from the accumulation of molecular damage that is not fully offset by resilience strategies. Such damage accumulation could therefore be considered a proxy measure of accelerated aging (Fig. 1). López-Otín et al. (2013) and Kennedy et al. (2014) have identified biological mechanisms of aging that can be traced in multiple organisms, including humans. These so-called "hallmarks" encompass biological processes such as proteostasis (i.e., protein homeostasis), adaptation to stress, nutrient sensing, genome maintenance, mitochondrial function, cellular senescence, metabolism, and inflammation. There is substantial evidence of a bidirectional relationship between inflammation and these mechanisms, meaning that the underlying processes can be adversely affected by inflammation, whereas defects in these processes can trigger an inflammatory response, potentially creating a vicious cycle that can contribute to accelerated aging. From an evolutionary perspective, we can hypothesize that preservation of effective proteostasis, which encompasses the maintenance of both the level and functionality

of the proteome, is essential to survival. In fact, virtually any type of biochemical pathway or stress response requires the integrity of proteins. Although we cover next the intimate relationship between proteostatic mechanisms, particularly the ISR, and inflammaging, details regarding the connection between the other mechanisms of aging and inflammation has been extensively reviewed elsewhere (Bektas et al. 2018; Ferrucci and Fabbri 2018; Franceschi et al. 2018; Furman et al. 2019).

The regulation of proteostasis involves evolutionarily conserved mechanisms that are interconnected and include the unfolded protein response (UPR) that senses and responds to misfolded protein accumulation in the endoplasmic reticulum (ER), the heat shock response (HSR) that regulates protein folding and degradation capacity, and the ISR that reprograms transcription and translation in response to stress (see Fig. 3). Broadly speaking, the ISR enables cells to pause protein synthesis to allow for sufficient time to deal with the accumulation of misfolded proteins, all while preserving the translation of proteins that play critical roles in promoting homeostasis, including cytokines and other proinflammatory mediators. Known stressors that trigger the ISR and its associated signaling stress-kinases (indicated here in parentheses) include the accumulation of misfolded proteins in the ER (PERK), amino acid deprivation (GCN2), iron deficiency and mitochondrial stress (HRI), or viral infection (PKR), although this list may very well grow as our knowledge of the complex mechanisms expands (Derisbourg et al. 2021a). Depending on the intensity and duration of the stress, ISR signaling enables the cell to either favor a return to homeostasis or apoptotic cell death. An important mediator of the stress-specific cellular response is ATF4, which becomes up-regulated following activation of the stress kinases and consequent phosphorylation of eukaryotic initiation factor 2α (eIF2α). ATF4 is a transcription factor that regulates the expression of genes specifically involved in survival responses, inducing the up-regulation of autophagy, the DNA-damage response, and inhibition of mTORC1 (Ameri and Harris 2008). However, if the stress is too

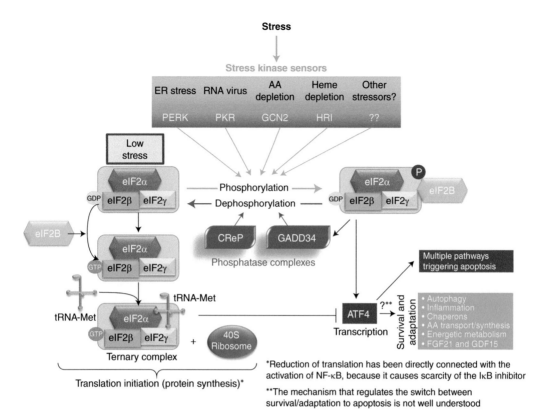

Figure 3. The integrated stress response. Translation initiation is controlled by the eIF2–GTP–Met-tRNAi ternary complex that interacts with the 40S ribosome to recognize the AUG start codon in mRNA (Derisbourg et al. 2021a). In metazoans, different types of stress are sensed, as are four different kinases—heme-regulated inhibitor (*HRI*), protein kinase R (*PKR*), general control nonderepressible 2 (*GCN2*), PKR-like ER kinase (*PERK*)—and possibly other kinases that are yet to be identified. Once activated, these kinases phosphorylate eIF2, which is no longer able to form the eIF2–GTP–Met-tRNAi ternary complex (Costa-Mattioli and Walter 2020), therefore slowing down or blocking translation. However, lowered ternary complex availability activates the transcription factor 4 (ATF4) that stimulates the transcription and translation of a subset of mRNAs that act as effectors of the ISR and enhance resilience responses. In the case of stresses that are too intense or prolonged in time, it can trigger apoptosis through different mechanisms. Of note, phosphorylate eIF2 also enhances the activity of the GADD34 phosphatase complex acting as a braking system that controls excessive ISR activation (Knowles et al. 2021).

intense or prolonged, exceeding the tolerance threshold of the cell, there is a shift toward apoptosis. The regulatory mechanisms that eventually shift the response toward cell death are not understood, but presumably involve a reaction to excessive damage accumulation. The intricate control of the ISR network through sophisticated transcriptional regulation is, in many ways, reminiscent of a subroutine in software programming and shows how a cell can mechanistically deal with stress and/or a crisis triggered by aging and inflammaging.

The link between ISR and inflammaging is supported by observations that dysregulation of the ISR is observed in many inflammaging-related disorders, including cancer, neurodegenerative disease, and metabolic syndrome (Ameri and Harris 2008). There is also emerging evidence that the ISR is up-regulated with aging and is involved in age-related diseases such as diabetes and cancer. Mechanistically, it is currently believed that the ISR activates the NF-κB transcriptional regulator (see further information in the next section) by slowing down the translation of its short-lived protein inhibitor IκB (Tam et al. 2012). This model is consistent with the observation that ISR activation leads to secretion of inflammatory cytokines, such as IL-1β and IL-6, factors that are directly related to NF-κB activity. Thus, inhibition of the ISR is a candidate mechanism for reducing inflammation. ISR inhibition has in fact been shown to extend survival in nematodes (Derisbourg et al. 2021b) and enhance cognitive function in aged mice (Krukowski et al. 2020), suggesting pharmacological modulation of the ISR may be a future therapeutic strategy for age-related chronic diseases characterized by inflammaging (Derisbourg et al. 2021a).

AGE-RELATED DYSBIOSIS AND INFLAMMAGING

Beyond the so-far-discussed intrinsic and extrinsic triggers of inflammaging, the gut microbiome and dysbiosis are newly emerging sources for age-associated chronic inflammation. There is evidence that changes in the gut microbiome and repeated chronic infections that become more prevalent with aging may contribute to systemic inflammation and activate the components of the ISR, especially in the most severe circumstances. For example, recent data suggest that *Shigella flexneri*, which primarily infects the gastrointestinal tract and, more relevant to aging, *Porphyromonas gingivalis*, the "keystone pathogen" of chronic oral inflammatory gum periodontitis, activate the ISR (Knowles et al. 2021). In a recent review, Ghosh et al. (2022) describe evidence indicating that the microbiome affects the host's metabolic, immune, and neurological functions in a reciprocal manner, as well as modifies the risk of diseases in general and age-related diseases in particular, many of which are linked to inflammation and inflammaging.

The diversity of the human gut microbiome is vast, with almost 2000 bacterial species (Almeida et al. 2019). Observational studies suggest that the degree of "diversity" is the most important characteristic of a "healthy microbiome," as problems occur when one bacterial species becomes dominant. Comparative analysis of microbiome profiles shows that some taxa of bacterial species are more prevalent in centenarians across various nationalities and geographies and reveals that a lower number of symbionts, such as the *Faecalibacterium* species, are associated with health in younger individuals. Moreover, there is a higher number of gut microbiota genes associated with xenobiotic degradation in long-lived older individuals (Rampelli et al. 2020). Other age-related changes in the microbiome include the loss of dominant commensal taxa (such as the health-associated genus *Bifidobacterium*) and an increase in other commensals, such as pathobionts *Streptococcus* and *Enterobacteriaceae*, which are associated with an age-related decline in health (Jeffery et al. 2016; Ghosh et al. 2020a). Studies examining cohorts of individuals, such as those enrolled in Ireland-based ELDERMET, have found similar changes that are characterized by loss of commensals and a gain of pathobionts, such as *Enterobacteriaceae* family members and disease-associated *Clostridium* species (Ghosh et al. 2022). Moreover, in examining 25 studies that investigated gut microbiome alterations in older individuals, Ghosh et al. (2022) identified a third group of commensal microbial markers (i.e., *Akkermansia, Barnesiellaceae, Butyricimonas, Butyrivibrio, Christensenellaceae, Odoribacter,* and *Oscillospira*), which increase with age but decrease in various age-related conditions. As such, these species appear to represent candidate biomarkers of healthy aging or physiological decline. For example, a decrease in *Akkermansia* has been associated with cognitive decline (Manderino et al. 2017), multiple age-related diseases/comorbidities (Singh et al. 2019), mortality among centenarians (Luan et al. 2020), and progeria (Bárcena et al. 2019). *Akkermansia* promotes the growth of butyrate producers (by producing acetate), which in turn decreases the loss of the colonic bilayer and hence reduce inflammation (Ghosh et al. 2022). *Akkermansia* also reduces the activation of innate B1a cells (preventing insulin resistance) (Bodogai et al. 2018), prevents cellular senescence (Shin et al. 2021), ameliorates progeroid symptoms (Bárcena et al. 2019), and reduces the risk of cardiometabolic disease in humans who are overweight or obese (Depommier et al. 2019), all factors known to increase inflammation. Furthermore, with regard to inflammation, a decrease in microbiome producers (such as *Blautia*, *Coprococcus*, *Dorea*, *Eubacterium*, *Faecalibacterium*, and *Roseburia*) of core short-chain fatty acids, which are known anti-inflammatory metabolites (Couto et al. 2020), has been associated with frailty (Ghosh et al. 2020a) and Alzheimer's disease (Haran et al. 2019). Of note, many of the unhealthy age-associated pathobionts mentioned result in metabolites that are connected to inflammation and oxidative stress, including trimethylamine (Lin et al. 2020), paracresol (Ghosh et al. 2022), and LPS (Awoyemi et al. 2018).

In addition to the beneficial effects of some microbial species against inflammation, evidence supports the premise that the microbiome can be an important contributor to inflammaging. Thevaranjan et al. (2017) performed a set of experiments in mice to identify connections between the microbiome profile and age-associated inflammatory changes. They found that mice maintained under germ-free conditions did not show an age-related increase in proinflammatory cytokine levels. However, co-housing germ-free mice with non-sterilely raised old mice but not young mice, increased proinflammatory cytokine levels. In TNF-α-deficient animals, age-associated microbiota changes were not observed, and the mutant mice were protected from age-associated inflammation. Finally, the investigators showed that age-associated microbiota changes in normal mice could be reversed by anti-TNF-α therapy by reducing TNF-α levels. Together, these findings suggest that inflammation is caused by both alterations in the microbiota and downstream consequences of the microbiota changes (Thevaranjan et al. 2017).

Last, lifestyle interventions such as the Mediterranean diet (Ghosh et al. 2020b), a diet rich in blueberries (Ntemiri et al. 2020), and many other diets including those that incorporate various prebiotic and microbial supplements, have been found to reduce inflammatory biomarkers or increase anti-inflammatory biomarkers. Such evidence indicates that modulation of the microbiome through dietary strategies may be one way to reduce inflammation and hence stave off physiological decline associated with aging (Ghosh et al. 2022). The connections between the microbiome and inflammation described

above have motivated clinical trials to manipulate the microbiome in older individuals to reduce inflammation. Examples include prebiotic administration to affect specific microbiota that influence inflammation, such as short-chain fatty acid producers (Chung et al. 2020), and direct microbial supplementation that targets gut inflammation in age-related conditions such as Alzheimer's disease (Leblhuber et al. 2018). In the future, microbiome manipulation focusing on inflammation may also include fecal microbiota transplantation (FMT), which to date has been primarily limited to clinical trials treating chronic *Clostridioides difficile* infection (Agrawal et al. 2016; Friedman-Korn et al. 2018). However, promising experiments in mice have demonstrated that FMT from young into old animals reversed age-associated inflammation in the central nervous system and retina (Parker et al. 2022) and also improved, in the old mice, peripheral and brain immunity and cognitive behavior impairments (Boehme et al. 2021).

IS REDUCING INFLAMMATION USEFUL?

Overwhelming observational evidence indicates that inflammation is a risk factor for chronic diseases, multimorbidity, disability, frailty, and mortality, prudently favoring inflammation suppression as a first choice of intervention to combat aging. Surprisingly, whether blocking inflammation prevents a decline or improves physical function in older individuals has not been definitively established, with a few exceptions that we review later in this section (Ferrucci and Fabbri 2018). From the data presented earlier in this work, it is reasonable to hypothesize that if inflammation is effectively targeted through interventions that selectively offset the deleterious effects of an inflammatory environment while retaining its critical role in the defense, repair, and regeneration of damaged macromolecules and cells, it would result in the expansion of health span and preservation of functional status in old age. Many different pharmacological and nonpharmacological strategies are currently available to reduce inflammation besides steroids. These include, salicylates (such as aspirin), propionic acid derivatives (such as Naproxen), acetic acid derivatives (such as Indomethacin), enolic acid (Oxicam) derivative (such as Piroxicam), anthranilic acid derivatives (such as Mefenamic), and selective COX-2 inhibitors (such as Celecoxib). Other drug classes have claimed to effectively reduce inflammation, including Losartan and Omega 3 fatty acids (in the form of fish oil). More recently, several monoclonal antibodies have been released that selectively block inflammatory mediators (cytokines) and chemokines and/or their receptors. Finally, new molecules that selectively block the NLRP3 inflammasome have been produced but will not be addressed here because of the lack of solid supporting data in animal models or humans.

In a prospective cohort comprised of 14,315 men (mean age 71 yr) who participated in the Physicians' Health Study I, a randomized controlled trial of aspirin (1982–1988) was conducted, with extended posttrial follow-up. Individuals who were regularly taking aspirin (at least 60 d/yr on average) were more likely than those that were not to self-report preserved mobility (Orkaby et al. 2022). In the ASPREE (aspirin in reducing events in the elderly) trial of 100 mg of aspirin daily versus placebo, 19,114 healthy adults aged 70+ yr (65+ yr if U.S. minority) in Australia and the United States were recruited. Over a median of 4.7 yr, incident disability in activities of daily living was similar in those receiving aspirin (776/9525) relative to placebo (787/9589). However, persistent disability in activities of daily living tended to be lower (nonsignificantly) in the aspirin group (Woods et al. 2021). The promising results of these studies is tempered by other studies that failed to demonstrate any effects of chronic aspirin administration on physical or cognitive functions and by a recent report from the ASPREE trial showing that the risk of a serious fall was significantly greater in the aspirin group (Barker et al. 2022). The ENERGIZE pilot randomized controlled trial failed to demonstrate any positive effect of Losartan and fish oil on plasma IL-6 and mobility in older persons (Pahor et al. 2020).

The Canakinumab Anti-Inflammatory Thrombosis Outcome Study (CANTOS) trial remains the strongest evidence that reducing inflammation prevents a "hard" medical outcome,

such as incident cardiovascular events (Ridker et al. 2017a). The CANTOS found that blocking IL-1 with the monoclonal antibody canakinumab significantly reduced cardiovascular events in individuals with established atherosclerotic disease who had already survived a myocardial infarction and had residual inflammatory risk. Interestingly, the protection was higher among those, who after receipt of the first dose, exhibited a decline in IL-6 and C-reactive protein. When reanalyzing the CANTOS database, canakinumab was also found to reduce the rate or incidence of lung cancer (Ridker et al. 2017b), anemia (Vallurupalli et al. 2020), hip or knee replacement (Schieker et al. 2020), and hospitalizations for heart failure (Everett et al. 2019), as well as to positively impact insulin resistance (Everett et al. 2018). These data strongly suggest that blockage of inflammation positively affects multiple chronic disease–associated health outcomes. By extension, we can hypothesize that this same approach would have beneficial effects on multiple health outcomes.

TNF-α triggers NF-κB, which, as discussed earlier, operates as a gate to many proinflammatory cytokines and inflammatory signals. There is therefore strong rationale to hypothesize that blocking TNF-α, especially in frail older persons who characteristically have an inflammatory component, will improve health outcomes and muscle function mobility in particular. In mice, pharmacological TNF-α blockade, with weekly subcutaneous injection of etanercept from 16 to 28 mo of age, prevented atrophy and loss of type II fibers and led to significant improvements in muscle function and life span (Sciorati et al. 2020). Other compounds that selectively block major inflammatory mediators, such as tocilizumab, sarilumab, and siltuximab, which interfere with IL-6 signaling; anakinra and rilonacept, which block IL-1 signaling; and infliximab and certolizumab pegol, which disrupt TNF-α signaling, to name a few, have also been tested extensively in overt inflammatory disease, such as rheumatoid arthritis or giant cell arteritis, with positive results thus far. Unfortunately, to date, none of these candidate therapeutics have been tested for their ability to prevent age-associated multimorbidity or risk of physical and cognitive disability.

It is important to recognize that "treating" inflammation is intrinsically complex, especially in "healthy" individuals. This is a particular concern if inflammation is blocked at a central hub of one of the different defensive mechanisms, a strategy employed by many of the agents used nowadays that were designed to fight overt inflammatory conditions. Because of such complexity, scientists have looked at nonpharmacological interventions to reduce inflammation and prevent related adverse health outcomes. There is some, albeit not overwhelming, evidence that physical activity and exercise can reduce inflammation (de Lemos Muller et al. 2019). In a randomized controlled trial in older persons, exercise reduced inflammation in adipose tissue as measured by the expression of proinflammatory cytokines, especially when paired with mega-3 supplementation (Čížková et al. 2020). A number of observational studies and intervention trials have also shown that adherence to the Mediterranean diet prevents chronic disease development (Salas-Salvadó et al. 2018). Indeed, dietary regimens based on the Mediterranean diet improve proinflammatory status and prevent mobility loss, cognitive decline, and frailty in older persons, the most severe and most dreaded consequences of aging (Milaneschi et al. 2011; Tanaka et al. 2018; Wang et al. 2018; Capurso et al. 2019; Tsigalou et al. 2020).

Looking to the future, more research on the specific causes and mechanisms that trigger inflammaging, as well as the defining features of inflammaging, will certainly provide clues about the most effective targets. Hopefully, such insights will direct us to new therapeutic mechanisms that are less prone to unwanted side-effects. For example, enhancing mitophagy via administration of Urolithin A or eliminating senescent cells through new senolytic drugs are emerging, promising approaches currently being tested in human trials.

REFERENCES

Agrawal A, Tay J, Ton S, Agrawal S, Gupta S. 2009. Increased reactivity of dendritic cells from aged subjects to self-antigen, the human DNA. *J Immunol* **182:** 1138–1145. doi:10.4049/jimmunol.182.2.1138

Agrawal M, Aroniadis OC, Brandt LJ, Kelly C, Freeman S, Surawicz C, Broussard E, Stollman N, Giovanelli A, Smith B, et al. 2016. The long-term efficacy and safety of fecal microbiota transplant for recurrent, severe, and complicated *Clostridium difficile* infection in 146 elderly individuals. *J Clin Gastroenterol* **50:** 403–407. doi:10.1097/MCG.0000000000000410

Alberro A, Iribarren-Lopez A, Sáenz-Cuesta M, Matheu A, Vergara I, Otaegui D. 2021. Inflammaging markers characteristic of advanced age show similar levels with frailty and dependency. *Sci Rep* **11:** 4358. doi:10.1038/s41598-021-83991-7

Almeida A, Mitchell AL, Boland M, Forster SC, Gloor GB, Tarkowska A, Lawley TD, Finn RD. 2019. A new genomic blueprint of the human gut microbiota. *Nature* **568:** 499–504. doi:10.1038/s41586-019-0965-1

Alpert A, Pickman Y, Leipold M, Rosenberg-Hasson Y, Ji X, Gaujoux R, Rabani H, Starosvetsky E, Kveler K, Schaffert S, et al. 2019. A clinically meaningful metric of immune age derived from high-dimensional longitudinal monitoring. *Nat Med* **25:** 487–495. doi:10.1038/s41591-019-0381-y

Alzeer J. 2022. Halalopathy: role of entropy in the aging process. *Am J Biomed Sci Res* **16:** 147–154. doi:10.34297/AJBSR.2022.16.002205

Ameri K, Harris AL. 2008. Activating transcription factor 4. *Int J Biochem Cell Biol* **40:** 14–21. doi:10.1016/j.biocel.2007.01.020

Awoyemi A, Trøseid M, Arnesen H, Solheim S, Seljeflot I. 2018. Markers of metabolic endotoxemia as related to metabolic syndrome in an elderly male population at high cardiovascular risk: a cross-sectional study. *Diabetol Metab Syndr* **10:** 59. doi:10.1186/s13098-018-0360-3

Banerjee D, Liou HC, Sen R. 2005. c-Rel-dependent priming of naive T cells by inflammatory cytokines. *Immunity* **23:** 445–458. doi:10.1016/j.immuni.2005.09.012

Bárcena C, Valdés-Mas R, Mayoral P, Garabaya C, Durand S, Rodríguez F, Fernández-García MT, Salazar N, Nogacka AM, Garatachea N, et al. 2019. Healthspan and lifespan extension by fecal microbiota transplantation into progeroid mice. *Nat Med* **25:** 1234–1242. doi:10.1038/s41591-019-0504-5

Barker AL, Morello R, Thao LTP, Seeman E, Ward SA, Sanders KM, Cumming RG, Pasco JA, Ebeling PR, Woods RL, et al. 2022. Daily low-dose aspirin and risk of serious falls and fractures in healthy older people: a substudy of the ASPREE randomized clinical trial. *JAMA Intern Med* **182:** 1289–1297. doi:10.1001/jamainternmed.2022.5028

Bektas A, Schurman SH, Sen R, Ferrucci L. 2018. Aging, inflammation and the environment. *Exp Gerontol* **105:** 10–18. doi:10.1016/j.exger.2017.12.015

Bektas A, Schurman SH, Franceschi C, Ferrucci L. 2020. A public health perspective of aging: do hyper-inflammatory syndromes such as COVID-19, SARS, ARDS, cytokine storm syndrome, and post-ICU syndrome accelerate short- and long-term inflammaging? *Immun Ageing* **17:** 23. doi:10.1186/s12979-020-00196-8

Ben-Sasson SZ, Hu-Li J, Quiel J, Cauchetaux S, Ratner M, Shapira I, Dinarello CA, Paul WE. 2009. IL-1 acts directly on CD4 T cells to enhance their antigen-driven expansion and differentiation. *Proc Natl Acad Sci* **106:** 7119–7124. doi:10.1073/pnas.0902745106

Ben-Sasson SZ, Caucheteux S, Crank M, Hu-Li J, Paul WE. 2011. IL-1 acts on T cells to enhance the magnitude of in vivo immune responses. *Cytokine* **56:** 122–125. doi:10.1016/j.cyto.2011.07.006

Bharath LP, Agrawal M, McCambridge G, Nicholas DA, Hasturk H, Liu J, Jiang K, Liu R, Guo Z, Deeney J, et al. 2020. Metformin enhances autophagy and normalizes mitochondrial function to alleviate aging-associated inflammation. *Cell Metab* **32:** 44–55.e6. doi:10.1016/j.cmet.2020.04.015

Bodogai M, O'Connell J, Kim K, Kim Y, Moritoh K, Chen C, Gusev F, Vaughan K, Shulzhenko N, Mattison JA, et al. 2018. Commensal bacteria contribute to insulin resistance in aging by activating innate B1a cells. *Sci Transl Med* **10:** eaat4271. doi:10.1126/scitranslmed.aat4271

Boehme M, Guzzetta KE, Bastiaanssen TFS, van de Wouw M, Moloney GM, Gual-Grau A, Spichak S, Olavarría-Ramírez L, Fitzgerald P, Morillas E, et al. 2021. Microbiota from young mice counteracts selective age-associated behavioral deficits. *Nat Aging* **1:** 666–676. doi:10.1038/s43587-021-00093-9

Boucher N, Dufeu-Duchesne T, Vicaut E, Farge D, Effros RB, Schächter F. 1998. CD28 expression in T cell aging and human longevity. *Exp Gerontol* **33:** 267–282. doi:10.1016/S0531-5565(97)00132-0

Britanova OV, Putintseva EV, Shugay M, Merzlyak EM, Turchaninova MA, Staroverov DB, Bolotin DA, Lukyanov S, Bogdanova EA, Mamedov IZ, et al. 2014. Age-related decrease in TCR repertoire diversity measured with deep and normalized sequence profiling. *J Immunol* **192:** 2689–2698. doi:10.4049/jimmunol.1302064

Brubaker AL, Rendon JL, Ramirez L, Choudhry MA, Kovacs EJ. 2013. Reduced neutrophil chemotaxis and infiltration contributes to delayed resolution of cutaneous wound infection with advanced age. *J Immunol* **190:** 1746–1757. doi:10.4049/jimmunol.1201213

Brueggeman JM, Zhao J, Schank M, Yao ZQ, Moorman JP. 2022. Trained immunity: an overview and the impact on COVID-19. *Front Immunol* **13:** 837524. doi:10.3389/fimmu.2022.837524

Cano-Gamez E, Soskic B, Roumeliotis TI, So E, Smyth DJ, Baldrighi M, Willé D, Nakic N, Esparza-Gordillo J, Larminie CGC, et al. 2020. Single-cell transcriptomics identifies an effectorness gradient shaping the response of CD4[+] T cells to cytokines. *Nat Commun* **11:** 1801. doi:10.1038/s41467-020-15543-y

Capurso C, Bellanti F, Lo Buglio A, Vendemiale G. 2019. The Mediterranean diet slows down the progression of aging and helps to prevent the onset of frailty: a narrative review. *Nutrients* **12:** 35. doi:10.3390/nu12010035

Cartwright TN, Worrell JC, Marchetti L, Dowling CM, Knox A, Kiely P, Mann J, Mann DA, Wilson CL. 2018. HDAC1 interacts with the p50 NF-κB subunit via its nuclear localization sequence to constrain inflammatory gene expression. *Biochim Biophys Acta Gene Regul Mech* **1861:** 962–970. doi:10.1016/j.bbagrm.2018.09.001

Chang LY, Li Y, Kaplan DE. 2017. Hepatitis C viraemia reversibly maintains subset of antigen-specific T-bet[+] tissue-like memory B cells. *J Viral Hepat* **24:** 389–396. doi:10.1111/jvh.12659

Chemin K, Gerstner C, Malmström V. 2019. Effector functions of CD4[+] T cells at the site of local autoimmune inflammation—lessons from rheumatoid arthritis. *Front Immunol* **10:** 353. doi:10.3389/fimmu.2019.00353

Chung WSF, Walker AW, Bosscher D, Garcia-Campayo V, Wagner J, Parkhill J, Duncan SH, Flint HJ. 2020. Relative abundance of the Prevotella genus within the human gut microbiota of elderly volunteers determines the inter-individual responses to dietary supplementation with wheat bran arabinoxylan-oligosaccharides. *BMC Microbiol* **20:** 283. doi:10.1186/s12866-020-01968-4

Čížková T, Štěpán M, Daďová K, Ondrůjová B, Sontáková L, Krauzová E, Matouš M, Koc M, Gojda J, Kračmerová J, et al. 2020. Exercise training reduces inflammation of adipose tissue in the elderly: cross-sectional and randomized interventional trial. *J Clin Endocrinol Metab* **105:** dgaa630.

Cleveland H, Jacobs G. 1999. Human choice: the genetic code for social development. *Futures* **31:** 959–970. doi:10.1016/S0016-3287(99)00055-5

Coleman MJ, Zimmerly KM, Yang XO. 2021. Accumulation of CD28[null] senescent T-cells is associated with poorer outcomes in Covid19 patients. *Biomolecules* **11:** 1425. doi:10.3390/biom11101425

Conway J, Duggal NA. 2021. Ageing of the gut microbiome: potential influences on immune senescence and inflammaging. *Ageing Res Rev* **68:** 101323. doi:10.1016/j.arr.2021.101323

Correia-Melo C, Birch J, Fielder E, Rahmatika D, Taylor J, Chapman J, Lagnado A, Carroll BM, Miwa S, Richardson G. 2019. Rapamycin improves healthspan but not inflammaging in *nfκb1[-/-]* mice. *Aging Cell* **18:** e12882. doi:10.1111/acel.12882

Cortegano I, Rodríguez M, Martín I, Prado MC, Ruíz C, Hortigüela R, Alía M, Vilar M, Mira H, Cano E, et al. 2017. Altered marginal zone and innate-like B cells in aged senescence-accelerated SAMP8 mice with defective IgG1 responses. *Cell Death Dis* **8:** e3000. doi:10.1038/cddis.2017.351

Costa-Mattioli M, Walter P. 2020. The integrated stress response: from mechanism to disease. *Science* **368:** eaat5314. doi:10.1126/science.aat5314

Couto MR, Gonçalves P, Magro F, Martel F. 2020. Microbiota-derived butyrate regulates intestinal inflammation: focus on inflammatory bowel disease. *Pharmacol Res* **159:** 104947. doi:10.1016/j.phrs.2020.104947

Davizon-Castillo P, McMahon B, Aguila S, Bark D, Ashworth K, Allawzi A, Campbell RA, Montenont E, Nemkov T, D'Alessandro A, et al. 2019. TNF-α-driven inflammation and mitochondrial dysfunction define the platelet hyperreactivity of aging. *Blood* **134:** 727–740. doi:10.1182/blood.2019000200

de Lemos Muller CH, Roberto de Matos J, Grigolo GB, Schroeder HT, Rodrigues-Krause J, Krauseet M. 2019. Exercise training for the elderly: inflammaging and the central role for HSP70. *J Sci Sport Exerc* **1:** 97–115. doi:10.1007/s42978-019-0015-6

Demaret J, Corroyer-Simovic B, Alidjinou EK, Goffard A, Trauet J, Miczek S, Vuotto F, Dendooven A, Huvent-Grelle D, Podvin J, et al. 2021. Impaired functional T-cell response to SARS-CoV-2 after two doses of BNT162b2 mRNA vaccine in older people. *Front Immunol* **12:** 778679. doi:10.3389/fimmu.2021.778679

Depommier C, Everard A, Druart C, Plovier H, Van Hul M, Vieira-Silva S, Falony G, Raes J, Maiter D, Delzenne NM, et al. 2019. Supplementation with *Akkermansia muciniphila* in overweight and obese human volunteers: a proof-of-concept exploratory study. *Nat Med* **25**: 1096–1103. doi:10.1038/s41591-019-0495-2

Derisbourg MJ, Hartman MD, Denzel MS. 2021a. Perspective: modulating the integrated stress response to slow aging and ameliorate age-related pathology. *Nat Aging* **1**: 760–768. doi:10.1038/s43587-021-00112-9

Derisbourg MJ, Wester LE, Baddi R, Denzel MS. 2021b. Mutagenesis screen uncovers lifespan extension through integrated stress response inhibition without reduced mRNA translation. *Nat Commun* **12**: 1678. doi:10.1038/s41467-021-21743-x

D'Souza SS, Zhang Y, Bailey JT, Fung ITH, Kuentzel ML, Chittur SV, Yang Q. 2021. Type I interferon signaling controls the accumulation and transcriptomes of monocytes in the aged lung. *Aging Cell* **20**: e13470.

Ehrhardt GR, Hijikata A, Kitamura H, Ohara O, Wang JY, Cooper MD. 2008. Discriminating gene expression profiles of memory B cell subpopulations. *J Exp Med* **205**: 1807–1817. doi:10.1084/jem.20072682

Elyahu Y, Hekselman I, Eizenberg-Magar I, Berner O, Strominger I, Schiller M, Mittal K, Nemirovsky A, Eremenko E, Vital A, et al. 2019. Aging promotes reorganization of the CD4 T cell landscape toward extreme regulatory and effector phenotypes. *Sci Adv* **5**: eaaw8330. doi:10.1126/sciadv.aaw8330

Everett BM, Donath MY, Pradhan AD, Thuren T, Pais P, Nicolau JC, Glynn RJ, Libby P, Ridker PM. 2018. Anti-inflammatory therapy with canakinumab for the prevention and management of diabetes. *J Am Coll Cardiol* **71**: 2392–2401. doi:10.1016/j.jacc.2018.03.002

Everett BM, Cornel JH, Lainscak M, Anker SD, Abbate A, Thuren T, Libby P, Glynn RJ, Ridker PM. 2019. Anti-inflammatory therapy with canakinumab for the prevention of hospitalization for heart failure. *Circulation* **139**: 1289–1299. doi:10.1161/CIRCULATIONAHA.118.038010

Ferrucci L, Fabbri E. 2018. Inflammageing: chronic inflammation in ageing, cardiovascular disease, and frailty. *Nat Rev Cardiol* **15**: 505–522. doi:10.1038/s41569-018-0064-2

Fielder E, Tweedy C, Wilson C, Oakley F, LeBeau FEN, Passos JF, Mann DA, von Zglinicki T, Jurk D. 2020. Anti-inflammatory treatment rescues memory deficits during aging in *nfkb1$^{-/-}$* mice. *Aging Cell* **19**: e13188. doi:10.1111/acel.13188

Franceschi C, Bonafè M, Valensin S, Olivieri F, De Luca M, Ottaviani E, De Benedictis G. 2000. Inflamm-aging: an evolutionary perspective on immunosenescence. *Ann NY Acad Sci* **908**: 244–254. doi:10.1111/j.1749-6632.2000.tb06651.x

Franceschi C, Salvioli S, Garagnani P, de Eguileor M, Monti D, Capri M. 2017. Immunobiography and the heterogeneity of immune responses in the elderly: a focus on inflammaging and trained immunity. *Front Immunol* **8**: 982. doi:10.3389/fimmu.2017.00982

Franceschi C, Garagnani P, Parini P, Giuliani C, Santoro A. 2018. Inflammaging: a new immune-metabolic viewpoint for age-related diseases. *Nat Rev Endocrinol* **14**: 576–590. doi:10.1038/s41574-018-0059-4

Frasca D, Romero M, Garcia D, Diaz A, Blomberg BB. 2021. Hyper-metabolic B cells in the spleens of old mice make antibodies with autoimmune specificities. *Immun Ageing* **18**: 9. doi:10.1186/s12979-021-00222-3

Friedman-Korn T, Livovsky DM, Maharshak N, Aviv Cohen N, Paz K, Bar-Gil Shitrit A, Goldin E, Koslowsky B. 2018. Fecal transplantation for treatment of *Clostridium difficile* infection in elderly and debilitated patients. *Dig Dis Sci* **63**: 198–203. doi:10.1007/s10620-017-4833-2

Fulop T, Larbi A, Dupuis G, Le Page A, Frost EH, Cohen AA, Witkowski JM, Franceschi C. 2018. Immunosenescence and inflamm-aging as two sides of the same coin: friends or foes? *Front Immunol* **8**: 1960. doi:10.3389/fimmu.2017.01960

Fulop T, Larbi A, Pawelec G, Khalil A, Cohen AA, Hirokawa K, Witkowski JM, Franceschi C. 2023. Immunology of aging: the birth of inflammaging. *Clin Rev Allergy Immunol* **64**: 109–122. doi:10.1007/s12016-021-08899-6

Furman D, Chang J, Lartigue L, Bolen CR, Haddad F, Gaudilliere B, Ganio EA, Fragiadakis GK, Spitzer MH, Douchet I, et al. 2017. Expression of specific inflammasome gene modules stratifies older individuals into two extreme clinical and immunological states. *Nat Med* **23**: 174–184. doi:10.1038/nm.4267

Furman D, Campisi J, Verdin E, Carrera-Bastos P, Targ S, Franceschi C, Ferrucci L, Gilroy DW, Fasano A, Miller GW, et al. 2019. Chronic inflammation in the etiology of disease across the life span. *Nat Med* **25**: 1822–1832. doi:10.1038/s41591-019-0675-0

García-García VA, Alameda JP, Page A, Casanova ML. 2021. Role of NF-κB in ageing and age-related diseases: lessons from genetically modified mouse models. *Cells* **10**: 1906. doi:10.3390/cells10081906

Ghoreschi K, Laurence A, Yang XP, Tato CM, McGeachy MJ, Konkel JE, Ramos HL, Wei L, Davidson TS, Bouladoux N, et al. 2010. Generation of pathogenic T$_H$17 cells in the absence of TGF-β signalling. *Nature* **467**: 967–971. doi:10.1038/nature09447

Ghosh TS, Das M, Jeffery IB, O'Toole PW. 2020a. Adjusting for age improves identification of gut microbiome alterations in multiple diseases. *eLife* **9**: e50240. doi:10.7554/eLife.50240

Ghosh TS, Rampelli S, Jeffery IB, Santoro A, Neto M, Capri M, Giampieri E, Jennings A, Candela M, Turroni S, et al. 2020b. Mediterranean diet intervention alters the gut microbiome in older people reducing frailty and improving health status: the NU-AGE 1-year dietary intervention across five European countries. *Gut* **69**: 1218–1228. doi:10.1136/gutjnl-2019-319654

Ghosh TS, Shanahan F, O'Toole PW. 2022. The gut microbiome as a modulator of healthy ageing. *Nat Rev Gastroenterol Hepatol* **19**: 565–584. doi:10.1038/s41575-022-00605-x

Gibson KL, Wu YC, Barnett Y, Duggan O, Vaughan R, Kondeatis E, Nilsson BO, Wikby A, Kipling D, Dunn-Walters DK. 2009. B-cell diversity decreases in old age and is correlated with poor health status. *Aging Cell* **8**: 18–25. doi:10.1111/j.1474-9726.2008.00443.x

Goronzy JJ, Weyand CM. 2012. Immune aging and autoimmunity. *Cell Mol Life Sci* **69**: 1615–1623. doi:10.1007/s00018-012-0970-0

Goronzy JJ, Weyand CM. 2013. Understanding immunosenescence to improve responses to vaccines. *Nat Immunol* **14:** 428–436. doi:10.1038/ni.2588

Grants JM, Wegrzyn J, Hui T, O'Neill K, Shadbolt M, Knapp DJHF, Parker J, Deng Y, Gopal A, Docking TR, et al. 2020. Altered microRNA expression links IL6 and TNF-induced inflammaging with myeloid malignancy in humans and mice. *Blood* **135:** 2235–2251. doi:10.1182/blood.2019003105

Hao Y, O'Neill P, Naradikian MS, Scholz JL, Cancro MP. 2011. A B-cell subset uniquely responsive to innate stimuli accumulates in aged mice. *Blood* **118:** 1294–1304. doi:10.1182/blood-2011-01-330530

Haran JP, Bhattarai SK, Foley SE, Dutta P, Ward DV, Bucci V, McCormick BA. 2019. Alzheimer's disease microbiome is associated with dysregulation of the anti-inflammatory P-glycoprotein pathway. *MBio* **10:** e00632-19. doi:10.1128/mBio.00632-19

Hashimoto K, Kouno T, Ikawa T, Hayatsu N, Miyajima Y, Yabukami H, Terooatea T, Sasaki T, Suzuki T, Valentine M, et al. 2019. Single-cell transcriptomics reveals expansion of cytotoxic CD4 T cells in supercentenarians. *Proc Natl Acad Sci* **116:** 24242–24251. doi:10.1073/pnas.1907883116

Hazeldine J, Harris P, Chapple IL, Grant M, Greenwood H, Livesey A, Sapey E, Lord JM. 2014. Impaired neutrophil extracellular trap formation: a novel defect in the innate immune system of aged individuals. *Aging Cell* **13:** 690–698. doi:10.1111/acel.12222

Hu Y, Chen Y, Chen Z, Zhang X, Guo C, Yu Z, Xu P, Sun L, Zhou X, Gong Y, et al. 2022. Dysregulated peripheral invariant natural killer T cells in plaque psoriasis patients. *Front Cell Dev Biol* **9:** 799560. doi:10.3389/fcell.2021.799560

Jeffery IB, Lynch DB, O'Toole PW. 2016. Composition and temporal stability of the gut microbiota in older persons. *ISME J* **10:** 170–182. doi:10.1038/ismej.2015.88

Joseph M, Wu Y, Dannebaum R, Rubelt F, Zlatareva I, Lorenc A, Du ZG, Davies D, Kyle-Cezar F, Das A, et al. 2022. Global patterns of antigen receptor repertoire disruption across adaptive immune compartments in COVID-19. *Proc Natl Acad Sci* **119:** e2201541119. doi:10.1073/pnas.2201541119

Jurk D, Wilson C, Passos JF, Oakley F, Correia-Melo C, Greaves L, Saretzki G, Fox C, Lawless C, Anderson R, et al. 2014. Chronic inflammation induces telomere dysfunction and accelerates ageing in mice. *Nat Commun* **5:** 4172. doi:10.1038/ncomms5172

Kaushik S, Tasset I, Arias E, Pampliega O, Wong E, Martinez-Vicente M, Cuervo AM. 2021. Autophagy and the hallmarks of aging. *Ageing Res Rev* **72:** 101468. doi:10.1016/j.arr.2021.101468

Kennedy BK, Berger SL, Brunet A, Campisi J, Cuervo AM, Epel ES, Franceschi C, Lithgow GJ, Morimoto RI, Pessin JE, et al. 2014. Geroscience: linking aging to chronic disease. *Cell* **159:** 709–713. doi:10.1016/j.cell.2014.10.039

Knowles A, Campbell S, Cross N, Stafford P. 2021. Bacterial manipulation of the integrated stress response: a new perspective on infection. *Front Microbiol* **12:** 645161. doi:10.3389/fmicb.2021.645161

Knox JJ, Buggert M, Kardava L, Seaton KE, Eller MA, Canaday DH, Robb ML, Ostrowski MA, Deeks SG, Slifka MK,

et al. 2017. T-bet⁺ B cells are induced by human viral infections and dominate the HIV gp140 response. *JCI Insight* **2:** e92943. doi:10.1172/jci.insight.92943

Kornete M, Piccirillo CA. 2012. Functional crosstalk between dendritic cells and Foxp3⁺ regulatory T cells in the maintenance of immune tolerance. *Front Immunol* **3:** 165. doi:10.3389/fimmu.2012.00165

Krukowski K, Nolan A, Frias ES, Boone M, Ureta G, Grue K, Paladini MS, Elizarraras E, Delgado L, Bernales S, et al. 2020. Small molecule cognitive enhancer reverses age-related memory decline in mice. *eLife* **9:** e62048. doi:10.7554/eLife.62048

Leblhuber F, Steiner K, Schuetz B, Fuchs D, Gostner JM. 2018. Probiotic supplementation in patients with Alzheimer's dementia—an explorative intervention study. *Curr Alzheimer Res* **15:** 1106–1113. doi:10.2174/1389200219666180813144834

Lee GH, Lee WW. 2016. Unusual CD4⁺CD28⁻ T cells and their pathogenic role in chronic inflammatory disorders. *Immune Netw* **16:** 322–329. doi:10.4110/in.2016.16.6.322

Lee KA, Flores RR, Jang IH, Saathoff A, Robbins PD. 2022. Immune senescence, immunosenescence and aging. *Front Aging* **3:** 900028. doi:10.3389/fragi.2022.900028

Le Garff-Tavernier M, Béziat V, Decocq J, Siguret V, Gandjbakhch F, Pautas E, Debré P, Merle-Beral H, Vieillard V. 2010. Human NK cells display major phenotypic and functional changes over the life span. *Aging Cell* **9:** 527–535. doi:10.1111/j.1474-9726.2010.00584.x

Levin EG, Lustig Y, Cohen C, Fluss R, Indenbaum V, Amit S, Doolman R, Asraf K, Mendelson E, Ziv A, et al. 2021. Waning immune humoral response to BNT162b2 COVID-19 vaccine over 6 months. *N Engl J Med* **385:** e84. doi:10.1056/NEJMoa2114583

Lin H, Liu T, Li X, Gao X, Wu T, Li P. 2020. The role of gut microbiota metabolite trimethylamine N-oxide in functional impairment of bone marrow mesenchymal stem cells in osteoporosis disease. *Ann Transl Med* **8:** 1009. doi:10.21037/atm-20-5307

Listì F, Candore G, Modica MA, Russo M, Di Lorenzo G, Esposito-Pellitteri M, Colonna-Romano G, Aquino A, Bulati M, Lio D, et al. 2006. A study of serum immunoglobulin levels in elderly persons that provides new insights into B cell immunosenescence. *Ann N Y Acad Sci* **1089:** 487–495. doi:10.1196/annals.1386.013

López-Otín C, Blasco MA, Partridge L, Serrano M, Kroemer G. 2013. The hallmarks of aging. *Cell* **153:** 1194–1217. doi:10.1016/j.cell.2013.05.039

Luan Z, Sun G, Huang Y, Yang Y, Yang R, Li C, Wang T, Tan D, Qi S, Jun C, et al. 2020. Metagenomics study reveals changes in gut microbiota in centenarians: a cohort study of Hainan centenarians. *Front Microbiol* **11:** 1474. doi:10.3389/fmicb.2020.01474

Manderino L, Carroll I, Azcarate-Peril MA, Rochette A, Heinberg L, Peat C, Steffen K, Mitchell J, Gunstad J. 2017. Preliminary evidence for an association between the composition of the gut microbiome and cognitive function in neurologically healthy older adults. *J Int Neuropsychol Soc* **23:** 700–705. doi:10.1017/S135561771700492

Marcos-Pérez D, Sánchez-Flores M, Maseda A, Lorenzo-López L, Millán-Calenti JC, Gostner JM, Fuchs D, Pásaro E, Laffon B, Valdiglesias V. 2018. Frailty in older adults is associated with plasma concentrations of inflammatory mediators but not with lymphocyte subpopulations. *Front Immunol* 9: 1056. doi:10.3389/fimmu.2018.01056

Milaneschi Y, Bandinelli S, Corsi AM, Lauretani F, Paolisso G, Dominguez LJ, Semba RD, Tanaka T, Abbatecola AM, Talegawkar SA, et al. 2011. Mediterranean diet and mobility decline in older persons. *Exp Gerontol* 46: 303–308. doi:10.1016/j.exger.2010.11.030

Mills KHG. 2023. IL-17 and IL-17-producing cells in protection versus pathology. *Nat Rev Immunol* 23: 38–54. doi:10.1038/s41577-022-00746-9

Mogilenko DA, Shchukina I, Artyomov MN. 2022. Immune ageing at single-cell resolution. *Nat Rev Immunol* 22: 484–498. doi:10.1038/s41577-021-00646-4

Naradikian MS, Myles A, Beiting DP, Roberts KJ, Dawson L, Herati RS, Bengsch B, Linderman SL, Stelekati E, Spolski R, et al. 2016. Cutting edge: IL-4, IL-21, and IFN-γ interact to govern T-bet and CD11c expression in TLR-activated B cells. *J Immunol* 197: 1023–1028. doi:10.4049/jimmunol.1600522

Netea MG, Quintin J, van der Meer JW. 2011. Trained immunity: a memory for innate host defense. *Cell Host Microbe* 9: 355–361. doi:10.1016/j.chom.2011.04.006

Nikolich-Žugich J. 2018. The twilight of immunity: emerging concepts in aging of the immune system. *Nat Immunol* 19: 10–19. doi:10.1038/s41590-017-0006-x

Nikolich-Zugich J, Knox KS, Rios CT, Natt B, Bhattacharya D, Fain MJ. 2020. SARS-CoV-2 and COVID-19 in older adults: what we may expect regarding pathogenesis, immune responses, and outcomes. *Geroscience* 42: 505–514. doi:10.1007/s11357-020-00186-0

Ntemiri A, Ghosh TS, Gheller ME, Tran TTT, Blum JE, Pellanda P, Vlckova K, Neto MC, Howell A, Thalacker-Mercer A, et al. 2020. Whole blueberry and isolated polyphenol-rich fractions modulate specific gut microbes in an in vitro colon model and in a pilot study in human consumers. *Nutrients* 12: 2800. doi:10.3390/nu12092800

Nussbaum L, Chen YL, Ogg GS. 2021. Role of regulatory T cells in psoriasis pathogenesis and treatment. *Br J Dermatol* 184: 14–24. doi:10.1111/bjd.19380

Ogawa K, Suzuki K, Okutsu M, Yamazaki K, Shinkai S. 2008. The association of elevated reactive oxygen species levels from neutrophils with low-grade inflammation in the elderly. *Immun Ageing* 5: 13. doi:10.1186/1742-4933-5-13

Orkaby AR, Dufour AB, Yang L, Sesso HD, Gaziano JM, Djousse L, Driver JA, Travison TG. 2022. Long-term aspirin use and self-reported walking speed in older men: the physicians' health study. *J Frailty Aging* 11: 12–17.

Pahor M, Guralnik JM, Anton SD, Ambrosius WT, Blair SN, Church TS, Espeland MA, Fielding RA, Gill TM, Glynn NW, et al. 2020. Impact and lessons from the lifestyle interventions and independence for elders (LIFE) clinical trials of physical activity to prevent mobility disability. *J Am Geriatr Soc* 68: 872–881. doi:10.1111/jgs.16365

Pang WW, Schrier SL, Weissman IL. 2017. Age-associated changes in human hematopoietic stem cells. *Semin Hematol* 54: 39–42. doi:10.1053/j.seminhematol.2016.10.004

Parker J, Romano S, Ansorge R, Aboelnour A, Le Gall G, Savva GM, Pontifex MG, Telatin A, Baker D, Jones E, et al. 2022. Fecal microbiota transfer between young and aged mice reverses hallmarks of the aging gut, eye, and brain. *Microbiome* 10: 68. doi:10.1186/s40168-022-01243-w

Pereira BI, De Maeyer RPH, Covre LP, Nehar-Belaid D, Lanna A, Ward S, Marches R, Chambers ES, Gomes DCO, Riddell NE, et al. 2020. Sestrins induce natural killer function in senescent-like CD8+ T cells. *Nat Immunol* 21: 684–694. doi:10.1038/s41590-020-0643-3

Povoleri GAM, Lalnunhlimi S, Steel KJA, Agrawal S, O'Byrne AM, Ridley M, Kordasti S, Frederiksen KS, Roberts CA, Taams LS. 2020. Anti-TNF treatment negatively regulates human CD4+ T-cell activation and maturation in vitro, but does not confer an anergic or suppressive phenotype. *Eur J Immunol* 50: 445–458. doi:10.1002/eji.201948190

Pritz T, Lair J, Ban M, Keller M, Weinberger B, Krismer M, Grubeck-Loebenstein B. 2015. Plasma cell numbers decrease in bone marrow of old patients. *Eur J Immunol* 45: 738–746. doi:10.1002/eji.201444878

Puchta A, Naidoo A, Verschoor CP, Loukov D, Thevaranjan N, Mandur TS, Nguyen PS, Jordana M, Loeb M, Xing Z, et al. 2016. TNF drives monocyte dysfunction with age and results in impaired anti-pneumococcal immunity. *PLoS Pathog* 12: e1005368. doi:10.1371/journal.ppat.1005368

Rampelli S, Soverini M, D'Amico F, Barone M, Tavella T, Monti D, Capri M, Astolfi A, Brigidi P, Biagi E, et al. 2020. Shotgun metagenomics of gut microbiota in humans with up to extreme longevity and the increasing role of xenobiotic degradation. *mSystems* 5: e00124-20. doi:10.1128/mSystems.00124-20

Ridker PM, Everett BM, Thuren T, MacFadyen JG, Chang WH, Ballantyne C, Fonseca F, Nicolau J, Koenig W, Anker SD, et al. 2017a. Antiinflammatory therapy with canakinumab for atherosclerotic disease. *N Engl J Med* 377: 1119–1131. doi:10.1056/NEJMoa1707914

Ridker PM, MacFadyen JG, Thuren T, Everett BM, Libby P, Glynn RJ, CANTOS Trial Group. 2017b. Effect of interleukin-1beta inhibition with canakinumab on incident lung cancer in patients with atherosclerosis: exploratory results from a randomised, double-blind, placebo-controlled trial. *Lancet* 390: 1833–1842.

Rodriguez IJ, Lalinde Ruiz N, Llano León M, Martínez Enríquez L, Montilla Velásquez MDP, Ortiz Aguirre JP, Rodríguez Bohórquez OM, Velandia Vargas EA, Hernández ED, Parra López CA. 2021. Immunosenescence study of T cells: a systematic review. *Front Immunol* 11: 604591. doi:10.3389/fimmu.2020.604591

Rubtsov AV, Rubtsova K, Fischer A, Meehan RT, Gillis JZ, Kappler JW, Marrack P. 2011. Toll-like receptor 7 (TLR7)–driven accumulation of a novel CD11c+ B-cell population is important for the development of autoimmunity. *Blood* 118: 1305–1315. doi:10.1182/blood-2011-01-331462

Rubtsova K, Rubtsov AV, Cancro MP, Marrack P. 2015. Age-associated B cells: a T-bet-dependent effector with roles in protective and pathogenic immunity. *J Immunol* 195: 1933–1937. doi:10.4049/jimmunol.1501209

Sabini E, O'Mahony A, Caturegli P. 2023. MyMD-1 improves health span and prolongs lifespan in old mice: a noninferiority study to rapamycin. *J Gerontol A Biol Sci Med Sci* 78: 227–235. doi:10.1093/gerona/glac142

Sakata-Kaneko S, Wakatsuki Y, Matsunaga Y, Usui T, Kita T. 2000. Altered Th1/Th2 commitment in human CD4+ T cells with ageing. *Clin Exp Immunol* 120: 267–273. doi:10.1046/j.1365-2249.2000.01224.x

Salas-Salvadó J, Becerra-Tomás N, García-Gavilán JF, Bulló M, Barrubés L. 2018. Mediterranean diet and cardiovascular disease prevention: what do we know? *Prog Cardiovasc Dis* **61:** 62–67. doi:10.1016/j.pcad.2018.04.006

Santoro A, Bientinesi E, Monti D. 2021. Immunosenescence and inflammaging in the aging process: age-related diseases or longevity? *Ageing Res Rev* **71:** 101422. doi:10.1016/j.arr.2021.101422

Sauce D, Dong Y, Campillo-Gimenez L, Casulli S, Bayard C, Autran B, Boddaert J, Appay V, Elbim C. 2017. Reduced oxidative burst by primed neutrophils in the elderly individuals is associated with increased levels of the CD16^{bright}/CD62L^{dim} immunosuppressive subset. *J Gerontol A Biol Sci Med Sci* **72:** 163–172. doi:10.1093/gerona/glw062

Sayed N, Huang Y, Nguyen K, Krejciova-Rajaniemi Z, Grawe AP, Gao T, Tibshirani R, Hastie T, Alpert A, Cui L, et al. 2021. An inflammatory aging clock (iAge) based on deep learning tracks multimorbidity, immunosenescence, frailty and cardiovascular aging. *Nat Aging* **1:** 598–615. doi:10.1038/s43587-021-00082-y

Schieker M, Conaghan PG, Mindeholm L, Praestgaard J, Solomon DH, Scotti C, Gram H, Thuren T, Roubenoff R, Ridker PM. 2020. Effects of interleukin-1β inhibition on incident hip and knee replacement: exploratory analyses from a randomized, double-blind, placebo-controlled trial. *Ann Intern Med* **173:** 509–515. doi:10.7326/M20-0527

Sciorati C, Gamberale R, Monno A, Citterio L, Lanzani C, De Lorenzo R, Ramirez GA, Esposito A, Manunta P, Manfredi AA, et al. 2020. Pharmacological blockade of TNFα prevents sarcopenia and prolongs survival in aging mice. *Aging (Albany NY)* **12:** 23497–23508. doi:10.18632/aging.202200

Selvarani R, Mohammed S, Richardson A. 2021. Effect of rapamycin on aging and age-related diseases—past and future. *Geroscience* **43:** 1135–1158. doi:10.1007/s11357-020-00274-1

Sen R, Smale ST. 2010. Selectivity of the NF-κB response. *Cold Spring Harb Perspect Biol* **2:** a000257.

Sharma R. 2021. Perspectives on the dynamic implications of cellular senescence and immunosenescence on macrophage aging biology. *Biogerontology* **22:** 571–587. doi:10.1007/s10522-021-09936-9

Shin J, Noh JR, Choe D, Lee N, Song Y, Cho S, Kang EJ, Go MJ, Ha SK, Chang DH, et al. 2021. Ageing and rejuvenation models reveal changes in key microbial communities associated with healthy ageing. *Microbiome* **9:** 240. doi:10.1186/s40168-021-01189-5

Shive C, Pandiyan P. 2022. Inflammation, immune senescence, and dysregulated immune regulation in the elderly. *Front Aging* **3:** 840827. doi:10.3389/fragi.2022.840827

Simell B, Vuorela A, Ekström N, Palmu A, Reunanen A, Meri S, Käyhty H, Väkeväinen M. 2011. Aging reduces the functionality of anti-pneumococcal antibodies and the killing of streptococcus pneumoniae by neutrophil phagocytosis. *Vaccine* **29:** 1929–1934. doi:10.1016/j.vaccine.2010.12.121

Singh H, Torralba MG, Moncera KJ, DiLello L, Petrini J, Nelson KE, Pieper R. 2019. Gastro-intestinal and oral microbiome signatures associated with healthy aging.

Geroscience **41:** 907–921. doi:10.1007/s11357-019-00098-8

Squarzoni S, Schena E, Sabatelli P, Mattioli E, Capanni C, Cenni V, D'Apice MR, Andrenacci D, Sarli G, Pellegrino V, et al. 2021. Interleukin-6 neutralization ameliorates symptoms in prematurely aged mice. *Aging Cell* **20:** e13285. doi:10.1111/acel.13285

Solá P, Mereu E, Bonjoch J, Casado M, Reina O, Blanco E, Esteller M, DiCroce L, Heyn H, Solanas G, et al. 2023. Targeting lymphoid-derived IL-17 signaling to delay skin aging. *Nat Aging* **3:** 688–704. doi:10.1038/s43587-023-00431-z

Songkiatisak P, Rahman SMT, Aqdas M, Sung MH. 2022. NF-κB, a culprit of both inflamm-ageing and declining immunity? *Immun Ageing* **19:** 20. doi:10.1186/s12979-022-00277-w

Tabibian-Keissar H, Hazanov L, Schiby G, Rosenthal N, Rakovsky A, Michaeli M, Shahaf GL, Pickman Y, Rosenblatt K, Melamed D, et al. 2016. Aging affects B-cell antigen receptor repertoire diversity in primary and secondary lymphoid tissues. *Eur J Immunol* **46:** 480–492. doi:10.1002/eji.201545586

Tam AB, Mercado EL, Hoffmann A, Niwa M. 2012. ER stress activates NF-κB by integrating functions of basal IKK activity, IRE1 and PERK. *PLoS ONE* **7:** e45078. doi:10.1371/journal.pone.0045078

Tanaka T, Talegawkar SA, Jin Y, Colpo M, Ferrucci L, Bandinelli S. 2018. Adherence to a Mediterranean diet protects from cognitive decline in the Invecchiare in Chianti study of aging. *Nutrients* **10:** 2007. doi:10.3390/nu10122007

Taniguchi K, Karin M. 2018. NF-κB, inflammation, immunity and cancer: coming of age. *Nat Rev Immunol* **18:** 309–324. doi:10.1038/nri.2017.142

Tavenier J, Rasmussen LJH, Houlind MB, Andersen AL, Panum I, Andersen O, Petersen J, Langkilde A, Nehlin JO. 2020. Alterations of monocyte NF-κB p65/RelA signaling in a cohort of older medical patients, age-matched controls, and healthy young adults. *Immun Ageing* **17:** 25. doi:10.1186/s12979-020-00197-7

Teissier T, Boulanger E, Cox LS. 2022. Interconnections between inflammageing and immunosenescence during ageing. *Cells* **11:** 359. doi:10.3390/cells11030359

Thevaranjan N, Puchta A, Schulz C, Naidoo A, Szamosi JC, Verschoor CP, Loukov D, Schenck LP, Jury J, Foley KP, et al. 2017. Age-associated microbial dysbiosis promotes intestinal permeability, systemic inflammation, and macrophage dysfunction. *Cell Host Microbe* **21:** 455–466.e4. doi:10.1016/j.chom.2017.03.002

Tilstra JS, Robinson AR, Wang J, Gregg SQ, Clauson CL, Reay DP, Nasto LA, St Croix CM, Usas A, Vo N, et al. 2012. NF-κB inhibition delays DNA damage-induced senescence and aging in mice. *J Clin Invest* **122:** 2601–2612. doi:10.1172/JCI45785

Tsigalou C, Konstantinidis T, Paraschaki A, Stavropoulou E, Voidarou C, Bezirtzoglou E. 2020. Mediterranean diet as a tool to combat inflammation and chronic diseases. An overview. *Biomedicines* **8:** 201.

Vallurupalli M, MacFadyen JG, Glynn RJ, Thuren T, Libby P, Berliner N, Ridker PM. 2020. Effects of interleukin-1β inhibition on incident anemia: exploratory analyses

Cite this article as *Cold Spring Harb Perspect Med* doi: 10.1101/cshperspect.a041197

from a randomized trial. *Ann Intern Med* **172**: 523–532. doi:10.7326/M19-2945

Verma N, Dimitrova M, Carter DM, Crevar CJ, Ross TM, Golding H, Khurana S. 2012. Influenza virus H1N1pdm09 infections in the young and old: evidence of greater antibody diversity and affinity for the hemagglutinin globular head domain (HA1 domain) in the elderly than in young adults and children. *J Virol* **86**: 5515–5522. doi:10.1128/JVI.07085-11

Walford RL. 1969. Immunologische aspekte des alterns [Immunologic aspects of aging]. *Klin Wochenschr* **47**: 599–605. doi:10.1007/BF01876949

Walker KA, Basisty N, Wilson DM 3rd, Ferrucci L. 2022. Connecting aging biology and inflammation in the omics era. *J Clin Invest* **132**: e158448. doi:10.1172/JCI158448

Wang S, Wang J, Kumar V, Karnell JL, Naiman B, Gross PS, Rahman S, Zerrouki K, Hanna R, Morehouse C, et al. 2018. IL-21 drives expansion and plasma cell differentiation of autoreactive CD11c^{hi}T-bet$^+$ B cells in SLE. *Nat Commun* **9**: 1758. doi:10.1038/s41467-018-03750-7

Wang Y, Hao Q, Su L, Liu Y, Liu S, Dong B. 2018. Adherence to the Mediterranean diet and the risk of frailty in old people: a systematic review and meta-analysis. *J Nutr Health Aging* **22**: 613–618. doi:10.1007/s12603-018-1020-x

Wendt K, Wilk E, Buyny S, Buer J, Schmidt RE, Jacobs R. 2006. Gene and protein characteristics reflect functional diversity of CD56^{dim} and CD56^{bright} NK cells. *J Leukoc Biol* **80**: 1529–1541. doi:10.1189/jlb.0306191

Weng N, Akbar AN, Goronzy J. 2009. CD28$^-$ T cells: their role in the age-associated decline of immune function. *Trends Immunol* **30**: 306–312. doi:10.1016/j.it.2009.03.013

Wenisch C, Patruta S, Daxböck F, Krause R, Hörl W. 2000. Effect of age on human neutrophil function. *J Leukoc Biol* **67**: 40–45. doi:10.1002/jlb.67.1.40

Woods RL, Espinoza S, Thao LTP, Ernst ME, Ryan J, Wolfe R, Shah RC, Ward SA, Storey E, Nelson MR, et al. 2021. Effect of aspirin on activities of daily living disability in community-dwelling older adults. *J Gerontol A Biol Sci Med Sci* **76**: 2007–2014. doi:10.1093/gerona/glaa316

Yang X, Wang X, Lei L, Sun L, Jiao A, Zhu K, Xie T, Liu H, Zhang X, Su Y, et al. 2021. Age-related gene alteration in naive and memory T cells using precise age-tracking model. *Front Cell Dev Biol* **8**: 624380. doi:10.3389/fcell.2020.624380

Yousefzadeh MJ, Flores RR, Zhu Y, Schmiechen ZC, Brooks RW, Trussoni CE, Cui Y, Angelini L, Lee KA, McGowan SJ, et al. 2021. An aged immune system drives senescence and ageing of solid organs. *Nature* **594**: 100–105. doi:10.1038/s41586-021-03547-7

Zhang L, Zhao J, Mu X, McGowan SJ, Angelini L, O'Kelly RD, Yousefzadeh MJ, Sakamoto A, Aversa Z, LeBrasseur NK, et al. 2021. Novel small molecule inhibition of IKK/NF-κB activation reduces markers of senescence and improves healthspan in mouse models of aging. *Aging Cell* **20**: e13486.

Mitochondrial Targeted Interventions for Aging

Sophia Z. Liu,[1] Ying Ann Chiao,[2] Peter S. Rabinovitch,[3] and David J. Marcinek[1]

[1]Department of Radiology, University of Washington, Seattle, Washington 98195, USA

[2]Aging and Metabolism Research Program, Oklahoma Medical Research Foundation, Oklahoma City, Oklahoma 73104, USA

[3]Department of Laboratory Medicine and Pathology, University of Washington, Seattle, Washington 98195, USA

Correspondence: dmarc@uw.edu

Changes in mitochondrial function play a critical role in the basic biology of aging and age-related disease. Mitochondria are typically thought of in the context of ATP production and oxidant production. However, it is clear that the mitochondria sit at a nexus of cell signaling where they affect metabolite, redox, and energy status, which influence many factors that contribute to the biology of aging, including stress responses, proteostasis, epigenetics, and inflammation. This has led to growing interest in identifying mitochondrial targeted interventions to delay or reverse age-related decline in function and promote healthy aging. In this review, we discuss the diverse roles of mitochondria in the cell. We then highlight some of the most promising strategies and compounds to target aging mitochondria in preclinical testing. Finally, we review the strategies and compounds that have advanced to clinical trials to test their ability to improve health in older adults.

MITOCHONDRIA IN AGING BIOLOGY

This is an exciting time to be studying mitochondria and aging, as there is now a well-established and important role for mitochondrial function in the biology of aging and age-related diseases. As a result, there is intensifying interest in developing strategies that target mitochondrial function to delay, slow, and reverse aging pathology and the decline in quality of life. Mitochondria play many roles in the cell and, despite this growing interest in mitochondrial targeted therapies, there is still a knowledge gap around the key aspects of mitochondrial function that drive aging and whether these are tissue specific or represent common mechanisms across multiple tissues. In this work, we will provide a brief overview of the roles that mitochondria play in the cell, their relationships to aging, and highlight some of the promising strategies being pursued to target mitochondria in preclinical studies and clinical trials. This is not meant to be a comprehensive review of the literature of mitochondria in aging biology, but instead we provide a brief background and highlight some of the most promising mitochondrial targeted interventions with clinical relevance for improving quality of life in our rapidly aging population (Fig. 1).

Mitochondria play a central role in cellular physiology and sit at the nexus integrating environmental and cell stressors with cell signaling

Cite this article as *Cold Spring Harb Perspect Med* doi: 10.1101/cshperspect.a041199

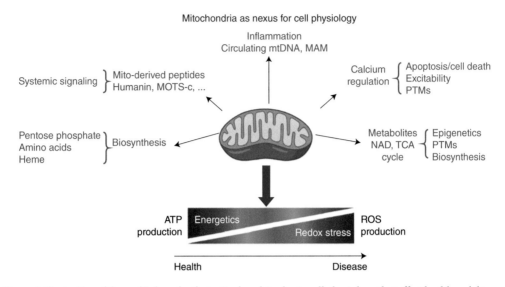

Figure 1. Illustration of the multiples roles that mitochondria play in cell physiology that affect health and disease.

and energetics that ultimately lead to adaptive or pathological responses. Mitochondria has traditionally been thought of in terms of cell ATP production or as the main source of oxidants in most cells. In fact, one of the earliest links between mitochondria and aging was proposed by Harman in 1972 (Harman 1972) when he implicated the mitochondria as the primary source of free radicals underlying the free radical theory of aging (Harman 1956). However, it is now clear that ATP production and redox homeostasis represent only a subset of the ways in which mitochondria communicate with the cytoplasm, nucleus, and the other cells to affect cellular health, and thus aging.

Mitochondrial Bioenergetics

Mitochondria are double-membrane organelles that originated evolutionarily through an endosymbiotic process where an alphaproteobacterium combined with a primitive eukaryotic cell (Sagan 1967). Most of the original bacterial genome has been transferred to the eukaryotic nucleus, but mitochondria maintain an independent circular genome that, in mammals, encodes for 13 protein subunits that are part of every complex of the electron transport system (ETS), except complex II, as well as mitochon-

drial tRNAs and ribosomal RNAs (Sanchez-Contreras et al. 2021). Mitochondria generate the majority of cellular ATP necessary to meet cell energy demands for growth, maintenance, stress response, and mechanical work through a process called oxidative phosphorylation. In the mitochondrial matrix carbohydrates, lipids, and amino acids are oxidized to generate NADH and $FADH_2$ through the tricarboxylic acid cycle (TCA) and β-oxidation. NADH and $FADH_2$ provide reducing equivalents (i.e., electrons) to the ETS located on the inner membrane of the mitochondria (Michal 1999) where they are used to pump protons from the matrix into the inner membrane space to generate a membrane potential that is used to drive ATP production as protons pass back into the matrix through the F1F0 ATP synthase (also known as complex V). ATP from the matrix is transported out of the matrix where it can be used in energy-consuming reactions by the cell in exchange for ADP, which is itself transported into the matrix by the adenine nucleotide transporter (ANT) (Nicholls and Ferguson 2002). The structure of the inner membrane, which is organized into tight folds called cristae that increase the membrane surface area for the inner membrane proteins that make up the complexes of the ETS, is critical for effective oxidative phos-

Cite this article as *Cold Spring Harb Perspect Med* doi: 10.1101/cshperspect.a041199

phorylation. In fact, swelling of the matrix and disorganized cristae is a common morphological sign of mitochondrial dysfunction (Taub et al. 2012).

Mitochondrial Redox Biology

Mitochondria are also a significant source of oxidants in most cells. During oxidative phosphorylation, electrons can leak from multiple sites in the ETS and react with molecular oxygen to form superoxide (Goncalves et al. 2015). Under typical conditions in most tissues, the primary sites of superoxide formation are from complex I and complex III of the ETS (Goncalves et al. 2015). Mitochondrial superoxide generation is membrane potential dependent, meaning that under conditions where membrane potential is high (e.g., normal respiratory function) but there is low ATP production, mitochondria generate more superoxide (Nicholls 2004). Inhibition or disruption of flux through the ETS can also lead to elevated superoxide production. In addition to the ETS, several matrix dehydrogenases can also generate superoxide, including pyruvate dehydrogenase, α-ketoglutarate dehydrogenase, and glutamate dehydrogenase; but under most conditions, these contribute less than the ETS sources to mitochondria oxidant production (Goncalves et al. 2015). Because superoxide is highly reactive and can induce oxidative damage to macromolecules, the mitochondria contain antioxidant systems to detoxify superoxide. Superoxide dismutase (SOD2 in the matrix and SOD1 in the inner membrane space) is a highly efficient enzyme that rapidly converts superoxide into hydrogen peroxide (H_2O_2). H_2O_2 is less reactive than superoxide and can travel greater distances within the matrix and cell. In the matrix, H_2O_2 is converted to water either by the glutathione (GSH) peroxidase system using GSH as an intermediate or the peroxiredoxin–thioredoxin system. Both systems rely on NADPH, which is linked to NAD in the matrix and the cytoplasm. In addition to their important role in detoxifying superoxide, these redox intermediates, Prx, Trx, GSH:GSSG, and H_2O_2, play important roles in redox signaling under-

lying stress response pathways (Rohrbach et al. 2006; Garcia et al. 2010; Mailloux et al. 2012). Disrupted redox homeostasis linked to mitochondrial dysfunction with age is associated with many of the hallmarks of aging in worms, mice, and humans.

Mitochondrial Metabolites in Aging

Mitochondria are also important regulators of intermediate metabolites that play an important role in regulating diverse cellular processes. In addition to their role in energy metabolism, TCA-cycle intermediates play key roles regulating gene expression and cell signaling that contribute to aging (Martínez-Reyes et al. 2016; Martínez-Reyes and Chandel 2020). Acetyl CoA is the common point of entry into the TCA for both pyruvate, following glycolysis, and fatty acids from β-oxidation and is also produced in the cytosol from citrate. It also contributes the acetyl group for acetylation of proteins and histones that drive epigenetic regulation of gene expression, both of which contribute to aging pathology. Elevating acetyl CoA in the brains of SAMP8 mice reduced brain aging (Currais et al. 2019). The concentration of α-ketoglutarate ([AKG] 2-oxoglutarate), the entry point for glutamate into the TCA cycle, also affects epigenetic regulation due to its role as a substrate for 2-oxoglutarate dioxygenases (Martínez-Reyes et al. 2016). AKG levels decrease in mammalian aging and alter epigenetics in multiple tissues. Elevating AKG levels reverses age-related pathology and cellular changes, including hearing loss, osteoporosis, and inflammation and extends lifespan in mouse models of aging (Asadi Shahmirzadi et al. 2020). Both fumarate and succinate, which are just upstream of AKG in the TCA, can also affect epigenetic regulation by inhibiting 2-oxoglutarate dehydrogenases (Ishii et al. 1998; Gallo et al. 2011; Edwards et al. 2013; Lima et al. 2022). NAD is a metabolic cofactor involved in multiple steps of the TCA cycle where it is reduced to NADH to provide electrons for complex I of the ETS. There is strong evidence that a decline in NAD levels with age is a driver of multiple age-related pathologies (Yoshino et al. 2018). This is due to its prolific role as a cofactor for enzymes involved in DNA damage response (PARP) and protein deacetylation (sirtuins). Defects in mitochondrial function, particularly in complex I activity, alter the NAD/NADH ratio and disrupt NAD homeostasis (Karamanlidis et al. 2013). Since defects in complex I function are common in aging tissues, this may contribute to reduced NAD with age (Karamanlidis et al. 2013). In a negative feedforward cycle, the decline in NAD further impairs mitochondrial function by leading to elevated acetylation though inhibition of sirtuin activity or increased pathological inflammation. This is supported by multiple reports showing that elevating NAD by supplementing with NAD precursors, nicotinamide riboside (NR) or nicotinamide mononucleotide (NMN), or inhibiting PARP activity to preserve NAD can prevent or reverse mitochondrial dysfunction and tissue degeneration (Ryu et al. 2016; Yoshino et al. 2018; Whitson et al. 2020; Romani et al. 2021). Given the systemic and prolific nature of the contribution of NAD and other TCA cycle metabolites to aging biology, maintaining metabolite homeostasis represents a potential mechanism by which preserved mitochondrial function could contribute to healthy aging.

Mitochondrial Calcium Homeostasis and Aging

Another important way in which mitochondria contribute to cell signaling is through their effect on calcium homeostasis. This effect is especially important in excitable cells like neurons and cardiac and skeletal muscle fibers. Mitochondria are typically in close physical association with the endoplasmic reticulum (ER)/sarcoplasmic reticulum, where they are poised to take up calcium upon release. This mitochondrial calcium uptake regulates mitochondrial ATP production by enhancing the activity of several dehydrogenases of the TCA cycle (Rossi et al. 2019). However, excessive calcium uptake also leads to elevated mitochondrial oxidant production and the opening of the mitochondrial permeability transition pore (mPTP) leading to the induction of cell death through apoptosis or necrosis. With age, mitochondria become more sensitized to

calcium uptake resulting in a lower threshold for mPTP opening and cell death (Picard et al. 2010; Zhang et al. 2020a). Elevated mitochondrial redox stress can also contribute to calcium-induced stress through redox-dependent posttranslation of the ryanodine receptor that leads to increased calcium leak from the ER (Andersson et al. 2011; Umanskaya et al. 2014). This dysregulation of calcium homeostasis contributes to cardiac and skeletal muscle dysfunction in aging mice, which can be prevented by reducing mitochondrial oxidant production by expressing mitochondrial catalase (mCAT)

Mitochondrial Quality Control in Aging

The mitochondrial unfolded protein response (mUPR) is typically discussed in the context of proteotoxic stress, but can also be initiated by other aspects of mitochondrial dysfunction such as impaired oxidative phosphorylation or elevated redox stress (Feng et al. 2001; Liu et al. 2005; Dell'agnello et al. 2007). When the mUPR is activated, the transcription factors ATF4 (ATF1 in *Caenorhabditis elegans*), ATF5, and CHOP are transported to the nucleus where they initiate transcription of multiple chaperones and proteases that act to restore proteostasis (Shpilka and Haynes 2018). Elevated mUPR is a key component of the beneficial effects of transient mitochondrial stress (hormesis) on aging and longevity induced by disruption of the electron transport chain or elevated redox stress early in life. Impaired regulation of the mUPR is associated with the loss of proteostasis in sarcopenia, Parkinson's (PD), and Alzheimer's disease (AD) (Ji et al. 2020; Urbina-Varela et al. 2020; Lin et al. 2022).

In the presence of more extreme mitochondrial stress, the cell mitochondria are engulfed by autophagosomes in a process called mitophagy. Depending on cell type, there are multiple mitophagy pathways that have been documented (Fivenson et al. 2017). The most common mitophagy pathway in mammals is the PINK/Parkin pathway. The process can be induced by decreasing membrane potential in damaged mitochondria, which activates PINK1 and phosphorylation of the E3 ubiquitin ligase Parkin, further activating ubiquitin-binding domains of autophagy liquid chromatography (LC) adaptor and the formation of autophagosome. The autophagosome then fuses with the lysosome resulting in formation of autophagosomes for degradation (Lazarou et al. 2015). Mitophagy can also occur in a ubiquitin-independent pathway where, upon mitochondrial stress, autophagy receptors are recruited to the outer mitochondrial membrane (OMM), which then recruit LC3 and autophagosomes to the mitochondria (Iorio et al. 2022). In addition, several mitophagy proteins also work in the PINK1/Parkin independent pathway, such as Ambra1, Nix, a member of Bcl-2 family, and FUNDC1 (Iorio et al. 2022).

Reduced mitophagy with age has been identified in many tissues, including mouse heart, brain, and skeletal muscle and is a contributor to neurodegenerative disease. Enhanced mitophagy to maintain mitochondrial quality control is a key aspect of the beneficial effects of exercise on skeletal muscle function (Zhang et al. 2020b). Interventions that elevate mitophagy, such as spermidine and urolithin a (discussed more below), also have been demonstrated to have a positive effect on skeletal muscle function and cognitive impairment in mouse models (Ryu et al. 2016; Fan et al. 2017; Schroeder et al. 2021). Maintaining mitochondrial quality control through efficient mitophagy is not only important to maintain well-functioning mitochondria, but also to prevent the release of mitochondrial components into the cytoplasm and circulation as damage-associated molecular patterns (DAMPs). mtDNA and other macromolecules released into the cytosol from improperly degraded mitochondria stimulate the release of proinflammatory cytokines through the activation of the NLRP3 inflammasome or the stimulator of interferon gene (STING) pathways (Zhang et al. 2019; Chen et al. 2021; Masumoto et al. 2021; Lin et al. 2022; Qiu et al. 2022).

Mitochondrial-Derived Peptides in Aging

Mitochondrial-derived peptides (MDPs) provide another example of systemic mitochondrial signaling to affect organismal health (Kim et al. 2021). Mammalian mtDNA is known to encode 13 mRNAs for proteins of the ETS, 22 tRNAs, and 2 rRNAs. In the last several years, the presence of several open reading frames that encode small peptides has been demonstrated. The two most well described MDPs are humanin and MOTS-c, although several other MDPs have been recently described (D'Souza et al. 2020; Miller et al. 2022). Both humanin and MOTS-c are involved in multiple signaling pathways and decline with age in rodents and humans (Yen et al. 2018). Humanin has been found to promote cell survival by inhibiting cytochrome c release by interacting with proapoptotic proteins, localizing to the lysosomal membrane and promote chaperone-mediated autophagy, and interact with the IGF-1 pathway (Xiao et al. 2016; Qin et al. 2018; Kim et al. 2022). At the organ and organismal scale, humanin may provide protection from cardiovascular disease, cognitive decline, and AD pathology. MOTS-c has been referred to as an exercise mimetic for its ability to improve metabolic phenotype and activate AMPK and NRF2 signaling in skeletal muscle (Yang et al. 2021). High-intensity exercise increased levels of MOTS-c in both skeletal muscle and plasma of humans. Both humanin and MOTS-c administered to aged mice improve function and reverse some pathological effects of aging.

MITOCHONDRIAL TARGETED THERAPIES

Antioxidants are the most well-studied class of compounds and supplements related to mitochondrial function and aging. As has been well documented, the effect of an antioxidant strategy in clinical trials has been mixed at best (Peternelj and Coombes 2011). A recent randomized trial with 35,000 healthy women aged 45 and above showed no beneficial effect with 10 yr vitamin E supplementation for cardiovascular health and total mortality (Lee et al. 2005). Similarly, the HOPE trial indicated a potential increased risk of heart failure in the vitamin E daily supplementation group (Lonn et al. 2005). These large epidemiology studies have challenged the idea that supplementation with antioxidants is universally beneficial. However, more targeted strategies to alter mitochondrial oxidative stress have shown some promise. Other approaches now include natural and pharmaceutical interventions that directly interact with components of the mitochondria or enhance mitochondrial quality and turnover.

Mitoquinone (MitoQ)

One strategy for mitochondrial targeted antioxidants takes advantage of the negative charge across the inner mitochondrial membrane (IMM) to deliver antioxidant agents to the mitochondrial matrix using triphenylphosphonium ion (TPP^+). The beneficial effects of these TPP^+-conjugated antioxidants have been demonstrated in preclinical models of aging and age-related diseases as described below. One of these antioxidants is MitoQ, which is a TPP^+-conjugated ubiquinone. MitoQ selectively concentrates in the mitochondria and prevents mitochondrial oxidative damage. It has been shown to prolong life span of SOD-deficient flies and improve pathology associated with antioxidant deficiency (Magwere et al. 2006). MitoQ shows beneficial effects in multiple models of neurodegeneration. In transgenic C. elegans with muscle-specific expression of human amyloid-β peptide (Aβ), a model of AD, MitoQ extends life span and improves health span of C. elegans while the ROS production, protein carbonyl content, and mtDNA damage burden remain unchanged (Ng et al. 2014). In in vitro models, MitoQ protects against Aβ-toxicity in primary neurons of amyloid precursor protein (APP) transgenic mice and in neuroblastoma cells treated with Aβ (Manczak et al. 2010). In vivo, 5-mo MitoQ treatment prevents cognitive decline and AD-like neuropathology in a widely used mouse model of AD (3xTg-AD mice), supporting the therapeutic benefits of MitoQ in AD (Mc-Manus et al. 2011). MitoQ treatment also shows neuroprotective effects in cell culture and mouse models of PD (Ghosh et al. 2010). In addition to its neuroprotective effects, MitoQ confers cardioprotection in multiple models of cardiovascular disease (Adlam et al. 2005; Graham et al. 2009; Supinski et al. 2009; Dare et al. 2015). MitoQ treatment reduces ischemia reperfusion (IR) injury in mouse and rat models of IR (Adlam et al. 2005; Mukhopadhyay et al. 2012; Dare et al. 2015). In

spontaneous hypertensive rats, 8-wk MitoQ treatment reduced systolic blood pressure and attenuated cardiac hypertrophy (Graham et al. 2009). Despite its promise in animal models, MitoQ showed no effect on the progression of PD symptoms over 12 mo (Snow et al. 2010). This is currently under investigation for age-related vascular dysfunction (NCT04851288, NCT02597023).

Skq1

Another TPP^+-conjugated antioxidant SkQ1 is a TPP^+-conjugated plastoquinone. SkQ1 treatment extends the life span of Podospora, Ceriodaphnia, Drosophila, female outbred SHR mice, male BALB/c, and C57Bl/6 mice (Anisimov et al. 2008, 2011). OXYS rats are a model of accelerated aging and develop a wide range of accelerated aging phenotypes, including cataract, retinopathy, and high blood pressure (Solov'eva et al. 1975). In senescence-accelerated OXYS rats, dietary SkQ1 treatment ameliorates age-related cataract and retinopathy (Neroev et al. 2008). Eye drops containing SkQ1 reverse cataract and retinopathy in young to middle-aged OXYS rats and prevent the development of uveitis and glaucoma in rabbit models (Neroev et al. 2008). In both Wistar and OXYS rats, 4-mo dietary SkQ1 treatment prevents the age-related declines in age-related biomarkers like growth hormone (GH) and insulin-like growth factor 1 (IGF-1) (Kolosova et al. 2012). In addition, studies also suggest that SkQ1 is protective against cardiac, renal, and brain IR injuries (Bakeeva et al. 2008). SkQO1 has shown some promise in clinical trials of dry eye syndrome (NCT02121301) but has not been tested for aging or age-related pathologies in humans.

MitoTEMPO

MitoTEMPO is a TPP^+-conjugated piperidine nitroxide (Trnka et al. 2008). In an ex vivo study, MitoTEMPO treatment enhances contractile function of hearts and aortic rings isolated from aged rats, normalizing the age-related impairments (Olgar et al. 2018). Ex vivo Mito-TEMPO treatment also attenuates age-related changes in electrical activities of aged rat cardiomyocytes and is associated with an antiarrhythmic benefit (Olgar et al. 2020). Moreover, in vivo treatment with MitoTEMPO is protective in multiple preclinical models of age-related cardiovascular diseases, including pressure-overload-induced heart failure, diabetic cardiomyopathy, and hypertension (Dikalova et al. 2010; Ni et al. 2016; Dey et al. 2018). In a mouse model of hind limb ischemia, MitoTEMPO treatment enhances mitochondrial function and attenuates the age-related decline in blood flow recovery in aged skeletal muscles (Miura et al. 2017). In addition, MitoTEMPO also ameliorates muscle wasting in mice with chronic kidney disease (Liu et al. 2020).

Due to the dependence on mitochondrial membrane potential for mitochondrial targeting, the delivery of TPP^+-conjugated antioxidants to mitochondria will be diminished when mitochondrial membrane potential is compromised in pathological conditions. Another limitation of these TPP^+-conjugated antioxidants is that they can inhibit mitochondrial respiration and disrupt mitochondrial membrane potential at high concentrations (Kelso et al. 2001; Antonenko et al. 2008; Pokrzywinski et al. 2016). These antioxidants have been shown to process pro-oxidant properties at high concentrations; therefore, extra precautions are needed to be taken to determine the optimal dosages that exert antioxidant effects but not pro-oxidant activities.

Astaxanthin

Astaxanthin (AX) is one of the most powerful carotenoid compounds and has gained special interest during recent decades due to its strong antioxidant activity, anti-inflammatory effects and potential to preserve health span with age (Kidd 2011). Its unique structure spanning the membrane bilayer can scavenge ROS in both inner and outer layers of membrane unlike other antioxidants act either at the inner (vitamin E and β-carotene) or outer membrane (vitamin C) (Kidd 2011; Vrolijk et al. 2015; Sztretye et al. 2019). In comparison with several other carotenoids (zeaxanthin, lutein, and lycopene), AX demonstrated the greatest reduction in lipid peroxidation while preserving membrane structure.

In addition, Kidd (2011) also reported AX-lowering plasma biomarkers of lipid peroxidation in humans. Furthermore, AX also exhibits unique benefits of improving fat oxidation, improving muscle fatigability, and enhancing exercise endurance in both aged mice and older adults. In preclinical studies, AX improved fat oxidation in mice through increased coimmunoprecipitation of fatty acyl transferase (FAT/CD36) with carnitine palmitoyltransferase I (CPTI), and AX reduced oxidative stress-induced modification of CPTI by hexanoyl-lysine adduct (HEL) (Ikeuchi et al. 2006; Aoi et al. 2008).

Astaxanthin has been consumed by humans as a supplement for 30 yr. There is growing evidence showing AX improves athletic performance and exercise capacity and reduces injury markers (Earnest et al. 2011; Djordjevic et al. 2012). Due to its benefits on muscle and cardiovascular health, AX as supplementation for more vulnerable populations such as older adults has gained more interest. A recent study that paired AX treatment with exercise training in older adults reported that adding AX supplementation improved muscle strength and muscle endurance in the tibialis anterior muscle compared with exercise alone (Liu et al. 2018). The improved muscle function in this group was associated with metabolic benefits of the AX supplementation, including improved fat oxidation during lower intensity exercise (Liu et al. 2021). These results point to a beneficial effect of AX supplementation to improve exercise-induced metabolic adaptation under low-intensity stimulus. Unfortunately, this study did not collect tissues to specifically measure differences in adaptive signaling associated with the functional improvements. The same study also reported sex-dependent increases in exercise efficiency and reduced CHO oxidation in older males, but not females. This study points to the value of clinical trials that combine exercise training with mitochondrial-targeted treatment, especially with nutraceutical supplements, to test strategies to enhance a healthy lifestyle in older populations.

There are many other natural products currently being investigated for their beneficial effects on mitochondrial and aging recently reviewed in detail (Liang et al. 2021). For example, a recent review of pipeline drugs for AD over the past 5 yr indicated 121 agents in 136 trials of AD therapies. Among those in phase 3: tricaprilin, ginkgo biloba, and ANAVEX2-73 (blarcamesine) were targeted for mitochondria dysfunction (Cummings et al. 2020). The mechanisms of action of these natural products are typically not straightforward and their functions are frequently defined by their effect on specific mitochondrial or cellular processes such as oxidative stress, as in the carotenoid astaxanthin discussed above, mitochondrial membrane potential, mitochondrial mitophagy, as in urolithin a discussed below, or biogenesis. One example of a compound derived from a plant-based natural product is J147. J147 is a derivative of curcumin, a plant-based compound with antioxidant and anti-inflammatory activities. J147 improves on the bioavailability of curcumin and possesses neurotrophic activity (Peterson and Popkin 1980). Due to its neurotrophic activity, studies with J147 have focused on neurodegenerative diseases. Several preclinical reports suggest a beneficial effect of J147 treatment in rodent models of AD (Kepchia et al. 2021). Recently, J147 has been demonstrated to target the ATP5A subunit of the mitochondrial ATP synthase (complex V) (Goldberg et al. 2018). Recently, J147 has been shown to inhibit the mitochondrial ATPsynthase, elevate mitochondrial membrane potential and ROS production, and modulate AMPK/mTOR signaling. The effect on membrane potential and ROS signaling appears to contribute to an effect of J147 treatment on calcium homeostasis that leads to altered downstream signaling (Kepchia et al. 2021). Like many of the natural-derived compounds the details of the mechanism of action of J147 on AD and aging remain to be worked out. However, based on data from rodent models of AD and the SAMP8 accelerated aging model, there is clear potential for J147 as a mitochondrial targeted strategy for extending health span (Prior et al. 2016; Kepchia et al. 2022). As a shared target for both aging and dementia, J147 is currently in phase I clinical trial (NCT03838185). This phase I clinical trial is intended to test the biosafety of this compound with a secondary goal of testing for a clinically meaningful effect on cognitive function among both young and old adults (Table 1).

Elamipretide

The Szeto–Schiller (SS) peptides are tetrapeptides with an alternating aromatic–cationic amino acids motif that were serendipitously found to preferentially concentrate in the IMM (Zhao et al. 2004; Doughan and Dikalov 2007; Bakeeva et al. 2008). Elamipretide, also referred to as SS-31 peptide, is the most studied member of the SS peptide family. It was later shown that the mitochondrial localization of elamipretide was conferred by its strong affinity with cardiolipin (CL), a phospholipid exclusively found in the mitochondrial membranes (Birk et al. 2014). The mitochondrial uptake of elamipretide is independent of the mitochondrial membrane potential, and, therefore, elamipretide can be taken up by depolarized mitochondria (Zhao et al. 2004; Doughan and Dikalov 2007). Originally thought to act as an ROS scavenger in the mitochondria, it is now clear that elamipretide reduces production of oxidants by the ETS (Szeto 2014; Birk et al. 2014). In vitro studies show that elamipretide increases oxygen consumption and ATP production in mitochondria (Birk et al. 2014). Its interaction with CL stabilizes cristae structure (Brown et al. 2014; Szeto 2014) and alters the charge distribution around the IMM (Mitchell et al. 2020). Recently it has been shown that elamipretide directly interacts with several proteins in the IMM, including the ANT, F1FO ATP synthase, and complexes I and III of the ETC (Chavez et al. 2020).

Studies have demonstrated the protective effects of elamipretide in cardiac aging and age-related cardiovascular disease. In mouse models of pressure-overload induced heart failure, elamipretide attenuates cardiac hypertrophy and improves cardiac function (Dai et al. 2011, 2012, 2013). The protective effects of elamipretide have also been demonstrated in a canine model of heart failure (Sabbah et al. 2012, 2016). In the canine model, 2-h elamipretide treatment improves ejection fraction, stroke volume, cardiac output, and left ventricle (LV) con-

Table 1. Rodent model ischemia reperfusion (IR) injury

Preclinical	Intervention	Model	Physiology/phenotype	References
	MitoQ	Transgenic *Caenorhabditis elegans* mode of Alzheimer's disease (AD)	Extends life span, delays Aβ-induced paralysis, but no change in ROS, protein carbonyl content, or mtDNA damage	Ng et al. 2014
		Wild-type and SOD-deficient flies	Prolongs life span only in SOD-deficient flies	Magwere et al. 2006
		AD mouse model	Protects against Aβ-toxicity	Manczak et al. 2010
		AD mouse model	Prevents cognitive decline	McManus et al. 2011
		Mouse model of Parkinson's disease (PD)	Neuroprotection effects	Ghosh et al. 2010
		Hypertension rat	Reduces systolic blood pressure and attenuates cardiac hypertrophy	Graham et al. 2009
	SkQ1	Accelerates aging mouse model	Accelerates aging mouse model	Neroev et al. 2008
		Accelerates aging rabbit model	Prevents the development of uveitis and glaucoma	Neroev et al. 2008
		Accelerates aging rat model	Prevents age-related decline in growth hormone (GH) and insulin-like growth factor 1 (IGF-1)	Kolosova et al. 2012
	MitoTEMPO	Aged rat	Enhances contractile function of hearts and aortic rings	Olgar et al. 2018
		Aged rat	Attenuates age-related changes in electrical activities; antiarrhythmic benefit	Olgar et al. 2020
		Aged mice under limb ischemia	Improves mitochondria function and blood flow in skeletal muscle	Miura et al. 2017
		Mice with chronic kidney disease (CKD)	Reduces muscle wasting	Liu et al. 2020
	Astaxanthin	Aged mice	Improves muscle fatigability, endurance, and fatty acid utilization	Ikeuchi et al. 2006
	J147	Rodent model of AD	Inhibits mitochondria ATP synthase; elevates membrane potential and ROS	Pior et al. 2016; Kepchia et al. 2018
	Elamipretide	Rodent model of heart failure (HF)	Reduces cardiac hypertrophy and improves cardiac function	Dai et al. 2011, 2012, 2013
		Canine model of HF	Ejection fraction, stroke volume, cardiac output, and left ventricle (LV) contractility	Sabbah et al. 2016
		Rodent model of IR injury	Preserves cardiac function after IR injury	Petri et al. 2006; Szeto et al. 2008
		Aged mice	8-wk reverse cardiac aging phonotype: hypertrophy, diastolic	Chiao et al. 2020

Continued

Table 1. *Continued*

Preclinical	Intervention	Model	Physiology/phenotype	References
		Rodent aging model	ATP production and fatigue resistance after 1 h single injection	Siegel et al. 2013
		Aged rodent	8-wk improvement in mitochondrial function, redox homeostasis, and exercise tolerance	Campbell et al. 2019
	Spermidine	Rodent aging model	4-wk supplementation improved autophagy; reduced of LV	Eisenberg et al. 2016
		Rodent stem cell	2-wk treatment maintain regeneration and reduced protein	Eisenberg et al. 2009
	Urolithin A (UA)	*C. elegans*	Extends life span and increases expression of mitogene and respiration capacity in aged	Ryu et al. 2016
		Rodent	Improves exercise tolerance in old mice and rat	

Clinical	Intervention	Model	Physiology response	References	Clinical trial #
	Humanin	Blood	Higher circulation level in children of centenarians compared to control	Yen et al. 2020	NCT03431844
	Elamipretide	Skeletal muscle	Improves mitochondria function (ATP_{max}) 2 h postinjection	Roshanravan et al. 2021	NCT02245620
		HF	Single infusion is safe	Daubert et al. 2017	NCT02388464
			High-dose ELAM-positive changes in LV volume		
		Barth syndrome	Improves 6 min walk and knee extensor strength at 36 wk	Reid et al. 2021	NCT03098797
		Atherosclerotic renal artery stenosis	Attenuates postprocedural hypoxia, increases renal blood flow, and improves kidney function	Saad et al. 2017	NCT01755858
		Mitochondrial myopathy	Increases 6 MWT after 5 d treatment, the improvement appears to be dose-dependent	Karaa et al. 2018, 2020	NCT03323749
		Reperfusion injury	Safe treatment is not associated with a decrease in myocardial infarct size	Chakrabarti et al. 2013; Gibson et al. 2016	NCT01572909
	AX	Skeletal muscle, metabolism	Improves fat oxidation at lower intensity exercise	Liu et al. 2021	NCT03368872
			Improves TA muscle strength and endurance	Liu et al. 2018	NCT03368872
			Improves strength, as well as improves endurance	Earnest et al. 2011	NCT01241877

Continued

Cite this article as *Cold Spring Harb Perspect Med* doi: 10.1101/cshperspect.a041199

Table 1. *Continued*

Clinical	Intervention	Model	Physiology response	References	Clinical trial #
			Astaxanthin (AX) improves athletic performance and exercise capacity, reduces injury markers	Djordjevic et al. 2012	NA
		Human blood	Lowers plasma biomarker of lipid peroxidation	Kidd et al. 2011	NCT01167205
	MitoQ	Early-onset AD mild cognitive impairment	Carotid artery, endothelial function, and brain blood flow	NA	NCT03514875
		PD	No effect on progression over 12 mo	Snow et al. 2010	NCT00329056
		Aging-related vascular dysfunction	Determines 3 mo mitoQ for endothelial function in older adults and the mechanisms		NCT04851288
	Tricaprilin	AD	Targets mitochondria dysfunction	NA	NCT05809908
	Ginkgo biloba	AD	Targets mitochondria dysfunction	NA	NCT03090516
	ANAVEX2-73	Mild cognitive impairment, due to AD or early-stage mild dementia	Target mitochondria dysfunction	NA	NCT03790709
	S-equol	AD	Positive results but not clinically significant ($p < 0.06$) that S-equol does not influence platelet mitochondria COX activity	Stancu et al. 2016	NCT02142777
					NCT03101085
	J147	Aging and dementia	Phase I safety trial, completed but results not published	NA	NCT03838185
	UA	Aging skeletal muscle	Improves muscle endurance after 2 mo	Liu et al. 2022	NCT03283462
			Beneficial for systemic metabolism and reduces inflammation after 4 mo		
		Aging skeletal muscle	4 wk supplementation elevates mitophage, mitochondrial biogenesis, and fatty acid oxidation gene expression	Andreux et al. 2019	NCT04160312
	Spermidine	Blood	Level reduced in older, but nonagenarian and centenarians remain the same level as middle-aged	Pucciarelli et al. 2012; Kiechi et al. 2018	NCT03378843
			Higher spermidine linked to increased survival		

tractility index (Sabbah et al. 2012) and 3-mo elamipretide treatment enhances ejection fraction and reduces LV end-diastolic pressure (Sabbah et al. 2016). Elamipretide also reduces cardiac IR injury and preserve cardiac function in various IR models (Petri et al. 2006; Szeto 2008). Recently, we have demonstrated that 8-wk elamipretide treatment reverses preexisting cardiac aging phenotypes, including cardiac hypertrophy, diastolic, and systolic dysfunction, in old C57/BL6J mice (Chiao et al. 2020; Pharaoh et al. 2023). Importantly, the improved cardiac function in old mice is accompanied by improved mitochondrial respiration, reduced oxidative damage, and normalized myofilament phosphorylation in the heart (Chiao et al. 2020). Elamipretide treatment is shown to improve mitochondrial respiration by reducing the age-related increase mitochondrial proton leak (Chiao et al. 2020), via a mechanism dependent on its interaction with ANT1 (Zhang et al. 2020a). A later study also found that combining elamipretide with NMN synergistically enhances the cardiac NAD$^+$ pool and improves cardiac function in old mice (Whitson et al. 2020).

In skeletal muscle, a single treatment with elamipretide increases the efficiency and magnitude of in vivo ATP production in old skeletal muscles and improves in vivo fatigue resistance after 1 h (Siegel et al. 2013), while 8-wk elamipretide treatment improves in vivo mitochondrial function, redox homeostasis, and exercise tolerance (Campbell et al. 2019) in aged mice. However, 4-mo daily treatment with elamipretide did not alter fatigue resistance, atrophy, and contractile properties of ex vivo extensor digitorum longus muscles, despite reduced mitochondrial redox stress (Sakellariou et al. 2016). These different results suggest a complex role for mitochondrial redox stress in aging muscle that may be dependent on the intact system integrating circulatory and nervous inputs into the muscle. In addition to the effects in aging heart and skeletal muscle noted above, elamipretide is protective in other models of age-associated diseases, including PD (Plecitá-Hlavatá et al. 2009), AD (Howitz et al. 2003), insulin resistance (Anderson et al. 2009), age-related vision decline (Alam et al. 2022), and kidney pathology (Sweetwyne et al. 2017) in preclinical models. Due to its promising results in preclinical studies, elamipretide has been the subject of multiple clinical trials.

In a clinical trial in older adults with low mitochondrial function (ATP$_{max}$ < 0.7 mM/sec and P/O < 1.9), a single elamipretide treatment improved in vivo maximum mitochondrial ATP production (ATP$_{max}$) in a hand muscle compared to placebo (Roshanravan et al. 2021). This positive effect on ATP$_{max}$ returned to placebo level by day 7 following treatment, consistent with 16 h half-time of elamipretide in human blood (Daubert et al. 2017). This acute response parallels that observed in aged mice and is consistent with the ability of elamipretide to reversibly bind to CL and restore mitochondrial ETS function. (Birk et al. 2013; Brown et al. 2014). A post hoc analysis revealed an elevation in first dorsal interosseous (FDI) muscle fatigue resistance 7 d after treatment. This separation between the effects on ATPmax and muscle endurance suggests that mitochondrial ATP production may not be the most important driver of muscle function and exercise tolerance with aging. This supports a complex role for the mitochondria involved in many different aspects of cell physiology outlined in the introduction of this review. In addition to the trial mentioned above for aging skeletal muscle, elamipretide is being tested in clinical phase I and phase II studies focused on mitochondrial myopathy, macular degeneration, cardiovascular, and renal disease population (Chakrabarti et al. 2013; Gibson et al. 2016; Daubert et al. 2017; Saad et al. 2017; Karaa et al. 2018, 2020; Hortmann et al. 2019; Butler et al. 2020; Reid Thompson et al. 2021).

Mitochondrial Quality Control

Mitophagy is impaired with increasing age- and age-related diseases. The decline in mitochondrial quality control and associated loss of mitochondrial function has been linked to slow walking speed and reduced muscle strength in older individuals (Picca et al. 2023). Improving mitochondrial biogenesis by restoring the level of mitophagy is associated with delaying the age-related decline in muscle health (Madeo et al. 2018).

Spermidine

Spermidine is a metabolic polyamine that is naturally present in food sources that acts as an autophagy inducer among other cellular activities (Pietrocola et al. 2016). Four weeks of spermidine treatment improved autophagic flux in aging cardiomyocytes and reduced pathology by promoting autophagosome turnover (Eisenberg et al. 2016). Support for induction of mitophagy as the mechanism of action of spermidine comes from results demonstrating that genetic inhibition of autophagy abolishes the life span extension in flies and worms (Eisenberg et al. 2009). Spermidine also has been reported to maintain regenerative function in aging muscle stem cells and reduced protein aggregates with 2 wk of treatment (García-Prat et al. 2016). Interest in spermidine as an aging intervention is supported by the observation that aging is associated with decline in tissue spermidine concentration in model organisms as well as humans (Madeo et al. 2018). Interestingly, a cross-sectional observation reported whole blood spermidine content decreased in older adults but remained at the level of young (middle-aged) among healthy nonagenarians and centenarians (Pucciarelli et al. 2012). Additional survey-based studies also reported reduced prevalence of heart failure related to consumption of spermidine intake linked to lower mortality (Kiechl et al. 2018) and that spermidine dietary intake was linked to a reduced risk for cognitive impairment in humans (Picca et al. 2023). These results support a potential role for spermidine in healthy aging and have led to more rigorous clinical trials testing spermidine in the context of healthy aging. A small pilot study suggested spermidine supplementation may have protective effects on cognitive function in older adults at risk for dementia (Wirth et al. 2018). A follow-up phase IIb study is ongoing (Wirth et al. 2022; NCT03094546).

Urolithin A

Urolithin A (UA) belongs to a family of urolithins produced in the colon following microbiota-mediated transformation of natural polyphenols ellagitannins (ETs) and ellagic acid (EA) (D'Amico et al. 2021). Natural compounds abundant in foods such as pomegranates, berries, and nuts. However, only 40% of older adults can convert the natural food source to UA due to variation in the gut microbiomes with age, health status, and dietary intake (D'Amico et al. 2021). Recent studies have demonstrated a mechanism where UA supplementation activates mitophagy pathways and induces mitochondrial biogenesis. In worms, UA supplementation extended life span dependent on autophagy genes *bec-1*, *sqst-1*, and *vps-34* and the mitophagy genes *pink-1*, *dct-1*, and *skn-1* expression (Ryu et al. 2016). In young worms, UA treatment unexpectedly reduced basal respiration, while maintaining maximum respiratory capacity, despite reduced mitochondrial content indicated by the lower mtDNA to nuclear DNA ratio. However, in aged worms, UA treatment led to increased expression of mitochondrial genes and preserved reserve respiratory capacity. This same study also demonstrated induction mitophagy-related genes, greater ubiquitination of mitochondrial proteins, and improved exercise tolerance in aged mice and rat models supporting a link between improved mitochondrial quality control through mitophagy and aging skeletal muscle function (Ryu et al. 2016).

A phase I study of safety and tolerability of UA supplementation showed 4 wk of UA supplementation in healthy sedentary older adults decreased plasma acylcarnitine level (Andreux et al. 2019). The study also demonstrated a direct impact of UA on elevated gene expression in skeletal muscle for genes associated with mitophagy, mitochondrial biogenesis, and fatty acid oxidation (Ryu et al. 2016). This study concluded UA supplementation is safe, bioavailable, and has a positive impact on mitochondria health. A follow-up, small-phase II clinical trial demonstrated that UA supplementation significantly improved the secondary end point of muscle endurance in two disparate muscles after 2 mo of treatment (FDI, primarily type II fiber; TA, primarily type I fiber) (Liu et al. 2022). Despite the absence of improvement in the primary endpoint, 6 min walk test, with UA, this study suggests that UW supplementation may directly improve aged skeletal muscle performance, even in the absence of exercise. Plasma levels of acylcarnitines, ceramides, and C-reactive protein were also decreased by UA at 4 mo, indicating beneficial effects of UA treatment on systemic metabolism and inflammation, despite the absence of an effect on muscle mitochondrial ATP production. These findings are consistent with the aforementioned phase I clinical study after 4-wk UA supplementation (Andreux et al. 2019) and indicate that UA warrants further study as a mitochondrial-targeted strategy to preserve function with age.

Mitochondrial Biogenesis

AMPK acts as a cellular energy sensor that works upstream to regulate signaling pathways that activate mitochondrial biogenesis, autophagy, and cellular stress. Aging-related decline of AMPK sensitivity activates cellular stress, impairs metabolic regulation, increases oxidative stress, and reduces autophagy, all of which contribute to age-related decline (Stancu 2015). AMPK can up-regulate both mitochondrial biogenesis and mitophagy to induce fragmentation of damaged mitochondria and recycling of damaged mitochondria to improve the mitochondrial pool. Indirect activators include any modulator that causes AMP or calcium accumulation, such as metformin, resveratrol, and curcumin. Metformin inhibits complex I of mitochondrial respiration leading to increased AMP/ATP ratio. Another category of AMPK activator was first identified by Abbott laboratories in 2006 (AICAR), which generates AMP mimetic compound AICAR monophosphate (ZMP), an allosteric activator of AMPK. Additionally, salicylate is a pro-drug form of aspirin. Aspirin is a derivative rapidly broken down to salicylate upon entering circulation, also resulting in activation of AMPK.

MITOCHONDRIAL-DERIVED PEPTIDES

One exciting class of compounds are the MDPs described above. Humanin was the first discovered MDP and has been shown to have strong neuroprotective effects against AD. It was initially cloned from the resilient occipital lobe of the brain of an AD patient and found that the peptide protected against amyloid-β toxicity in neuronal cells (Yen et al. 2020). In humans, the cerebrospinal fluid level of humanin is reduced in AD patients (Yen et al. 2020). The circulating level in children of centenarians also showed higher levels of humanin compared with age-matched controls (Yen et al. 2020). The clinical trial registry clinicaltrials.gov indicates that at least one study has been completed to investigate the level of humanin in myocardium tissue and blood in relation to early complication occurrence and frequency after cardiac operation (NCT03431844).

After the initial discovery of humanin, seven additional MDPs, SHLPs1-6, and MOTS-c have been discovered (Miller et al. 2022). SHLPs, small humanin-like peptides, are encoded from the 16S rRNA region, and, at least for SHLP2-3, share some biological function with humanin. MOTS-c has also been characterized as an aging modulator and has found to decline in the circulation of middle-aged and older adults compared to younger controls. Importantly, the same study also reported MOTS-c was highest in aged human skeletal muscle suggesting it was tissue specific (D'Souza et al. 2020). As noted above MOTS-c treatment reproduces some of the benefical effects of exercise, and both humanin and MOTS-c have promise as potential interventions to preserve health span.

CONCLUSION

As stated at the beginning of this review, this is an exciting time to be working at the intersection between mitochondrial biology and aging due to the rapid development of new strategies and increasing interest and ability to conduct clinical trials focused on aspects of healthy aging. The aforementioned compounds, while not a comprehensive review of every mitochondrial-targeted compound in the literature, highlight promising new targets and strategies to capitalize on the important role for mitochondria in healthy aging. The greater appreciation of the diverse and complex roles of mitochondria in regulating cell health in aging is leading to a growth in strategies focused on improving mitochondrial health rather than the more typical targeting of specific enzymes or pathways. Given the multiple points of intersection between mitochondria and aging biology, these more wholistic approaches to mitochondrial health present new opportunities to identify new interventions, but also create a cycle where these new interventions provide new insights into the mitochondrial mechanisms of aging. These factors combined with growing interest from industry in aging is creating an environment likely to lead to breakthroughs in mitochondrial-targeted interventions for healthy aging in the next several years.

REFERENCES

Adlam VJ, Harrison JC, Porteous CM, James AM, Smith RA, Murphy MP, Sammut IA. 2005. Targeting an antioxidant to mitochondria decreases cardiac ischemia-reperfusion injury. *FASEB J* **19:** 1088–1095. doi:10.1096/fj.05-3718 com

Alam NM, Douglas RM, Prusky GT. 2022. Treatment of age-related visual impairment with a peptide acting on mitochondria. *Dis Model Mech* **15:** dmm048256.

Anderson EJ, Lustig ME, Boyle KE, Woodlief TL, Kane DA, Lin CT, Price JW, Kang L, Rabinovitch PS, Szeto HH, et al. 2009. Mitochondrial H_2O_2 emission and cellular redox state link excess fat intake to insulin resistance in both rodents and humans. *J Clin Invest* **119:** 573–581. doi:10 .1172/JCI37048

Andersson DC, Betzenhauser MJ, Reiken S, Meli AC, Umanskaya A, Xie W, Shiomi T, Zalk R, Lacampagne A, Marks AR. 2011. Ryanodine receptor oxidation causes intracellular calcium leak and muscle weakness in aging. *Cell Metab* **14:** 196–207. doi:10.1016/j.cmet.2011 .05.014

Andreux PA, Blanco-Bose W, Ryu D, Burdet F, Ibberson M, Aebischer P, Auwerx J, Singh A, Rinsch C. 2019. The mitophagy activator urolithin A is safe and induces a molecular signature of improved mitochondrial and cellular health in humans. *Nat Metab* **1:** 595–603. doi:10 .1038/s42255-019-0073-4

Anisimov VN, Bakeeva LE, Egormin PA, Filenko OF, Isakova EF, Manskikh VN, Mikhelson VM, Panteleeva AA, Pasyukova EG, Pilipenko DI, et al. 2008. Mitochondria-targeted plastoquinone derivatives as tools to interrupt execution of the aging program. 5: SkQ1 prolongs lifespan and prevents development of traits of senescence. *Biochemistry (Mosc)* **73:** 1329–1342. doi:10.1134/S000 6297908120055

Anisimov VN, Egorov MV, Krasilshchikova MS, Lyamzaev KG, Manskikh VN, Moshkin MP, Novikov EA, Popovich IG, Rogovin KA, Shabalina IG, et al. 2011. Effects of the mitochondria-targeted antioxidant SkQ1 on lifespan of rodents. *Aging (Albany NY)* **3:** 1110–1119. doi:10.18632/ aging.100404

Antonenko YN, Avetisyan AV, Bakeeva LE, Chernyak BV, Chertkov VA, Domnina LV, Ivanova OY, Izyumov DS, Khailova LS, Klishin SS, et al. 2008. Mitochondria-targeted plastoquinone derivatives as tools to interrupt execution of the aging program. 1: Cationic plastoquinone derivatives: synthesis and in vitro studies. *Biochemistry Biokhimiia* **73:** 1273–1287. doi:10.1134/S00062979081 20018

Aoi W, Naito Y, Takanami Y, Ishii T, Kawai Y, Akagiri S, Kato Y, Osawa T, Yoshikawa T. 2008. Astaxanthin improves muscle lipid metabolism in exercise via inhibitory effect of oxidative CPT I modification. *Biochem Biophys Res Commun* **366:** 892–897. doi:10.1016/j.bbrc.2007.12 .019

Asadi Shahmirzadi A, Edgar D, Liao CY, Hsu YM, Lucanic M, Asadi Shahmirzadi A, Wiley CD, Gan G, Kim DE, Kasler HG, et al. 2020. α-Ketoglutarate, an endogenous metabolite, extends lifespan and compresses morbidity in aging mice. *Cell Metab* **32:** 447–456.e6. doi:10.1016/j .cmet.2020.08.004

Bakeeva LE, Barskov IV, Egorov MV, Isaev NK, Kapelko VI, Kazachenko AV, Kirpatovsky VI, Kozlovsky SV, Lakomkin VL, Levina SB, et al. 2008. Mitochondria-targeted plastoquinone derivatives as tools to interrupt execution of the aging program. 2: Treatment of some ROS- and age-related diseases (heart arrhythmia, heart infarctions, kidney ischemia, and stroke). *Biochemistry (Mosc)* **73:** 1288–1299. doi:10.1134/S000629790812002X

Birk AV, Chao WM, Bracken WC, Warren JD, Szeto HH. 2013. Targeting mitochondrial cardiolipin and the cytochrome *c*/cardiolipin complex to promote electron transport and optimize mitochondrial ATP synthesis. *Br J Pharmacol* **171:** 2017–2028. doi:10.1111/bph.12468

Birk AV, Chao WM, Bracken C, Warren JD, Szeto HH. 2014. Targeting mitochondrial cardiolipin and the cytochrome *c*/cardiolipin complex to promote electron transport and optimize mitochondrial ATP synthesis. *Br J Pharmacol* **171:** 2017–2028. doi:10.1111/bph.12468

Brown DA, Hale SL, Baines CP, del Rio CL, Hamlin RL, Yueyama Y, Kijtawornrat A, Yeh ST, Frasier CR, Stewart LM, et al. 2014. Reduction of early reperfusion injury with the mitochondria-targeting peptide Bendavia. *J Cardiovasc Pharmacol Therapeut* **19:** 121–132. doi:10.1177/ 1074248413508003

Butler J, Khan MS, Anker SD, Fonarow GC, Kim RJ, Nodari S, O'Connor CM, Pieske B, Pieske-Kraigher E, Sabbah HN, et al. 2020. Effects of elamipretide on left ventricular function in patients with heart failure with reduced ejection fraction: the PROGRESS-HF phase 2 trial. *J Card Fail* **26:** 429–437. doi:10.1016/j.cardfail.2020.02.001

Campbell MD, Duan J, Samuelson AT, Gaffrey MJ, Merrihew GE, Egertson JD, Wang L, Bammler TK, Moore RJ, White CC, et al. 2019. Improving mitochondrial function with SS-31 reverses age-related redox stress and improves exercise tolerance in aged mice. *Free Radic Biol Med* **134:** 268–281. doi:10.1016/j.freeradbiomed.2018.12.031

Chakrabarti AK, Feeney K, Abueg C, Brown DA, Czyz E, Tendera M, Janosi A, Giugliano RP, Kloner RA, Weaver WD, et al. 2013. Rationale and design of the EMBRACE STEMI study: a phase 2a, randomized, double-blind, placebo-controlled trial to evaluate the safety, tolerability and efficacy of intravenous Bendavia on reperfusion injury in patients treated with standard therapy including primary percutaneous coronary intervention and stenting for ST-segment elevation myocardial infarction. *Am Heart J* 165: 509–514.e7. doi:10.1016/j.ahj.2012.12.008

Chavez JD, Tang X, Campbell MD, Reyes G, Kramer PA, Stuppard R, Keller A, Zhang H, Rabinovitch PS, Marcinek DJ, et al. 2020. Mitochondrial protein interaction landscape of SS-31. *Proc Natl Acad Sci* 117: 15363–15373. doi:10.1073/pnas.2002250117

Chen MY, Ye XJ, He XH, Ouyang DY. 2021. The signaling pathways regulating NLRP3 inflammasome activation. *Inflammation* 44: 1229–1245. doi:10.1007/s10753-021-01439-6

Chiao YA, Zhang H, Sweetwyne M, Whitson J, Ting YS, Basisty N, Pino LK, Quarles E, Nguyen NH, Campbell MD, et al. 2020. Late-life restoration of mitochondrial function reverses cardiac dysfunction in old mice. *eLife* 9: e55513. doi:10.7554/eLife.55513

Cummings J, Lee G, Ritter A, Sabbagh M, Zhong K. 2020. Alzheimer's disease drug development pipeline: 2020. *Alzheimers Dement (N Y)* 6: e12050.

Currais A, Huang L, Goldberg J, Petrascheck M, Ates G, Pinto-Duarte A, Shokhirev MN, Schubert D, Maher P. 2019. Elevating acetyl-CoA levels reduces aspects of brain aging. *eLife* 8: e47866. doi:10.7554/eLife.47866

Dai DF, Chen T, Szeto H, Nieves-Cintrón M, Kutyavin V, Santana LF, Rabinovitch PS. 2011. Mitochondrial targeted antioxidant peptide ameliorates hypertensive cardiomyopathy. *J Am Coll Cardiol* 58: 73–82. doi:10.1016/j.jacc.2010.12.044

Dai DF, Hsieh EJ, Liu Y, Chen T, Beyer RP, Chin MT, MacCoss MJ, Rabinovitch PS. 2012. Mitochondrial proteome remodelling in pressure overload-induced heart failure: the role of mitochondrial oxidative stress. *Cardiovasc Res* 93: 79–88. doi:10.1093/cvr/cvr274

Dai DF, Hsieh EJ, Chen T, Menendez LG, Basisty NB, Tsai L, Beyer RP, Crispin DA, Shulman NJ, Szeto HH, et al. 2013. Global proteomics and pathway analysis of pressure-overload-induced heart failure and its attenuation by mitochondrial-targeted peptides. *Circulation Heart Failure* 6: 1067–1076. doi:10.1161/CIRCHEARTFAILURE.113.000406

D'Amico D, Andreux PA, Valdés P, Singh A, Rinsch C, Auwerx J. 2021. Impact of the natural compound urolithin A on health, disease, and aging. *Trends Mol Med* 27: 687–699. doi:10.1016/j.molmed.2021.04.009

Dare AJ, Logan A, Prime TA, Rogatti S, Goddard M, Bolton EM, Bradley JA, Pettigrew GJ, Murphy MP, Saeb-Parsy K. 2015. The mitochondria-targeted anti-oxidant MitoQ decreases ischemia-reperfusion injury in a murine syngeneic heart transplant model. *J Heart Lung Transplant* 34: 1471–1480. doi:10.1016/j.healun.2015.05.007

Daubert MA, Yow E, Dunn G, Marchev S, Barnhart H, Douglas PS, O'Connor C, Goldstein S, Udelson JE, Sabbah HN. 2017. Novel mitochondria-targeting peptide in heart failure treatment: a randomized, placebo-controlled trial of elamipretide. *Circ Heart Fail* 10: e004389. doi:10.1161/CIRCHEARTFAILURE.117.004389

Dell'agnello C, Leo S, Agostino A, Szabadkai G, Tiveron C, Zulian A, Prelle A, Roubertoux P, Rizzuto R, Zeviani M. 2007. Increased longevity and refractoriness to Ca^{2+}-dependent neurodegeneration in Surf1 knockout mice. *Hum Mol Genet* 16: 431–444. doi:10.1093/hmg/ddl477

Dey S, DeMazumder D, Sidor A, Foster DB, O'Rourke B. 2018. Mitochondrial ROS drive sudden cardiac death and chronic proteome remodeling in heart failure. *Circ Res* 123: 356–371. doi:10.1161/CIRCRESAHA.118.312708

Dikalova AE, Bikineyeva AT, Budzyn K, Nazarewicz RR, McCann L, Lewis W, Harrison DG, Dikalov SI. 2010. Therapeutic targeting of mitochondrial superoxide in hypertension. *Circ Res* 107: 106–116. doi:10.1161/CIRCRESAHA.109.214601

Djordjevic B, Baralic I, Kotur-Stevuljevic J, Stefanovic A, Ivanisevic J, Radivojevic N, Andjelkovic M, Dikic N. 2012. Effect of astaxanthin supplementation on muscle damage and oxidative stress markers in elite young soccer players. *J Sports Med Phys Fitness* 52: 382–392.

Doughan AK, Dikalov SI. 2007. Mitochondrial redox cycling of mitoquinone leads to superoxide production and cellular apoptosis. *Antioxid Redox Signal* 9: 1825–1836. doi:10.1089/ars.2007.1693

D'Souza RF, Woodhead JST, Hedges CP, Zeng N, Wan J, Kumagai H, Lee C, Cohen P, Cameron-Smith D, Mitchell CJ, et al. 2020. Increased expression of the mitochondrial derived peptide, MOTS-c, in skeletal muscle of healthy aging men is associated with myofiber composition. *Aging (Albany NY)* 12: 5244–5258. doi:10.18632/aging.102944

Earnest CP, Lupo M, White KM, Church TS. 2011. Effect of astaxanthin on cycling time trial performance. *Int J Sports Med* 32: 882–888. doi:10.1055/s-0031-1280779

Edwards CB, Copes N, Brito AG, Canfield J, Bradshaw PC. 2013. Malate and fumarate extend lifespan in *Caenorhabditis elegans*. *PLoS ONE* 8: e58345. doi:10.1371/journal.pone.0058345

Eisenberg T, Knauer H, Schauer A, Büttner S, Ruckenstuhl C, Carmona-Gutierrez D, Ring J, Schroeder S, Magnes C, Antonacci L, et al. 2009. Induction of autophagy by spermidine promotes longevity. *Nat Cell Biol* 11: 1305–1314. doi:10.1038/ncb1975

Eisenberg T, Abdellatif M, Schroeder S, Primessnig U, Stekovic S, Pendl T, Harger A, Schipke J, Zimmermann A, Schmidt A, et al. 2016. Cardioprotection and lifespan extension by the natural polyamine spermidine. *Nat Med* 22: 1428–1438. doi:10.1038/nm.4222

Fan J, Yang X, Li J, Shu Z, Dai J, Liu X, Li B, Jia S, Kou X, Yang Y, et al. 2017. Spermidine coupled with exercise rescues skeletal muscle atrophy from D-gal-induced aging rats through enhanced autophagy and reduced apoptosis via AMPK-FOXO3a signal pathway. *Oncotarget* 8: 17475–17490. doi:10.18632/oncotarget.15728

Feng J, Bussière F, Hekimi S. 2001. Mitochondrial electron transport is a key determinant of life span in *Caenorhabditis elegans*. *Dev Cell* 1: 633–644. doi:10.1016/S1534-5807(01)00071-5

Fivenson EM, Lautrup S, Sun N, Scheibye-Knudsen M, Stevnsner T, Nilsen H, Bohr VA, Fang EF. 2017. Mitophagy in neurodegeneration and aging. *Neurochem Int* 109: 202–209. doi:10.1016/j.neuint.2017.02.007

Gallo M, Park D, Riddle DL. 2011. Increased longevity of some *C. elegans* mitochondrial mutants explained by activation of an alternative energy-producing pathway. *Mech Ageing Dev* 132: 515–518. doi:10.1016/j.mad.2011.08.004

Garcia J, Han D, Sancheti H, Yap LP, Kaplowitz N, Cadenas E. 2010. Regulation of mitochondrial glutathione redox status and protein glutathionylation by respiratory substrates. *J Biol Chem* **285:** 39646–39654. doi:10.1074/jbc.M110.164160

García-Prat L, Martínez-Vicente M, Perdiguero E, Ortet L, Rodríguez-Ubreva J, Rebollo E, Ruiz-Bonilla V, Gutarra S, Ballestar E, Serrano AL, et al. 2016. Autophagy maintains stemness by preventing senescence. *Nature* **529:** 37–42. doi:10.1038/nature16187

Ghosh A, Chandran K, Kalivendi SV, Joseph J, Antholine WE, Hillard CJ, Kanthasamy A, Kanthasamy A, Kalyanaraman B. 2010. Neuroprotection by a mitochondria-targeted drug in a Parkinson's disease model. *Free Radic Biol Med* **49:** 1674–1684. doi:10.1016/j.freeradbiomed.2010.08.028

Gibson CM, Giugliano RP, Kloner RA, Bode C, Tendera M, Jánosi A, Merkely B, Godlewski J, Halaby R, Korjian S, et al. 2016. EMBRACE STEMI study: a phase 2a trial to evaluate the safety, tolerability, and efficacy of intravenous MTP-131 on reperfusion injury in patients undergoing primary percutaneous coronary intervention. *Eur Heart J* **37:** 1296–1303. doi:10.1093/eurheartj/ehv597

Goldberg J, Currais A, Prior M, Fischer W, Chiruta C, Ratliff E, Daugherty D, Dargusch R, Finley K, Esparza-Moltó PB, et al. 2018. The mitochondrial ATP synthase is a shared drug target for aging and dementia. *Aging Cell* **17:** e12715. doi:10.1111/acel.12715

Goncalves RL, Quinlan CL, Perevoshchikova IV, Hey-Mogensen M, Brand MD. 2015. Sites of superoxide and hydrogen peroxide production by muscle mitochondria assessed ex vivo under conditions mimicking rest and exercise. *J Biol Chem* **290:** 209–227. doi:10.1074/jbc.M114.619072

Graham D, Huynh NN, Hamilton CA, Beattie E, Smith RA, Cochemé HM, Murphy MP, Dominiczak AF. 2009. Mitochondria-targeted antioxidant MitoQ$_{10}$ improves endothelial function and attenuates cardiac hypertrophy. *Hypertension* **54:** 322–328. doi:10.1161/HYPERTENSIONAHA.109.130351

Harman D. 1956. Aging: a theory based on free radical and radiation chemistry. *J Gerontol* **11:** 298–300. doi:10.1093/geronj/11.3.298

Harman D. 1972. The biologic clock: the mitochondria? *J Am Geriatr Soc* **20:** 145–147. doi:10.1111/j.1532-5415.1972.tb00787.x

Hortmann M, Robinson S, Mohr M, Mauler M, Stallmann D, Reinöhl J, Duerschmied D, Peter K, Carr J, Gibson CM, et al. 2019. The mitochondria-targeting peptide elamipretide diminishes circulating HtrA2 in ST-segment elevation myocardial infarction. *Eur Heart J Acute Cardiovasc Care* **8:** 695–702. doi:10.1177/2048872617710789

Howitz KT, Bitterman KJ, Cohen HY, Lamming DW, Lavu S, Wood JG, Zipkin RE, Chung P, Kisielewski A, Zhang LL, et al. 2003. Small molecule activators of sirtuins extend *Saccharomyces cerevisiae* lifespan. *Nature* **425:** 191–196. doi:10.1038/nature01960

Ikeuchi M, Koyama T, Takahashi J, Yazawa K. 2006. Effects of astaxanthin supplementation on exercise-induced fatigue in mice. *Biol Pharm Bull* **29:** 2106–2110. doi:10.1248/bpb.29.2106

Iorio R, Celenza G, Petricca S. 2022. Mitophagy: molecular mechanisms, new concepts on parkin activation and the emerging role of AMPK/ULK1 axis. *Cells* **11:** 30. doi:10.3390/cells11010030

Ishii N, Fujii M, Hartman PS, Tsuda M, Yasuda K, Senoo-Matsuda N, Yanase S, Ayusawa D, Suzuki K. 1998. A mutation in succinate dehydrogenase cytochrome b causes oxidative stress and ageing in nematodes. *Nature* **394:** 694–697. doi:10.1038/29331

Ji T, Zhang X, Xin Z, Xu B, Jin Z, Wu J, Hu W, Yang Y. 2020. Does perturbation in the mitochondrial protein folding pave the way for neurodegeneration diseases? *Ageing Res Rev* **57:** 100997. doi:10.1016/j.arr.2019.100997

Karaa A, Haas R, Goldstein A, Vockley J, Weaver WD, Cohen BH. 2018. Randomized dose-escalation trial of elamipretide in adults with primary mitochondrial myopathy. *Neurology* **90:** e1212–e1221. doi:10.1212/WNL.0000000000005255

Karaa A, Haas R, Goldstein A, Vockley J, Cohen BH. 2020. A randomized crossover trial of elamipretide in adults with primary mitochondrial myopathy. *J Cachexia Sarcopenia Muscle* **11:** 909–918. doi:10.1002/jcsm.12559

Karamanlidis G, Lee CF, Garcia-Menendez L, Kolwicz SC Jr, Suthammarak W, Gong G, Sedensky MM, Morgan PG, Wang W, Tian R. 2013. Mitochondrial complex I deficiency increases protein acetylation and accelerates heart failure. *Cell Metab* **18:** 239–250. doi:10.1016/j.cmet.2013.07.002

Kelso GF, Porteous CM, Coulter CV, Hughes G, Porteous WK, Ledgerwood EC, Smith RA, Murphy MP. 2001. Selective targeting of a redox-active ubiquinone to mitochondria within cells: antioxidant and antiapoptotic properties. *J Biol Chem* **276:** 4588–4596. doi:10.1074/jbc.M009093200

Kepchia D, Currais A, Dargusch R, Finley K, Schubert D, Maher P. 2021. Geroprotective effects of Alzheimer's disease drug candidates. *Aging (Albany NY)* **13:** 3269–3289. doi:10.18632/aging.202631

Kepchia D, Huang L, Currais A, Liang Z, Fischer W, Maher P. 2022. The Alzheimer's disease drug candidate J147 decreases blood plasma fatty acid levels via modulation of AMPK/ACC1 signaling in the liver. *Biomed Pharmacother* **147:** 112648. doi:10.1016/j.biopha.2022.112648

Kidd P. 2011. Astaxanthin, cell membrane nutrient with diverse clinical benefits and anti-aging potential. *Altern Med Rev* **16:** 355–364.

Kiechl S, Pechlaner R, Willeit P, Notdurfter M, Paulweber B, Willeit K, Werner P, Ruckenstuhl C, Iglseder B, Weger S, et al. 2018. Higher spermidine intake is linked to lower mortality: a prospective population-based study. *Am J Clin Nutr* **108:** 371–380. doi:10.1093/ajcn/nqy102

Kim SJ, Miller B, Kumagai H, Silverstein AR, Flores M, Yen K. 2021. Mitochondrial-derived peptides in aging and age-related diseases. *Geroscience* **43:** 1113–1121. doi:10.1007/s11357-020-00262-5

Kim SJ, Devgan A, Miller B, Lee SM, Kumagai H, Wilson KA, Wassef G, Wong R, Mehta HH, Cohen P, et al. 2022. Humanin-induced autophagy plays important roles in skeletal muscle function and lifespan extension. *Biochim Biophys Acta Gen Subj* **1866:** 130017. doi:10.1016/j.bbagen.2021.130017

Kolosova NG, Stefanova NA, Muraleva NA, Skulachev VP. 2012. The mitochondria-targeted antioxidant SkQ1 but not N-acetylcysteine reverses aging-related biomarkers in rats. *Aging (Albany NY)* **4:** 686–694. doi:10.18632/aging .100493

Lazarou M, Sliter DA, Kane LA, Sarraf SA, Wang C, Burman JL, Sideris DP, Fogel AI, Youle RJ. 2015. The ubiquitin kinase PINK1 recruits autophagy receptors to induce mitophagy. *Nature* **524:** 309–314. doi:10.1038/nature14893

Lee IM, Cook NR, Gaziano JM, Gordon D, Ridker PM, Manson JE, Hennekens CH, Buring JE. 2005. Vitamin E in the primary prevention of cardiovascular disease and cancer: the women's health study: a randomized controlled trial. *JAMA* **294:** 56–65. doi:10.1001/jama.294.1 .56

Liang Z, Currais A, Soriano-Castell D, Schubert D, Maher P. 2021. Natural products targeting mitochondria: emerging therapeutics for age-associated neurological disorders. *Pharmacol Ther* **221:** 107749. doi:10.1016/j.pharmthera .2020.107749

Lima T, Li TY, Mottis A, Auwerx J. 2022. Pleiotropic effects of mitochondria in aging. *Nat Aging* **2:** 199–213. doi:10 .1038/s43587-022-00191-2

Lin MM, Liu N, Qin ZH, Wang Y. 2022. Mitochondrial-derived damage-associated molecular patterns amplify neuroinflammation in neurodegenerative diseases. *Acta Pharmacol Sin* **43:** 2439–2447. doi:10.1038/s41401-022-00879-6

Liu X, Jiang N, Hughes B, Bigras E, Shoubridge E, Hekimi S. 2005. Evolutionary conservation of the *clk-1*-dependent mechanism of longevity: loss of *mclk1* increases cellular fitness and lifespan in mice. *Genes Dev* **19:** 2424–2434. doi:10.1101/gad.1352905

Liu SZ, Ali AS, Campbell MD, Kilroy K, Shankland EG, Roshanravan B, Marcinek DJ, Conley KE. 2018. Building strength, endurance, and mobility using an astaxanthin formulation with functional training in elderly. *J Cachexia Sarcopenia Muscle* **9:** 826–833. doi:10.1002/jcsm.12318

Liu Y, Perumal E, Bi X, Wang Y, Ding W. 2020. Potential mechanisms of uremic muscle wasting and the protective role of the mitochondria-targeted antioxidant Mito-TEMPO. *Int Urol Nephrol* **52:** 1551–1561. doi:10.1007/ s11255-020-02508-9

Liu SZ, Valencia AP, VanDoren MP, Shankland EG, Roshanravan B, Conley KE, Marcinek DJ. 2021. Astaxanthin supplementation enhances metabolic adaptation with aerobic training in the elderly. *Physiol Rep* **9:** e14887.

Liu S, D'Amico D, Shankland E, Bhayana S, Garcia JM, Aebischer P, Rinsch C, Singh A, Marcinek DJ. 2022. Effect of urolithin A supplementation on muscle endurance and mitochondrial health in older adults: a randomized clinical trial. *JAMA Netw Open* **5:** e2144279. doi:10.1001/ja manetworkopen.2021.44279

Lonn E, Bosch J, Yusuf S, Sheridan P, Pogue J, Arnold JM, Ross C, Arnold A, Sleight P, Probstfield J, et al. 2005. Effects of long-term vitamin E supplementation on cardiovascular events and cancer: a randomized controlled trial. *JAMA* **293:** 1338–1347. doi:10.1001/jama.293.11 .1338

Madeo F, Eisenberg T, Pietrocola F, Kroemer G. 2018. Spermidine in health and disease. *Science* **359:** eaan2788. doi:10.1126/science.aan2788

Magwere T, West M, Riyahi K, Murphy MP, Smith RA, Partridge L. 2006. The effects of exogenous antioxidants on lifespan and oxidative stress resistance in *Drosophila melanogaster*. *Mech Ageing Dev* **127:** 356–370. doi:10 .1016/j.mad.2005.12.009

Mailloux RJ, Adjeitey CN, Xuan JY, Harper ME. 2012. Crucial yet divergent roles of mitochondrial redox state in skeletal muscle *vs.* brown adipose tissue energetics. *FASEB J* **26:** 363–375. doi:10.1096/fj.11-189639

Manczak M, Mao P, Calkins MJ, Cornea A, Reddy AP, Murphy MP, Szeto HH, Park B, Reddy PH. 2010. Mitochondria-targeted antioxidants protect against amyloid-β toxicity in Alzheimer's disease neurons. *J Alzheimers Dis* **20:** S609–S631. doi:10.3233/JAD-2010-100564

Martínez-Reyes I, Chandel NS. 2020. Mitochondrial TCA cycle metabolites control physiology and disease. *Nat Commun* **11:** 102. doi:10.1038/s41467-019-13668-3

Martínez-Reyes I, Diebold LP, Kong H, Schieber M, Huang H, Hensley CT, Mehta MM, Wang T, Santos JH, Woychik R, et al. 2016. TCA cycle and mitochondrial membrane potential are necessary for diverse biological functions. *Mol Cell* **61:** 199–209. doi:10.1016/j.molcel.2015.12.002

Masumoto J, Zhou W, Morikawa S, Hosokawa S, Taguchi H, Yamamoto T, Kurata M, Kaneko N. 2021. Molecular biology of autoinflammatory diseases. *Inflamm Regen* **41:** 33. doi:10.1186/s41232-021-00181-8

McManus MJ, Murphy MP, Franklin JL. 2011. The mitochondria-targeted antioxidant MitoQ prevents loss of spatial memory retention and early neuropathology in a transgenic mouse model of Alzheimer's disease. *J Neurosci* **31:** 15703–15715. doi:10.1523/JNEUROSCI.0552-11 .2011

Michal G. 1999. *Biochemical pathways*. Wiley, New York.

Miller B, Kim SJ, Kumagai H, Yen K, Cohen P. 2022. Mitochondria-derived peptides in aging and healthspan. *J Clin Invest* **132:** e158449. doi:10.1172/JCI158449

Mitchell W, Ng EA, Tamucci JD, Boyd KJ, Sathappa M, Coscia A, Pan M, Han X, Eddy NA, May ER, et al. 2020. The mitochondria-targeted peptide SS-31 binds lipid bilayers and modulates surface electrostatics as a key component of its mechanism of action. *J Biol Chem* **295:** 7452–7469. doi:10.1074/jbc.RA119.012094

Miura S, Saitoh SI, Kokubun T, Owada T, Yamauchi H, Machii H, Takeishi Y. 2017. Mitochondrial-targeted antioxidant maintains blood flow, mitochondrial function, and redox balance in old mice following prolonged limb ischemia. *Int J Mol Sci* **18:** 1897. doi:10.3390/ijms 18091897

Mukhopadhyay P, Horváth B, Zsengeller Z, Batkai S, Cao Z, Kechrid M, Holovac E, Erdelyi K, Tanchian G, Liaudet L, et al. 2012. Mitochondrial reactive oxygen species generation triggers inflammatory response and tissue injury associated with hepatic ischemia-reperfusion: therapeutic potential of mitochondrially targeted antioxidants. *Free Radic Biol Med* **53:** 1123–1138. doi:10.1016/j.freerad biomed.2012.05.036

Neroev VV, Archipova MM, Bakeeva LE, Fursova A, Grigorian EN, Grishanova AY, Iomdina EN, Ivashchenko Zh N, Katargina LA, Khoroshilova-Maslova IP, et al. 2008. Mitochondria-targeted plastoquinone derivatives as tools to interrupt execution of the aging program. 4: Age-related eye disease. SkQ1 returns vision to blind animals. *Bio-*

chemistry (Mosc) **73:** 1317–1328. doi:10.1134/S0006 297908120043

Ng LF, Gruber J, Cheah IK, Goo CK, Cheong WF, Shui G, Sit KP, Wenk MR, Halliwell B. 2014. The mitochondria-targeted antioxidant MitoQ extends lifespan and improves healthspan of a transgenic *Caenorhabditis elegans* model of Alzheimer disease. *Free Radic Biol Med* **71:** 390–401. doi:10.1016/j.freeradbiomed.2014.03.003

Ni R, Cao T, Xiong S, Ma J, Fan GC, Lacefield JC, Lu Y, Le Tissier S, Peng T. 2016. Therapeutic inhibition of mitochondrial reactive oxygen species with mito-TEMPO reduces diabetic cardiomyopathy. *Free Radic Biol Med* **90:** 12–23. doi:10.1016/j.freeradbiomed.2015.11.013

Nicholls DG. 2004. Mitochondrial membrane potential and aging. *Aging Cell* **3:** 35–40. doi:10.1111/j.1474-9728.2003.00079.x

Nicholls DG, Ferguson SJ. 2002. *Bioenergetics 3*. Academic, London.

Olgar Y, Degirmenci S, Durak A, Billur D, Can B, Kayki-Mutlu G, Arioglu-Inan EE, Turan B. 2018. Aging related functional and structural changes in the heart and aorta: MitoTEMPO improves aged-cardiovascular performance. *Exp Gerontol* **110:** 172–181. doi:10.1016/j.exger.2018.06.012

Olgar Y, Billur D, Tuncay E, Turan B. 2020. MitoTEMPO provides an antiarrhythmic effect in aged-rats through attenuation of mitochondrial reactive oxygen species. *Exp Gerontol* **136:** 110961. doi:10.1016/j.exger.2020.110961

Peternelj TT, Coombes JS. 2011. Antioxidant supplementation during exercise training: beneficial or detrimental? *Sports Med* **41:** 1043–1069. doi:10.2165/11594400-000000000-00000

Peterson LG, Popkin MK. 1980. Neuropsychiatric effects of chemotherapeutic agents for cancer. *Psychosomatics* **21:** 141–153. doi:10.1016/S0033-3182(80)73711-8

Petri S, Kiaei M, Damiano M, Hiller A, Wille E, Manfredi G, Calingasan NY, Szeto HH, Beal MF. 2006. Cell-permeable peptide antioxidants as a novel therapeutic approach in a mouse model of amyotrophic lateral sclerosis. *J Neurochem* **98:** 1141–1148. doi:10.1111/j.1471-4159.2006.04018.x

Pharaoh G, Kamat V, Kannan S, Stuppard RS, Whitson J, Martin-Perez M, Qian WJ, MacCoss MJ, Villen J, Rabinovitch P, et al. 2023. Elamipretide improves ADP sensitivity in aged mitochondria by increasing uptake through the adenine nucleotide translocator (ANT). *Geroscience* doi:10.1007/s11357-023-00861-y

Picard M, Ritchie D, Wright KJ, Romestaing C, Thomas MM, Rowan SL, Taivassalo T, Hepple RT. 2010. Mitochondrial functional impairment with aging is exaggerated in isolated mitochondria compared to permeabilized myofibers. *Aging Cell* **9:** 1032–1046. doi:10.1111/j.1474-9726.2010.00628.x

Picca A, Triolo M, Wohlgemuth SE, Martenson MS, Mankowski RT, Anton SD, Marzetti E, Leeuwenburgh C, Hood DA. 2023. Relationship between mitochondrial quality control markers, lower extremity tissue composition, and physical performance in physically inactive older adults. *Cells* **12:** 183. doi:10.3390/cells12010183

Pietrocola F, Pol J, Vacchelli E, Rao S, Enot DP, Baracco EE, Levesque S, Castoldi F, Jacquelot N, Yamazaki T, et al. 2016. Caloric restriction mimetics enhance anticancer immunosurveillance. *Cancer Cell* **30:** 147–160. doi:10.1016/j.ccell.2016.05.016

Plecitá-Hlavatá L, Ježek J, Jezek P. 2009. Pro-oxidant mitochondrial matrix-targeted ubiquinone MitoQ$_{10}$ acts as anti-oxidant at retarded electron transport or proton pumping within complex I. *Int J Biochem Cell Biol* **41:** 1697–1707. doi:10.1016/j.biocel.2009.02.015

Pokrzywinski KL, Biel TG, Kryndushkin D, Rao VA. 2016. Therapeutic targeting of the mitochondria initiates excessive superoxide production and mitochondrial depolarization causing decreased mtDNA integrity. *PLoS ONE* **11:** e0168283. doi:10.1371/journal.pone.0168283

Prior M, Goldberg J, Chiruta C, Farrokhi C, Kopynets M, Roberts AJ, Schubert D. 2016. Selecting for neurogenic potential as an alternative for Alzheimer's disease drug discovery. *Alzheimers Dement* **12:** 678–686. doi:10.1016/j.jalz.2016.03.016

Pucciarelli S, Moreschini B, Micozzi D, De Fronzo GS, Carpi FM, Polzonetti V, Vincenzetti S, Mignini F, Napolioni V. 2012. Spermidine and spermine are enriched in whole blood of nona/centenarians. *Rejuvenation Res* **15:** 590–595. doi:10.1089/rej.2012.1349

Qin Q, Mehta H, Yen K, Navarrete G, Brandhorst S, Wan J, Delrio S, Zhang X, Lerman LO, Cohen P, et al. 2018. Chronic treatment with the mitochondrial peptide humanin prevents age-related myocardial fibrosis in mice. *Am J Physiol Heart Circ Physiol* **315:** H1127–H1136. doi:10.1152/ajpheart.00685.2017

Qiu Y, Huang Y, Chen M, Yang Y, Li X, Zhang W. 2022. Mitochondrial DNA in NLRP3 inflammasome activation. *Int Immunopharmacol* **108:** 108719. doi:10.1016/j.intimp.2022.108719

Reid Thompson W, Hornby B, Manuel R, Bradley E, Laux J, Carr J, Vernon HJ. 2021. A phase 2/3 randomized clinical trial followed by an open-label extension to evaluate the effectiveness of elamipretide in Barth syndrome, a genetic disorder of mitochondrial cardiolipin metabolism. *Genet Med* **23:** 471–478. doi:10.1038/s41436-020-01006-8

Rohrbach S, Gruenler S, Teschner M, Holtz J. 2006. The thioredoxin system in aging muscle: key role of mitochondrial thioredoxin reductase in the protective effects of caloric restriction? *Am J Physiol Regul Integr Comp Physiol* **291:** R927–R935. doi:10.1152/ajpregu.00890.2005

Romani M, Sorrentino V, Oh CM, Li H, de Lima TI, Zhang H, Shong M, Auwerx J. 2021. NAD$^+$ boosting reduces age-associated amyloidosis and restores mitochondrial homeostasis in muscle. *Cell Rep* **34:** 108660. doi:10.1016/j.celrep.2020.108660

Roshanravan B, Liu SZ, Ali AS, Shankland EG, Goss C, Amory JK, Robertson HT, Marcinek DJ, Conley KE. 2021. In vivo mitochondrial ATP production is improved in older adult skeletal muscle after a single dose of elamipretide in a randomized trial. *PLoS ONE* **16:** e0253849. doi:10.1371/journal.pone.0253849

Rossi A, Pizzo P, Filadi R. 2019. Calcium, mitochondria and cell metabolism: a functional triangle in bioenergetics. *Biochim Biophys Acta Mol Cell Res* **1866:** 1068–1078. doi:10.1016/j.bbamcr.2018.10.016

Ryu D, Mouchiroud L, Andreux PA, Katsyuba E, Moullan N, Nicolet-Dit-Félix AA, Williams EG, Jha P, Lo Sasso G, Huzard D, et al. 2016. Urolithin A induces mitophagy and prolongs lifespan in *C. elegans* and increases muscle function in rodents. *Nat Med* **22**: 879–888. doi:10.1038/nm.4132

Saad A, Herrmann SMS, Eirin A, Ferguson CM, Glockner JF, Bjarnason H, McKusick MA, Misra S, Lerman LO, Textor SC. 2017. Phase 2a clinical trial of mitochondrial protection (Elamipretide) during stent revascularization in patients with atherosclerotic renal artery stenosis. *Circ Cardiovasc Interv* **10**: e005487. doi:10.1161/CIRCINTERVENTIONS.117.005487

Sabbah HN, Wang M, Zhang K, Gupta RC, Rastogi S. 2012. Acute intravenous infusion of Bendavia (MTP-131), a novel mitochondria-targeting peptide, improves left ventricular systolic function in dogs with advanced heart failure. *Circulation* **126**: A15385.

Sabbah HN, Gupta RC, Kohli S, Wang M, Hachem S, Zhang K. 2016. Chronic therapy with elamipretide (MTP-131), a novel mitochondria-targeting peptide, improves left ventricular and mitochondrial function in dogs with advanced heart failure. *Circ Heart Failure* **9**: e002206. doi:10.1161/CIRCHEARTFAILURE.115.002206

Sagan L. 1967. On the origin of mitosing cells. *J Theor Biol* **14**: 255–274. doi:10.1016/0022-5193(67)90079-3

Sakellariou GK, Pearson T, Lightfoot AP, Nye GA, Wells N, Giakoumaki II, Vasilaki A, Griffiths RD, Jackson MJ, McArdle A. 2016. Mitochondrial ROS regulate oxidative damage and mitophagy but not age-related muscle fiber atrophy. *Sci Rep* **6**: 33944. doi:10.1038/srep33944

Sanchez-Contreras M, Sweetwyne MT, Kohrn BF, Tsantilas KA, Hipp MJ, Schmidt EK, Fredrickson J, Whitson JA, Campbell MD, Rabinovitch PS, et al. 2021. A replication-linked mutational gradient drives somatic mutation accumulation and influences germline polymorphisms and genome composition in mitochondrial DNA. *Nucleic Acids Res* **49**: 11103–11118. doi:10.1093/nar/gkab901

Schroeder S, Hofer SJ, Zimmermann A, Pechlaner R, Dammbrueck C, Pendl T, Marcello GM, Pogatschnigg V, Bergmann M, Müller M, et al. 2021. Dietary spermidine improves cognitive function. *Cell Rep* **35**: 108985. doi:10.1016/j.celrep.2021.108985

Shpilka T, Haynes CM. 2018. The mitochondrial UPR: mechanisms, physiological functions and implications in ageing. *Nat Rev Mol Cell Biol* **19**: 109–120. doi:10.1038/nrm.2017.110

Siegel MP, Kruse SE, Percival JM, Goh J, White CC, Hopkins HC, Kavanagh TJ, Szeto HH, Rabinovitch PS, Marcinek DJ. 2013. Mitochondrial-targeted peptide rapidly improves mitochondrial energetics and skeletal muscle performance in aged mice. *Aging Cell* **12**: 763–771. doi:10.1111/acel.12102

Snow BJ, Rolfe FL, Lockhart MM, Frampton CM, O'Sullivan JD, Fung V, Smith RA, Murphy MP, Taylor KM, Protect Study G. 2010. A double-blind, placebo-controlled study to assess the mitochondria-targeted antioxidant MitoQ as a disease-modifying therapy in Parkinson's disease. *Mov Disord* **25**: 1670–1674. doi:10.1002/mds.23148

Solov'eva NA, Morozkova TS, Salganik RI. 1975. Development of a rat subline with symptoms of hereditary galactosemia and study of its biochemical characteristics. *Genetika* **11**: 63–71.

Stancu AL. 2015. AMPK activation can delay aging. *Discoveries (Craiova)* **3**: e53. doi:10.15190/d.2015.45

Supinski GS, Murphy MP, Callahan LA. 2009. MitoQ administration prevents endotoxin-induced cardiac dysfunction. *Am J Physiol Regul Integr Comp Physiol* **297**: R1095–R1102. doi:10.1152/ajpregu.90902.2008

Sweetwyne MT, Pippin JW, Eng DG, Hudkins KL, Chiao YA, Campbell MD, Marcinek DJ, Alpers CE, Szeto HH, Rabinovitch PS, et al. 2017. The mitochondrial-targeted peptide, SS-31, improves glomerular architecture in mice of advanced age. *Kidney Int* **91**: 1126–1145. doi:10.1016/j.kint.2016.10.036

Szeto HH. 2008. Mitochondria-targeted cytoprotective peptides for ischemia-reperfusion injury. *Antioxid Redox Signal* **10**: 601–620. doi:10.1089/ars.2007.1892

Szeto HH. 2014. First-in-class cardiolipin-protective compound as a therapeutic agent to restore mitochondrial bioenergetics. *Br J Pharmacol* **171**: 2029–2050. doi:10.1111/bph.12461

Sztretye M, Dienes B, Gönczi M, Czirják T, Csernoch L, Dux L, Szentesi P, Keller-Pintér A. 2019. Astaxanthin: a potential mitochondrial-targeted antioxidant treatment in diseases and with aging. *Oxid Med Cell Longev* **2019**: 3849692. doi:10.1155/2019/3849692

Taub PR, Ramirez-Sanchez I, Ciaraldi TP, Perkins G, Murphy AN, Naviaux R, Hogan M, Maisel AS, Henry RR, Ceballos G, et al. 2012. Alterations in skeletal muscle indicators of mitochondrial structure and biogenesis in patients with type 2 diabetes and heart failure: effects of epicatechin rich cocoa. *Clin Transl Sci* **5**: 43–47. doi:10.1111/j.1752-8062.2011.00357.x

Trnka J, Blaikie FH, Smith RA, Murphy MP. 2008. A mitochondria-targeted nitroxide is reduced to its hydroxylamine by ubiquinol in mitochondria. *Free Radic Biol Med* **44**: 1406–1419. doi:10.1016/j.freeradbiomed.2007.12.036

Umanskaya A, Santulli G, Xie W, Andersson DC, Reiken SR, Marks AR. 2014. Genetically enhancing mitochondrial antioxidant activity improves muscle function in aging. *Proc Natl Acad Sci* **111**: 15250–15255. doi:10.1073/pnas.1412754111

Urbina-Varela R, Castillo N, Videla LA, Del Campo A. 2020. Impact of mitophagy and mitochondrial unfolded protein response as new adaptive mechanisms underlying old pathologies: sarcopenia and non-alcoholic fatty liver disease. *Int J Mol Sci* **21**: 7704. doi:10.3390/ijms21207704

Vrolijk MF, Opperhuizen A, Jansen EH, Godschalk RW, Van Schooten FJ, Bast A, Haenen GR. 2015. The shifting perception on antioxidants: the case of vitamin E and β-carotene. *Redox Biol* **4**: 272–278. doi:10.1016/j.redox.2014.12.017

Whitson JA, Bitto A, Zhang H, Sweetwyne MT, Coig R, Bhayana S, Shankland EG, Wang L, Bammler TK, Mills KF, et al. 2020. SS-31 and NMN: two paths to improve metabolism and function in aged hearts. *Aging Cell* **19**: e13213. doi:10.1111/acel.13213

Wirth M, Benson G, Schwarz C, Köbe T, Grittner U, Schmitz D, Sigrist SJ, Bohlken J, Stekovic S, Madeo F, et al. 2018. The effect of spermidine on memory performance in older adults at risk for dementia: a randomized controlled trial. *Cortex* **109**: 181–188. doi:10.1016/j.cortex.2018.09.014

Wirth M, Schwarz C, Benson G, Horn N, Buchert R, Lange C, Köbe T, Hetzer S, Maglione M, Michael E, et al. 2022.

Correction: effects of spermidine supplementation on cognition and biomarkers in older adults with subjective cognitive decline (SmartAge)—study protocol for a randomized controlled trial. *Alzheimers Res Ther* **14:** 81. doi:10.1186/s13195-022-01012-9

Xiao J, Kim SJ, Cohen P, Yen K. 2016. Humanin: functional interfaces with IGF-I. *Growth Horm IGF Res* **29:** 21–27. doi:10.1016/j.ghir.2016.03.005

Yang B, Yu Q, Chang B, Guo Q, Xu S, Yi X, Cao S. 2021. MOTS-c interacts synergistically with exercise intervention to regulate PGC-1α expression, attenuate insulin resistance and enhance glucose metabolism in mice via AMPK signaling pathway. *Biochim Biophys Acta Mol Basis Dis* **1867:** 166126. doi:10.1016/j.bbadis.2021.166126

Yen K, Wan J, Mehta HH, Miller B, Christensen A, Levine ME, Salomon MP, Brandhorst S, Xiao J, Kim SJ, et al. 2018. Humanin prevents age-related cognitive decline in mice and is associated with improved cognitive age in humans. *Sci Rep* **8:** 14212. doi:10.1038/s41598-018-32616-7

Yen K, Mehta HH, Kim SJ, Lue Y, Hoang J, Guerrero N, Port J, Bi Q, Navarrete G, Brandhorst S, et al. 2020. The mitochondrial derived peptide humanin is a regulator of lifespan and healthspan. *Aging (Albany NY)* **12:** 11185–11199. doi:10.18632/aging.103534

Yoshino J, Baur JA, Imai SI. 2018. NAD$^+$ intermediates: the biology and therapeutic potential of NMN and NR. *Cell Metab* **27:** 513–528. doi:10.1016/j.cmet.2017.11.002

Zhang X, Wu X, Hu Q, Wu J, Wang G, Hong Z, Ren J; Lab for Trauma and Surgical Infections. 2019. Mitochondrial DNA in liver inflammation and oxidative stress. *Life Sci* **236:** 116464. doi:10.1016/j.lfs.2019.05.020

Zhang H, Alder NN, Wang W, Szeto H, Marcinek DJ, Rabinovitch PS. 2020a. Reduction of elevated proton leak rejuvenates mitochondria in the aged cardiomyocyte. *eLife* **9:** e60827. doi:10.7554/eLife.60827

Zhang Y, Oliveira AN, Hood DA. 2020b. The intersection of exercise and aging on mitochondrial protein quality control. *Exp Gerontol* **131:** 110824. doi:10.1016/j.exger.2019.110824

Zhao K, Zhao GM, Wu D, Soong Y, Birk AV, Schiller PW, Szeto HH. 2004. Cell-permeable peptide antioxidants targeted to inner mitochondrial membrane inhibit mitochondrial swelling, oxidative cell death, and reperfusion injury. *J Biol Chem* **279:** 34682–34690. doi:10.1074/jbc.M402999200

Biological Restraints on Indefinite Survival

Jan Vijg[1] and Steven N. Austad[2]

[1]Department of Genetics, Albert Einstein College of Medicine, Bronx, New York 10461, USA

[2]Protective Life Endowed Chair in Healthy Aging Research, Department of Biology, The University of Alabama at Birmingham, Birmingham, Alabama 35233, USA

Correspondence: jan.vijg@einsteinmed.edu; austad@uab.edu

Multiple observations that organismal life span can be extended by nutritional, genetic, or pharmacological intervention has raised the prospect of transforming medicine with the goal of slowing, stopping, or even reversing age-associated disease and maintaining or restoring health and resilience in the increasing numbers of elderly across the world. The potential for such an enterprise is supported in theory by plant and animal models of negligible senescence, most notably the small, freshwater organism *Hydra* spp. The existence of some very long-lived species, including bowhead whale, Greenland shark, and giant tortoises, suggests that increased healthy life spans in humans, significantly higher than the current known maximum life span of about 120 years, may be possible. Here we discuss the biological restraints on human life extension based on the evolutionary basis of aging and our current genetic and molecular insights into the processes responsible for age-related loss of function and increased disease risk.

While life is eternal and has existed on our planet for nearly 4 billion years, most individual life forms have to deal with limits. Throughout human history, mortality, one of those limits, has always been difficult to accept. This goes back to the more than 5000-year-old *Epic of Gilgamesh* in which the hero sets out to conquer death but fails. Likewise, according to the Bible, there was no aging and death when Adam and Eve still lived in paradise. Only after they had committed the original sin, they brought God's curse of death upon themselves and every other living thing as well. But also in real life, humans have always tried to cheat death. China's powerful first Emperor, Qin Shi Huang, refused to accept his mortality, always seeking the fabled elixir of life. He died nevertheless and left us his immortalized terracotta army at his tomb close to his capital city of Xianyang (close to current Xi'an).

Interestingly, things have not changed a great deal since those days. Quests for immortality are still common, most of them easily recognizable as quackery, but scientists contemplating technology's power to conquer aging and death play an increasingly important role as part of new, well-funded private research organizations (Eisenstein 2022). Most notably in this respect is the concept of "longevity escape velocity," the idea that life span will be manufactured by medical technology faster than the rising risk of death due to aging (de Grey 2004). Rather than seeking immortality through elixirs of life, rejuvenation is now often considered possible through regeneration (e.g., by turning somatic cells back into partially undifferentiated stem cells) (de Magalhães and Ocampo 2022).

Meanwhile, demographic studies suggest that our prospects of breaking through the limits of human life span have not really gotten much better since Qin Shi Huang's crude attempts (Colchero et al. 2021). What has dramatically improved, however, is health span. Owing to the explosion of new technology in the nineteenth century the two great killers of the past (i.e., famine and infectious diseases) have been largely tamed, at least in technologically developed countries. And over the last decades, progress in medical research has greatly increased our capacity to optimize the health of older people, resulting in significantly improved survival of the oldest old. However, more recently, we have begun to see diminishing returns of these efforts, with improvements in survival with age rapidly declining after age 100. Indeed, while the number of centenarians has exploded over the last 30 years, their mortality rate of ~50% per year has not changed (Modig et al. 2017). After steadily rising since reliable data have become available in the 1950s, the maximum reported age at death has not increased since the 1990s (Dong et al. 2016). Subsequent extreme value statistical analyses from large data sets of elderly individuals indicates that improvement in the human life span, defined by us as the oldest known person, has ceased (Gbari et al. 2017; Einmahl et al. 2019). Indeed, the world's oldest known person ever is still Jeanne Calment, who died in 1997 at the age of 122 years, 164 days (Allard et al. 1998). No other person, before or since, is known to have reached even the age of 120 years.

Conclusions that the limits of human life span has been reached are somewhat clouded by two issues. First, life expectancy at birth steadily increased from a mere 50 years in the most developed countries in 1900 to over 80 years in most developed countries today. This long-term pattern led some authors to conclude that life span itself is fluid and perhaps even malleable (Oeppen and Vaupel 2002). However, it should be noted that, most recently, that is, since 2010, the rise in life expectancy has decelerated or even reversed slightly in many developed nations (Cardona and Bishai 2018). This pattern was evident even before the appearance of COVID-19, which accentuated that reversal.

Second, experimental laboratory populations of worms, flies, and mice have had their life spans increased, sometimes dramatically. In the nematode, *Caenorhabditis elegans*, for instance, genetic mutations and environmental manipulation have increased median and maximum longevity nearly 10-fold (Shmookler Reis et al. 2009). Survival of individual laboratory mice of standard genetic backgrounds eating standard mouse diets seldom exceeds 3 years, but a single mutation in the growth hormone receptor produced a mouse that lived almost 5 years (Pilcher 2003). Moreover, in worms and flies, the typical age-related increase in mortality has been found to slow, stop, or even decrease at later ages (Curtsinger et al. 1992). Various attempts have been made to extrapolate these findings of a mortality "plateau" at the oldest ages to human population studies. Most notably, from studying data on all inhabitants of Italy aged 105 and older, it has been concluded that human mortality rate reached a plateau after the age of 105, suggesting there may be no theoretical limit to human longevity (Barbi et al. 2018). However, even if this were true (it has been disputed [Gavrilov and Gavrilova 2019]), the probability of survival at this age is so low that the influence of such a mortality plateau on maximum human life span would be miniscule (Beltrán-Sánchez et al. 2018).

Of what, if any, relevance are studies of short-lived, genetically modified laboratory species to the future of human longevity? Are there other species, species with longer life spans or that fail to show signs of aging without genetic manipulation, that might be more relevant? Here we will review the biological restraints on indefinite survival. First, we will discuss the evolutionary logic underlying species-specific limits to life span with a focus on possible exceptions in terms of organisms that show negligible senescence.

Cite this article as *Cold Spring Harb Perspect Med* doi: 10.1101/cshperspect.a041200

"Senescence" we should emphasize as we use the term is synonymous with "aging," the widespread decline in physiological function that is associated with increasing age. It is not shorthand for cellular senescence, a different concept entirely. We will then discuss the possible primary mechanisms of aging that prevent extended species life span. Finally, we will consider the biomedical advances needed to break through the basic biology that underlies current limits to human life span.

EVOLUTIONARY BASIS OF LIMITED LONGEVITY

Mathematical modeling of evolutionary processes has revealed that aging exists because of the decline in the force of natural selection after the age of first reproduction due to unavoidable environmentally imposed death (Rose 1991). Indeed such modeling led W.D. Hamilton to conclude that senescence "cannot be avoided by any conceivable organism" (Hamilton 1966) and that conclusion was widely accepted in the evolutionary biology community, at least for organisms where there was a clear distinction between somatic and germ lines. However, that strong statement was eventually challenged and alternative models parameterized differently were developed that allowed for organisms that do not undergo senescence, or even do the reverse, display negative senescence, that is, improve survival and reproduction with increasing age (Baudisch 2005). At some point, however, mathematical models need to be validated against the real world, and, in fact, organisms that escape aging were devilishly difficult to discover. Even the exquisitely well-studied bacterium *Escherichia coli*, which had always been assumed not to age was discovered to do so (Rang et al. 2011). In fact, the only reasonably well-documented species not observed to undergo signs of senescence appear to be cnidarians in the genus *Hydra* (Martínez 1998; Schaible et al. 2015).

Recently, however, a number of other species, generally those that live exceptionally long lives, have been claimed to undergo "negligible senescence," a useful term, but one that disguises an important distinction. That distinction is between species that age very slowly such as Greenland sharks, which may live several centuries (Nielsen et al. 2016), and those that do not age at all. In practical terms, it is a distinction between species that grow old but do so slowly, and those that show no signs of senescence at all. Such species would remain eternally youthful, in other words, the very grail of human aspirations. To the extent that non-aging species exist, particularly if they are widespread, it would give some credence to the possibility that we will break the limits of human longevity and perhaps create eternal youth for ourselves.

EVIDENCE FOR THE ABSENCE OF SENESCENCE

The astronomer Carl Sagan often said that extraordinary claims (in science) require extraordinary evidence. Eternal youth in any species would be an extraordinary claim, so what sort of extraordinary evidence would validate such a claim? We feel that three legs are required to support that particular stool. First, there must be evidence from survival patterns. Senescence is often measured as the rate of increase in mortality with age. The most common method is to evaluate the Gompertz exponent, which is the slope of a line relating age to the logarithm of age-specific mortality (Finch 1990). The shallower the slope, the slower the aging. A slope of zero indicates the absence of mortality senescence. So no increase in mortality rate with age is one important bit of supportive evidence. It is necessary but not sufficient. The other aspect of demographic senescence is reproductive rate. A non-aging organism should also display no decrease in reproductive rate with increasing age. Finally, there is physical or physiological evidence. Non-aging organisms should show no signs of deteriorating physical capabilities with increasing age.

As noted above, the poster children for lack of senescence are laboratory populations of species of the cnidarian genus, *Hydra*, small, freshwater animals consisting of a base, stalk, and mouth surrounded by tentacles. In the laboratory, they reproduce primarily by budding. We emphasize *laboratory populations* to make the point that in the real world of nature, there is no such thing as immortality. Environmental dangers are omnipresent, whether they are predators, pathogens, poisons, famine, or climatic catastrophe. The laboratory environment minimizes or eliminates such hazards and thus may reveal the *potential* for immortality. It is this potential that *Hydra* provides the strongest evidence to support. Martínez found no increase in mortality, or decrease in budding rates in several groups of *Hydra vulgaris* over 4 years (Martínez 1998). That study was later followed by Schaible and colleagues (including Martínez), who evaluated mortality rates of hundreds of *Hydra* of three strains and two species in two different laboratories for up to 8 years. They also observed no increase in mortality or decrease in budding rate over that period (Schaible et al. 2015). Despite these results, a legitimate question is whether 8 years is sufficient time to detect senescence in *Hydra*, if it exists. For an animal that develops in weeks and reproduces several times per month, it would seem like this should be sufficient time, but it is difficult to be certain. It is too bad that no physical or physiological function assays were done over this time as they would confirm whether *Hydra* really achieve something approaching eternal youth. Assays such as spontaneous contraction rate, prey capture ability, and regeneration rate, which have been used in other *Hydra* studies (Yoshida et al. 2006), could have made a most compelling case for eternal youth.

Other species with at least some claim to lacking senescence include the so-called immortal jellyfish, *Turritopsis nutricula*, another cnidarian with the unique life history feature that, under stress, it can reverse developmental stages from a fully independent, sexually mature jellyfish-like adult back to its juvenile *Hydra*-like state, then develop once again back to its adult stage (Piraino et al. 1996). From this unique life history feature, it has developed the reputation (and nickname) of potential immortality, although no reports exist that it can make these transformations an unlimited (or even large) number of times.

Other claims for the absence of senescence are based virtually entirely on long life, some-

times combined with information that the animals are still reproductively active at later ages. Greenland sharks have developed such a reputation despite the fact that no mortality trajectories with age are available. Recently though, two papers have reported no age-related increase in mortality in multiple species of turtles. Da Silva and colleagues take direct aim at Hamilton's claim that, due to evolutionary dynamics, senescence is inescapable, by analyzing mortality data from zoo populations of 52 turtle and tortoise species (da Silva et al. 2022). They find that approximately three-quarters of those species exhibit mortality patterns statistically consistent with an absence of senescence in a Gompertzian sense and that a few additional species display mortality senescence but at lower rates than humans. How compellingly does this challenge Hamilton's claim? To state the obvious, evolutionary hypotheses should be critically evaluated in the environments in which evolution occurred (i.e., in nature). Da Silva and colleagues do point out that evidence from separate studies carried out in nature on three of the species they analyzed, all provided evidence for senescence. The most thorough of these field studies, a 24-year field study of more than 1000 painted turtles (*Chrysemys picta*), found evidence for both mortality senescence and reproductive senescence. Importantly, in that study, although egg production increased slightly with age, egg quality decreased, so that fewer eggs actually hatched in older females. So merely counting egg production in older individuals is not sufficient. Overall Darwinian fitness indeed declined with age (Warner et al. 2016).

A related question is how to interpret Gompertzian slopes. Does a shallower slope inevitably suggest slower aging or could there be contextual factors that need be considered? For an example of how context matters, consider that American women in the year 1900 showed a slower rise in mortality with age than they did in the year 2000 (Fig. 1; Bell and Miller 2005), yet this hardly suggests that women aged more slowly in 1900. Life expectancy was 30 years longer in 2000 and women were healthier at every age. The difference in slope simply reflects a bigger change in early life relative to later life mortality over the twentieth

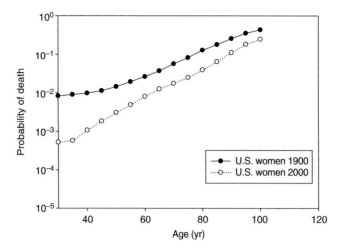

Figure 1. Age-specific mortality in American women in 1900 and 2000 (Bell and Miller 2005). Note the lower Gompertz slope in 1900. Clearly this does not represent slower aging. Life expectancy among American women in 1900 was 49 years and in 2000 was over 79 years. Women were healthier in 2000 at all ages. The change in slope reflects greater progress in reducing mortality at younger compared with older ages.

century. Considering both Gompertz slope and another survival metric, in this case life expectancy (although it could have been a number of others), helps interpret the plot. To help interpret the Gompertz slopes in da Silva et al., we note that life expectancies of many of the turtle species seem low in zoos. In a number of species, reported life expectancies are shorter than the age of first reproduction, which would be unusual in iteroparous species and none of the species show greater-than-human life expectancies. So whether the Gompertz slopes indicate lack of senescence or a high rate of nonsenescent deaths throughout life is not clear.

A second study by Reinke and colleagues reports mortality patterns generated from individual mark-capture data from long-term field studies of 77 species of turtles, tortoises as well as other ectothermic vertebrates, including crocodiles, snakes, lizards, frogs, and salamanders (Reinke et al. 2022). They also report apparent lack of mortality senescence in a number of species, again, particularly among the turtles. While provocative, particularly so as these are studies from nature, there is still no evidence on reproductive senescence or its absence or on changes in physical function with age. One limitation of both of these papers is the small number of an-

imals alive at later ages, where senescence would be the most evident if it exists. Determining age-specific mortality rate with confidence requires a significant number of individuals of the age in question. One thing is clear, however, irrespective of these published survival patterns. Even in the longest-lived giant tortoise species, individuals do not maintain eternal youth. They eventually become aged. Harriet, a Galápagos tortoise reputedly 170 years old at her death in 2006 succumbed to a heart attack, and Jonathan, supposedly the oldest currently living terrestrial vertebrate at an estimated age somewhere between 160 and 190 years has been blind from cataracts, has lost his olfactory sense, and consequently has had to be fed by hand since 2015 (Austad 2022). If the fountain of youth is to be found, it may not be among the oldest turtles.

To be sure, both studies are of considerable interest, but both also fall short of demonstrating a lack of senescence in any of the species in question.

PRIMARY MECHANISMS SETTING LIMITS TO LIFE

In spite of challenges posed by seemingly immortal or very slowly aging species, the decline in the force of natural selection after the age of first reproduction remains the best explanation of why we age. This would lead to the accumulation in the germline of mutations not subject to purifying selection because they are acting only late in life (Medawar 1952). However, this tells us little about the nature of the mechanisms that ultimately determine life span of a species. If aging is caused by late-acting genetic variants accumulating by genetic drift, why are there so many similarities in aging phenotypes among individuals of the same species, and even between species? It was George Williams who first came up with the idea that such late-acting gene variants have important functions at an early age, driving their selection through fitness effects (Williams 1957). His argument was that genes, or in fact genetic variants, can have beneficial effects at a young age, which is why they have been selected during evolution, but adverse effects at later ages. To illustrate this "pleiotropic gene theory of aging," Williams himself provided an example in the form of a hypothetical gene variant positively selected during evolution because it had a favorable effect on bone calcification in the developmental period. However, as a side effect it produced depositions of calcium in the arterial walls. Because the adverse effect of calcium deposition in the arteries only shows up late in life, evolution would not select against this hypothetical gene variant.

At the time it was not realized that many if not most genes have multiple functions. But by now many examples of pleiotropic genes or gene regulatory pathways have been identified. For example, pathways that cause inflammation, a hallmark of aging that has been found to be associated with multiple diseases, from arthritis, cardiovascular disease and cancer to diabetes mellitus, chronic kidney disease, non-alcoholic fatty liver disease, and autoimmune and neurodegenerative disorders, must have been selected because aggressive immune response protects the young against infection (Finch 2010).

Other pleiotropic pathways are those that are part of the somatotropic axis. Growth and reproduction are obviously under positive selection because they enhance fitness. However, they

have multiple late-acting adverse effects, as was dramatically illustrated by the discovery, first in the nematode worm, that weak mutations that dampen such activities increase life span. Inhibiting insulin/IGF-1 signaling in worms, flies, and mice extends life span, as mentioned earlier, sometimes to a very large extent, at least in the worm (Kenyon 2005). Dampening the somatotropic axis intertwines with the paradigm for all interventions in aging: dietary restriction (DR) (Brown-Borg 2015).

As expected, there is a price tag on this increased longevity and it has to be paid in the wild under natural conditions (Jenkins et al. 2004). While trade-offs in the control of longevity remain incompletely understood (Maklakov and Chapman 2019), it is highly unlikely that interventions in normal patterns of growth and reproduction will provide a rational strategy to extend limits to life span.

With the exceptions mentioned, the observed life span gains by dampening growth and reproduction in organisms more complex than worms are modest and appear to diminish with complexity (Vijg and Campisi 2008). For DR, it also remains difficult to distinguish between a true life span effect or the amelioration of an artificially unhealthy diet in laboratory animals (Wolf 2021). This is especially true for the various inbred mouse and rat strains, as suggested by the possible absence of a DR effect in wild mice (Harper et al. 2006).

While interventions in the many pleiotropic pathways associated with early fitness have the potential to increase health span with modest gains in mean life span, they are likely not a good strategy to extend species-specific life span limits. For that purpose we need to closely examine the pathways that allow a species to maintain its somatic tissues for long periods of time. According to Kirkwood's disposable soma theory (Kirkwood 1977), life span is the product of a balance between investments in growth and reproduction on the one hand and somatic maintenance on the other. If this is true, we may be able to intervene in the sources of the wear and tear that require somatic maintenance or possibly manipulate the somatic maintenance pathways themselves. However, the main problem here is that there are not just a few cellular defense systems, but a great many.

In his imperfectness model, Gladyshev argues that aging is a consequence of numerous forms of damage collectively termed the deleteriome (Gladyshev 2016). While in an organism such as *Hydra* such damage could be diluted out by the processes of continuous cell division and selection, explaining its potential immortality (above), in organisms with fully differentiated nonrenewable cells and structures, this same damage will accumulate and cause aging. As the processes that generate these deleteriomes are under genetic regulation, different species will have different capabilities to deal with them, which may explain their different life spans. It is tempting to speculate that evolution used loci involved in somatic maintenance to change life span over time, such as the delayed aging and longer life spans that developed in insular opossums as compared to those on the mainland due to greatly reduced exposure to predation (Austad 1993). This increase in life span from 31 to 45 months in a short time span (i.e., over 4000–5000 years of separation) is difficult to explain from systematically eliminating the late-life adverse effects from genes critical for maintaining early-life fitness.

It has been argued that somatic DNA damage would be central to this deleteriome and affects most, if not all, aspects of the aging phenotype, making it a potentially unifying cause of aging (Schumacher et al. 2021). Advances in sequencing technology have now provided ample evidence that one of the consequences of DNA damage, somatic mutations, accumulate in most if not all human and animal tissues with age (Zhang and Vijg 2018), at a rate that was found to be tissue-specific (Fig. 2). Moreover, in primary fibroblasts from different rodent species, an inverse correlation has been found between mutation burden induced by the same dose of a mutagen and maximum life span (Zhang et al. 2021). This finding has now been extended to a much broader range of species (Cagan et al. 2022).

Also, the capability of DNA repair to remove DNA damage correlates with life span (Tian et al. 2019), something that has been suggested since the 1970s (Hart and Setlow 1974). Because the DNA of the genome is the central repository of all functional information, with somatic muta-

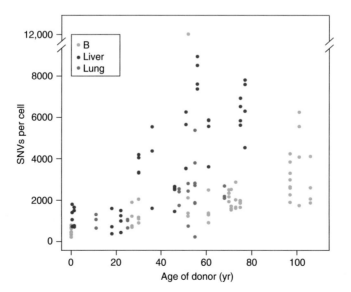

Figure 2. The number of single-nucleotide variants (SNVs) per cell as a function of age in human B lymphocytes, liver hepatocytes, and lung bronchial cells. (Figure created from data in Zhang et al. 2019, Brazhnik et al. 2020, and Huang et al. 2022.)

tions both inevitable and irreversible, the possibility cannot be ruled out that interventions at that level, if at all possible, would be sufficient to modify species-specific life span. However, it remains unclear whether somatic mutations or DNA damage in general are a key causal factor in age-related functional decline and disease apart from cancer. Moreover, genome maintenance and its regulation are extremely complex, making it highly unlikely that interventions at that level will emerge soon.

CONCLUSIONS AND FUTURE PROSPECTS

Based on demographic data, there is now strong evidence that human life span has a practical natural limit. As death rates reach the annual level of 30%–50%, as is the case at extreme old age, it becomes pointless to speculate on an unlimited life span without significant amelioration of the fundamental aging processes. A natural limit to a species' life span is in keeping with Hamilton's conclusion that senescence cannot be avoided due to the decline in force of natural selection after the age of first reproduction. Exceptions to this rule, most notably *Hydra*, are explained from a continuous state of cell renewal similar to embryos. For all other examples of extremely long-lived species, the evidence for a lack of senescence is inconclusive. Breaking through the glass ceiling of evolution's iron law that has given each species a formidable repertoire of late-acting adverse genetic variants, some of which have beneficial effects critical to early life, seems a bridge too far even for the twenty-first century's powerful technology.

The immediate conclusion that can be drawn from this is that the focus of geroscience should be on improving health span, which, in contrast to radical life extension, is testable. Indeed, this has already been very successful in adding life to years, and while there is evidence for diminishing returns (Dong et al. 2016), new geroscience approaches may well reinitiate further improvements (Kaeberlein et al. 2015). For instance, it is by no means clear that we have yet discovered the optimal lifestyle interventions to preserve and prolong health and certain drugs currently in early phase clinical trials may be capable of de-

laying the onset of groups of diseases simultaneously (DeVito et al. 2022).

To substantially delay the aging process that caps maximum life span extension in our species, it will be necessary to mimic evolution, but then in real time, to eliminate the multiple causes of aging while retaining early fitness and species' identity. This would require approaches to increase cellular defense, which in view of the utter complexity of the deleteriome seems beyond our current technological capacity, although what the future holds is, of course, unknown.

ACKNOWLEDGMENTS

This work was supported by National Institutes of Health (NIH) grants AG058811, AG057434, AG050886, and the Glenn Foundation for Medical Research to S.N.A. and NIH grants AG017242, CA180126, AG047200, AG038072, ES029519, HL145560, AG056278, and the Glenn Foundation for Medical Research to J.V. We thank Dr. Shixiang Sun for preparing Figure 2.

REFERENCES

Allard M, Lebre V, Robine JM. 1998. *Jeanne Calment: from Van Gogh's time to ours.* W.H. Freeman, New York.

Austad SN. 1993. Retarded senescence in an insular population of Virginia opossums. *J Zool* **229:** 695–708. doi:10.1111/j.1469-7998.1993.tb02665.x

Austad SN. 2022. *Methuselah's zoo: what nature can teach us about living longer, healthier lives.* MIT Press, Cambridge, MA.

Barbi E, Lagona F, Marsili M, Vaupel JW, Wachter KW. 2018. The plateau of human mortality: demography of longevity pioneers. *Science* **360:** 1459–1461. doi:10.1126/science.aat3119

Baudisch A. 2005. Hamilton's indicators of the force of selection. *Proc Natl Acad Sci* **102:** 8263–8268. doi:10.1073/pnas.0502155102

Bell FC, Miller ML. 2005. *Life tables for the United States Social Security Area 1900–2100 (SSA Pub. No. 11-11536).* Social Security Administration, Washington, DC.

Beltrán-Sánchez H, Austad SN, Finch CE. 2018. Comment on "The plateau of human mortality: demography of longevity pioneers." *Science* **361:** eaav1200. doi:10.1126/science.aav1200

Brazhnik K, Sun S, Alani O, Kinkhabwala M, Wolkoff AW, Maslov AY, Dong X, Vijg J. 2020. Single-cell analysis reveals different age-related somatic mutation profiles between stem and differentiated cells in human liver. *Sci Adv* **6**: eaax2659. doi:10.1126/sciadv.aax2659

Brown-Borg HM. 2015. The somatotropic axis and longevity in mice. *Am J Physiol Endocrinol Metab* **309**: E503–E510. doi:10.1152/ajpendo.00262.2015

Cagan A, Baez-Ortega A, Brzozowska N, Abascal F, Coorens THH, Sanders MA, Lawson ARJ, Harvey LMR, Bhosle S, Jones D, et al. 2022. Somatic mutation rates scale with lifespan across mammals. *Nature* **604**: 517–524. doi:10.1038/s41586-022-04618-z

Cardona C, Bishai D. 2018. The slowing pace of life expectancy gains since 1950. *BMC Public Health* **18**: 151. doi:10.1186/s12889-018-5058-9

Colchero F, Aburto JM, Archie EA, Boesch C, Breuer T, Campos FA, Collins A, Conde DA, Cords M, Crockford C, et al. 2021. The long lives of primates and the "invariant rate of ageing" hypothesis. *Nat Commun* **12**: 3666. doi:10.1038/s41467-021-23894-3

Curtsinger JW, Fukui HH, Townsend DR, Vaupel JW. 1992. Demography of genotypes: failure of the limited life-span paradigm in *Drosophila melanogaster*. *Science* **258**: 461–463. doi:10.1126/science.1411541

da Silva R, Conde DA, Baudisch A, Colchero F. 2022. Slow and negligible senescence among testudines challenge evolutionary theories of senescence. *Science* **376**: 1466–1470. doi:10.1126/science.abl7811

de Grey ADNJ. 2004. Escape velocity: why the prospect of extreme human life extension matters now. *PLoS Biol* **2**: e817.

de Magalhães JP, Ocampo A. 2022. Cellular reprogramming and the rise of rejuvenation biotech. *Trends Biotechnol* **40**: 639–642. doi:10.1016/j.tibtech.2022.01.011

DeVito LM, Barzilai N, Cuervo AM, Niederhofer LJ, Milman S, Levine M, Promislow D, Ferrucci L, Kuchel GA, Mannick J, et al. 2022. Extending human healthspan and longevity: a symposium report. *Ann NY Acad Sci* **1507**: 70–83. doi:10.1111/nyas.14681

Dong X, Milholland B, Vijg J. 2016. Evidence for a limit to human lifespan. *Nature* **538**: 257–259. doi:10.1038/nature19793

Einmahl JJ, Einmahl JHJ, de Haan L. 2019. Limits to human life span through extreme value theory. *J Am Stat Assoc* **114**: 1075–1080. doi:10.1080/01621459.2018.1537912

Eisenstein M. 2022. Rejuvenation by controlled reprogramming is the latest gambit in anti-aging. *Nat Biotechnol* **40**: 144–146. doi:10.1038/d41587-022-00002-4

Finch CE. 1990. *Longevity, senescence, and the genome*. University of Chicago Press, Chicago.

Finch CE. 2010. Evolution in health and medicine Sackler colloquium: evolution of the human lifespan and diseases of aging: roles of infection, inflammation, and nutrition. *Proc Natl Acad Sci* **107**: 1718–1724. doi:10.1073/pnas.0909606106

Gavrilov LA, Gavrilova NS. 2019. New trend in old-age mortality: Gompertzialization of mortality trajectory. *Gerontology* **65**: 451–457. doi:10.1159/000500141

Gbari S, Poulain M, Dal L, Denuit M. 2017. Extreme value analysis of mortality at the oldest ages: a case study based on individual ages at death. *North Am Actuar J* **21**: 397–416. doi:10.1080/10920277.2017.1301260

Gladyshev VN. 2016. Aging: progressive decline in fitness due to the rising deleteriome adjusted by genetic, environmental, and stochastic processes. *Aging Cell* **15**: 594–602. doi:10.1111/acel.12480

Hamilton WD. 1966. The moulding of senescence by natural selection. *J Theor Biol* **12**: 12–45. doi:10.1016/0022-5193(66)90184-6

Harper JM, Leathers CW, Austad SN. 2006. Does caloric restriction extend life in wild mice? *Aging Cell* **5**: 441–449. doi:10.1111/j.1474-9726.2006.00236.x

Hart RW, Setlow RB. 1974. Correlation between deoxyribonucleic acid excision-repair and life-span in a number of mammalian species. *Proc Natl Acad Sci* **71**: 2169–2173. doi:10.1073/pnas.71.6.2169

Huang Z, Sun S, Lee M, Maslov AY, Shi M, Waldman S, Marsh A, Siddiqui T, Dong X, Peter Y, et al. 2022. Single-cell analysis of somatic mutations in human bronchial epithelial cells in relation to aging and smoking. *Nat Genet* **54**: 492–498. doi:10.1038/s41588-022-01035-w

Jenkins NL, McColl G, Lithgow GJ. 2004. Fitness cost of extended lifespan in *Caenorhabditis elegans*. *Proc Biol Sci* **271**: 2523–2526. doi:10.1098/rspb.2004.2897

Kaeberlein M, Rabinovitch PS, Martin GM. 2015. Healthy aging: the ultimate preventative medicine. *Science* **350**: 1191–1193. doi:10.1126/science.aad3267

Kenyon C. 2005. The plasticity of aging: insights from long-lived mutants. *Cell* **120**: 449–460. doi:10.1016/j.cell.2005.02.002

Kirkwood TB. 1977. Evolution of ageing. *Nature* **270**: 301–304. doi:10.1038/270301a0

Maklakov AA, Chapman T. 2019. Evolution of ageing as a tangle of trade-offs: energy versus function. *Proc Biol Sci* **286**: 20191604.

Martínez DE. 1998. Mortality patterns suggest lack of senescence in hydra. *Exp Gerontol* **33**: 217–225. doi:10.1016/S0531-5565(97)00113-7

Medawar PB. 1952. *An unsolved problem in biology*. H.K. Lewis, London.

Modig K, Andersson T, Vaupel J, Rau R, Ahlbom A. 2017. How long do centenarians survive? Life expectancy and maximum lifespan. *J Intern Med* **282**: 156–163. doi:10.1111/joim.12627

Nielsen J, Hedeholm RB, Heinemeier J, Bushnell PG, Christiansen JS, Olsen J, Ramsey CB, Brill RW, Simon M, Steffensen KF, et al. 2016. Eye lens radiocarbon reveals centuries of longevity in the Greenland shark (*Somniosus microcephalus*). *Science* **353**: 702–704. doi:10.1126/science.aaf1703

Oeppen J, Vaupel JW. 2002. Demography. Broken limits to life expectancy. *Science* **296**: 1029–1031. doi:10.1126/science.1069675

Pilcher HR. 2003. Money for old mice. *Nature* doi:10.1038/news030915-13

Piraino S, Boero F, Aeschbach B, Schmid V. 1996. Reversing the life cycle: medusae transforming into polyps and cell transdifferentiation in *Turritopsis nutricula* (Cnidaria, Hydrozoa). *Biol Bull* **190**: 302–312. doi:10.2307/1543022

Rang CU, Peng AY, Chao L. 2011. Temporal dynamics of bacterial aging and rejuvenation. *Curr Biol* **21**: 1813–1816. doi:10.1016/j.cub.2011.09.018

Reinke BA, Cayuela H, Janzen FJ, Lemaître JF, Gaillard JM, Lawing AM, Iverson JB, Christiansen DG, Martínez-Solano I, Sánchez-Montes G, et al. 2022. Diverse aging rates in ectothermic tetrapods provide insights for the evolution of aging and longevity. *Science* **376:** 1459–1466. doi:10.1126/science.abm0151

Rose MR. 1991. *Evolutionary biology of aging*. Oxford University Press, Oxford.

Schaible R, Scheuerlein A, Dańko MJ, Gampe J, Martínez DE, Vaupel JW. 2015. Constant mortality and fertility over age in *Hydra*. *Proc Natl Acad Sci* **112:** 15701–15706. doi:10.1073/pnas.1521002112

Schumacher B, Pothof J, Vijg J, Hoeijmakers JHJ. 2021. The central role of DNA damage in the ageing process. *Nature* **592:** 695–703. doi:10.1038/s41586-021-03307-7

Shmookler Reis RJ, Bharill P, Tazearslan C, Ayyadevara S. 2009. Extreme-longevity mutations orchestrate silencing of multiple signaling pathways. *Biochim Biophys Acta* **1790:** 1075–1083. doi:10.1016/j.bbagen.2009.05.011

Tian X, Firsanov D, Zhang Z, Cheng Y, Luo L, Tombline G, Tan R, Simon M, Henderson S, Steffan J, et al. 2019. SIRT6 is responsible for more efficient DNA double-strand break repair in long-lived species. *Cell* **177:** 622–638.e22. doi:10.1016/j.cell.2019.03.043

Vijg J, Campisi J. 2008. Puzzles, promises and a cure for ageing. *Nature* **454:** 1065–1071. doi:10.1038/nature07216

Warner DA, Miller DA, Bronikowski AM, Janzen FJ. 2016. Decades of field data reveal that turtles senesce in the wild. *Proc Natl Acad Sci* **113:** 6502–6507. doi:10.1073/pnas.1600035113

Williams GC. 1957. Pleiotropy, natural selection, and the evolution of senescence. *Evolution (NY)* **11:** 398–411. doi:10.1111/j.1558-5646.1957.tb02911.x

Wolf AM. 2021. Rodent diet aids and the fallacy of caloric restriction. *Mech Ageing Dev* **200:** 111584. doi:10.1016/j.mad.2021.111584

Yoshida K, Fujisawa T, Hwang JS, Ikeo K, Gojobori T. 2006. Degeneration after sexual differentiation in hydra and its relevance to the evolution of aging. *Gene* **385:** 64–70. doi:10.1016/j.gene.2006.06.031

Zhang L, Vijg J. 2018. Somatic mutagenesis in mammals and its implications for human disease and aging. *Annu Rev Genet* **52:** 397–419. doi:10.1146/annurev-genet-120417-031501

Zhang L, Dong X, Lee M, Maslov AY, Wang T, Vijg J. 2019. Single-cell whole-genome sequencing reveals the functional landscape of somatic mutations in B lymphocytes across the human lifespan. *Proc Natl Acad Sci* **116:** 9014–9019. doi:10.1073/pnas.1902510116

Zhang L, Dong X, Tian X, Lee M, Ablaeva J, Firsanov D, Lee SG, Maslov AY, Gladyshev VN, Seluanov A, et al. 2021. Maintenance of genome sequence integrity in long- and short-lived rodent species. *Sci Adv* **7:** eabj3284. doi:10.1126/sciadv.abj3284

Cite this article as *Cold Spring Harb Perspect Med* doi: 10.1101/cshperspect.a041200

Resistance and Resilience to Alzheimer's Disease

Caitlin S. Latimer,[1] Katherine E. Prater,[2] Nadia Postupna,[1] and C. Dirk Keene[1]

[1]Department of Laboratory Medicine and Pathology, University of Washington School of Medicine, Seattle 98195, Washington, USA

[2]Department of Neurology, University of Washington, Seattle 98195, Washington, USA

Correspondence: caitlinl@uw.edu

Dementia is a significant public health crisis; the most common underlying cause of age-related cognitive decline and dementia is Alzheimer's disease neuropathologic change (ADNC). As such, there is an urgent need to identify novel therapeutic targets for the treatment and prevention of the underlying pathologic processes that contribute to the development of AD dementia. Although age is the top risk factor for dementia in general and AD specifically, these are not inevitable consequences of advanced age. Some individuals are able to live to advanced age without accumulating significant pathology (resistance to ADNC), whereas others are able to maintain cognitive function despite the presence of significant pathology (resilience to ADNC). Understanding mechanisms of resistance and resilience will inform therapeutic strategies to promote these processes to prevent or delay AD dementia. This article will highlight what is currently known about resistance and resilience to AD, including our current understanding of possible underlying mechanisms that may lead to candidate preventive and treatment interventions for this devastating neurodegenerative disease.

Dementia is a significant public health crisis, with the number of individuals living with dementia currently around 50 million worldwide, and expected to increase to 82 million in 2030 and 152 million in 2050 (World Health Organization 2019). Although there are a number of underlying pathologic processes associated with dementia, the most common cause of age-related cognitive decline and dementia is Alzheimer's disease (AD), a progressive neurodegenerative disease characterized by the accumulation in the brain of extracellular plaques composed principally of amyloid β (Aβ) and intracellular neurofibrillary tangles (NFTs) composed of hyperphosphorylated tau (pTau). These pathologies, which are collectively referred to as AD neuropathologic change (ADNC), can be identified across multiple characteristic brain regions (Maurer et al. 1997; Brettschneider et al. 2015) and are thought to subserve neuronal dysfunction and eventually neuron loss. AD severity is determined neuropathologically by the extent of involvement of the brain by these pathologic changes, and the more extensive they are, the more pronounced the neurodegeneration and the greater the likelihood that an individual will clinically present with dementia during life (Hyman et al. 2012; Montine et al. 2012; Nelson et al. 2012).

Age is the principal risk factor for dementia in general and ADNC specifically. The prevalence of AD progressively increases with advancing age, affecting more than 30% of persons age

Cite this article as *Cold Spring Harb Perspect Med* doi: 10.1101/cshperspect.a041201

85 or older (Alzheimer's Association 2020), but AD and dementia are not inevitable consequences of advanced age. Rather, a number of studies indicate a growing diversity of genetic, environmental, and lifestyle modifiers that may influence an individual's risk for developing AD and dementia with age (Chen et al. 2019; Wang et al. 2019). Studies have shown that although many people harbor some, often low, level of ADNC by late midlife (Braak et al. 2011), this is not universal and not everybody will eventually develop this pathology. The phenomenon of reaching advanced age without accumulating significant amounts of AD-related pathology is termed "resistance to AD" (Arenaza-Urquijo and Vemuri 2018). Some mechanisms responsible for this resistance may be specific to AD pathogenesis, whereas others may reflect a better general state of brain health or even an overall slower aging process. Similar to somatic aging, the rate of brain aging can vary across individuals and is determined by a multitude of factors related to genetics, environment, and lifestyle.

Among people who do develop ADNC, there is also a significant variability in the degree of cognitive impairment related to the level of pathology present (Crystal et al. 1988; Katzman et al. 1988). For a given amount of pathological burden, there exists a close to normal distribution of cognitive presentation, with the majority of cases presenting with an average level of impairment, and the rest forming the "tails" at either end. Thus, some individuals with intermediate levels of AD pathological burden, which is considered sufficient explanation for dementia by current consensus guidelines (Montine et al. 2016), show marked cognitive impairment, whereas a separate subset maintain high levels of cognitive functioning, and the rest present somewhere in between, demonstrating decline from their baseline functioning, but not to the point of necessitating constant care-giver support. The ability to maintain normal cognition despite a significant burden of AD pathology is termed "resilience to AD" (Arenaza-Urquijo and Vemuri 2018). According to several reports, up to 30% of older individuals with normal cognition harbor sufficient plaque and tangle pathology to meet diagnostic criteria for intermediate or high level of ADNC (Riley et al. 2005; Schneider et al. 2009; Corrada et al. 2012). Compared to symptomatic individuals with similar levels of ADNC, these subjects show relative preservation of neuron numbers, synaptic integrity, and axonal markers (Perez-Nievas et al. 2013; Boros et al. 2017; Walker et al. 2022), and lower levels of inflammation (Barroeta-Espar et al. 2019) and oxidative stress (Walker et al. 2022). To date, the protective mechanisms responsible for these differences remain largely unknown.

As late-life dementia, and AD in particular, remain among the most pressing public health concerns, discovering protective mechanisms that can slow or prevent the development of ADNC and/or delay the onset of cognitive decline is of paramount importance. In this work, we explore what is currently understood regarding resistance and resilience to ADNC, beginning with definitions of these concepts and their caveats in the context of ADNC. This is followed by a summary of modifying factors that are associated with varying degrees of resistance and resilience to ADNC and the possible mechanisms that upon further investigation may uncover unexplored pathways toward the identification of candidate preventive and treatment interventions.

ALZHEIMER'S DISEASE

Clinical Diagnosis

Alzheimer's disease has traditionally been defined based on both the clinical symptoms (dementia) and the pathologic features (McKhann et al. 1984, 2011). A clinical diagnosis of AD requires integration of the patient's presenting signs and symptoms, the evolution of those symptoms over time, and the absence of other potential contributing causes. AD typically begins with memory-predominant cognitive decline, particularly an inability to generate new memories. These changes can be characterized using several well-established psychometric tests that interrogate diverse cognitive domains to determine which, and to what extent, each is affected (Knopman et al. 2001). Although memory loss is the most common presenting symptom in AD, this is neither unique to AD nor is it always the dominantly affected domain. Less common presentations of AD can preferentially involve other aspects of cognition, including executive function or language. Regardless of the presenting symptoms, AD is progressive; the patient will continue to decline over time, typically extending across multiple cognitive domains beyond those at presentation, resulting in a significant loss of a patient's sense of self and ability to function independently.

Pathologic Diagnosis

There are a number of other neurodegenerative diseases that clinically overlap with AD and can be challenging to effectively exclude when assessing an individual with dementia. Therefore, a diagnosis of AD is truly clinical–pathologic and relies on an assessment of the underlying postmortem pathology for confirmation. The defining neuropathologic features of AD include extracellular plaques of Aβ protein, intracellular tangles comprised of pTau, and neuritic plaques that include pTau-positive dystrophic neurites entangled within Aβ plaques (Montine et al. 2012). The presence of these changes is collectively referred to as AD neuropathologic change (ADNC) and complete evaluation requires not only their identification, but also an assessment of the burden and extent of pathology.

Aβ pathology derives from abnormal cleavage of the amyloid precursor protein (APP), which forms fibrils that are prone to aggregation and ultimately deposits in the neural parenchyma as plaques. This pathology occurs in aging as well as in AD, although usually to a lesser extent (Dickson et al. 1992; Thal et al. 2002). However, the more extensive the Aβ pathology the more likely it is associated with cognitive impairment. Aβ plaques are theorized to deposit first in the cerebrum, beginning in the neocortex, followed by limbic structures (i.e., hippocampus), and later the deep grey matter nuclei (i.e., basal ganglia). Only in more advanced disease do infratentorial structures (brainstem and cerebellum) become involved (Thal et al. 2002). Aβ plaques have a number of different morphologies, but most simply can be characterized as diffuse or neuritic. The latter is defined as an Aβ plaque character-

ized by the inclusion of dystrophic neurites containing pTau (Tomlinson et al. 1968). Although Aβ plaque distribution across the brain is an important metric for all types of plaques, neuritic plaques are further characterized by their cerebral cortical density (Mirra et al. 1991; Mirra 1997).

Neurofibrillary tangles (NFTs) form from the hyperphosphorylation and fibrillization of the protein tau within neurons. Like Aβ plaques, NFTs appear to follow a stereotypical progression throughout the brain, first characterized by Braak and Braak (1991) as generally beginning in limbic structures, specifically the entorhinal cortex, hippocampus, and medial temporal lobe, and later progressing into the neocortex (Braak et al. 2006). The most advanced stages of NFT pathology involve highly specialized areas of the brain—the primary motor and sensory cortex. The extent of NFT pathology correlates with severity of cognitive impairment (Nelson et al. 2012).

To generate an overall ADNC score of not, low, intermediate, or high, the extent of brain involvement of Aβ plaques and NFTs, along with the burden (density) of cortical neuritic plaques, are considered together following published guidelines (Montine et al. 2012). The more severe the ADNC (intermediate or high), the more likely that the individual had a clinical history of cognitive decline and carried a clinical diagnosis of AD. However, the features of ADNC are also found to varying degrees in the absence of cognitive symptoms, including exceptional examples of cognitively intact individuals with high ADNC (Latimer et al. 2019).

RESISTANCE AND RESILIENCE

Defining Resistance and Resilience

Over the years, several different terms have been used to describe the phenomenon of surviving to advanced age without developing AD dementia, including cognitive reserve, brain reserve, brain maintenance, and compensation (Katzman et al. 1988; Stern 2002, 2009; Mortimer et al. 2003; Nyberg et al. 2012). Although these terms were helpful to begin the discussion of resistance and resilience to AD, in some cases they define only a possible mechanism behind resistance and resilience. Although an initial lack of consistent terminology limited research progress, more recently a number of publications have proposed definitions and a framework for applying these concepts (Arenaza-Urquijo and Vemuri 2018; Montine et al. 2019).

The neuropathological definition of ADNC has helped advance studies of resistance and resilience to AD. Incorporating the pathological definition allows for the exclusion of individuals with other neurodegenerative diseases on the basis of the underlying pathology, and it also allows for the distinction to be made between those who never develop the pathology of AD and those who maintain cognitive function in the face of significant ADNC. Although both of these types of individuals remain dementia-free and clinically may be indistinguishable, the striking differences in the neuropathologic findings between these two groups suggest that there may be multiple pathways to preventing AD dementia. The "resistance" pathway results in prevention of the pathology necessary to cause the clinical symptoms of AD, whereas the "resilience" pathways lead to an ability to cope with the presence of ADNC (Fig. 1).

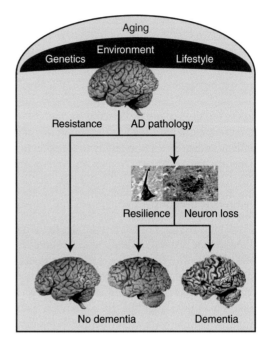

Figure 1. In the context of aging, a number of modifying factors, including genetic, environmental, and lifestyle influences, contribute to the risk of Alzheimer's disease (AD) and dementia. If no AD pathology develops and there is no history of dementia, this is termed "resistance to ADNC." However, if AD pathology does develop but there is no history of dementia, this is termed "resilience to ADNC." Conversely, if neuron loss occurs in the context of AD pathology, this is typically associated with dementia.

Caveats of Current Definitions

Two major factors prevent the full definition of resistance and resilience and remain topics of ongoing research in several fields of AD. The first relates to how cognitive impairment is defined and thereby how to determine the presence of dementia. There are certain normative psychometric scores, below which is considered consistent with a diagnosis of dementia. But there are numerous types of cognitive tests that assess different cognitive domains. Further, any single individual may test well within a range considered cognitively normal but that represents a decline in their personal performance. One could argue that as long as an individual is maintaining a level of mental fitness that allows for the continued performance of activities of daily living, this can still be considered cognitively intact for the purposes of successful aging. Indeed, the genetic, environmental, or lifestyle factors that provided

this individual with particularly high mental acuity could represent mechanisms of resistance or resilience. Although convenient, using the same cutoff test score for the diagnosis of cognitive decline without considering prior personal performance ignores the fact that the severity of the underlying pathological process needed to reach that specific cutoff score can vary significantly between individuals and is, at least in theory, directly proportional to the individual's prior cognitive performance. A full discussion of defining cognitive function and dementia is beyond the scope of this article, but one should consider these caveats when conceptualizing and modeling resistance and resilience to ADNC, which by definition requires some assessment of cognitive status.

In addition to challenges in finding agreed-upon metrics to detect dementia, there are not accepted criteria for thresholds of pathologic peptide burden for resistance and resilience states. There are currently no definitive criteria for what constitutes an absolute maximum pathologic burden for resistance to ADNC, but large cohort studies have provided some guidance. For resistance, the 2012 NIA-AA guidelines for the neuropathologic assessment of Alzheimer's disease describe a "low" level of ADNC that is not considered an adequate explanation for cognitive impairment or dementia, and therefore individuals with a low degree of ADNC without cognitive impairment above a certain (but not agreed upon) age would be considered resistant to developing ADNC to the degree necessary for causing cognitive consequences (Montine et al. 2012). For resilience, using these same 2012 guidelines, "intermediate" and "high" ADNC are a pathologic burden that is considered "sufficient explanation for dementia," and therefore an individual who remains cognitively intact with this level of ADNC can be considered resilient to ADNC. However, as two of the three parameters used in these guidelines are largely based on the spread of AD pathology throughout the brain, they do not address whether the local burden of pathology in any given brain region plays a role in defining the burden of ADNC and are potentially insensitive to define resilience. Although ADNC is specific in terms of the type of pathologies that are present and where in the brain they are located, the overlap between latent or preclinical disease versus true resilience is uncertain. Thus, more stringent (higher thresholds for pathology) criteria for resilience lead to increased probability that a given level of pathology is indicative of true resilience. Quantitative measures across brain regions provide opportunities to understand the role of local pathologic burden, in addition to regional distribution, to dementia and therefore add potential to derive more precise threshold values to define resilience. Further, ADNC may be influenced by the presence of other neuropathologies that are common in the aging brain, including Lewy bodies, phosphorylated TDP-43, vascular brain injury, and glial proteinopathies. The presence of any of these copathologies confounds the definitions of AD, resilience, and resistance. A clear definition of ADNC that accounts for the level of pathology needed for cognitive decline, the amount of pathology in addition to spread, and how to account for copathologies will be important next steps toward more fully defining resistance and resilience to AD.

Research is ongoing to help inform processes to develop biologically and clinically relevant definitions of resistance and resilience. However, using the definitions we have outlined here, a number of interesting studies shed some light on potential mechanisms of resistance and resilience in AD.

Mechanisms of Resistance and Resilience to Alzheimer's Disease

The mechanisms that underlie an individual's ability to either resist the development of ADNC or to tolerate significant ADNC burden and live to advanced age without significant cognitive decline are currently unknown. This is therefore an area of intense research interest because understanding mechanisms of resistance and resilience to ADNC could provide a roadmap to potential preventive strategies or treatments for those that are unable to evade ADNC and its consequences. To this end, identification of the factors that appear to modify an individual's risk of developing ADNC and dementia are an important first step to understanding the mechanisms that underlie resistance and resilience. Many such factors have been identified in the literature, and they fall generally into the categories of genetic risk and modifiable mediators

Genetic Mediators of Resistance and Resilience

Although early-onset familial forms of AD are caused by mutations in genes that encode proteins involved in the processing of the APP, including the *APP* gene itself as well as *presenilin 1* and *presenilin 2*, such mutations are rare and not thought to play a significant role in the development of AD for most individuals (Bird 1993; Bertram and Tanzi 2012). Unlike early-onset AD, there does not appear to be a single genetic cause of the more prevalent, late-onset AD. Instead, a variety of loci have been identified that each carry some generally small level of increased risk (Lambert et al. 2009, 2013; Seshadri et al. 2010; Hollingworth et al. 2011; Naj et al. 2011; Escott-Price et al. 2015). The strongest known genetic risk factor that promotes late-onset AD in white people, and therefore imparts a lack of resistance, is the presence of the *APOE*-ε4 allele (Seshadri et al. 2010; Lambert et al. 2013; Serrano-Pozo et al. 2021; Bellenguez et al. 2022). In contrast, the presence of the *APOE*-ε2 allele has a strong negative association with AD dementia in similar cohorts (Seshadri et al. 2010; Serrano-Pozo et al. 2021). The *APOE*-ε2 allele is hypothesized to be protective and therefore potentially confers a genetic resistance or resilience to ADNC. The strength of the association with *APOE*-ε4 and *APOE*-ε2 has been repeatedly demonstrated through multiple large genome-wide association studies (GWASs; Seshadri et al. 2010; Lambert et al. 2013; Bellenguez et al. 2022). Although *APOE* genotype provides the strongest risk and potential protection for late-onset/sporadic AD, many other genetic risk factors have been identified through ever larger GWAS analyses, revealing the complex nature of genetic influence on whether an individual will develop AD or develop a resistance or resilience phenotype, should they live to advanced age.

Genetic risk variants that have been identified can be categorized according to the cellular/tissue pathways that are involved in a number of different processes linked to AD including lipid homeostasis/cholesterol metabolism, innate immunity, endocytosis, cytoskeletal changes, and apoptosis (Medway and Morgan 2014). Similarly, researchers have identified several variants that may drive cognitive resilience to the presence of pathology in genes associated with cellular responses to stress, cell-cycle regulation, angiogenesis, heme biosynthesis, and synaptic plasticity (Mukherjee et al. 2012; Hohman et al. 2017; Ramanan et al. 2021). In particular, these studies have been focused on resilience to Aβ pathology, and newer research will ideally focus on additional factors that may drive ADNC-related cognitive decline and pathology (Serrano-Pozo et al. 2021). One study of resistance to ADNC identified a

genetic variant that can confer protection and is involved in the biological pathways associated with cellular responses to stress (Lu et al. 2014). Further studies are needed, particularly in the oldest old, to identify additional genetic variants associated with either resistance or resilience to AD as it is increasingly apparent that a large set of genes, each with small effect on promoting resistance or resilience, will be found, rather than a single large genetic factor. These sets of genes are compiled to generate values that predict overall heritable risk, called polygenic risk scores (PRS), and allow researchers to better understand the overall effect of a set of genes encompassing a complex set of biological pathways related to disease or resistance and resilience to disease (Escott-Price et al. 2015; Huq et al. 2021). We anticipate that over the next few years researchers will develop PRS associated with resistance and resilience to AD using similar approaches that have led to the identification of risk genes for late-onset AD (Escott-Price et al. 2015; Huq et al. 2021).

Modifiable Mediators of Resistance and Resilience

One of the principal goals of studying resistance and resilience to ADNC is to identify potentially modifiable environmental and lifestyle factors that delay development of ADNC or promote one's ability tolerate its detrimental effects on cognition. There are a multitude of potentially modifiable life-course factors that may impact ADNC development or tolerance with strong evidence implicating education, physical activity, diet, and social interaction. The association between education and AD risk in particular has long been studied (Zhang et al. 1990; Ott et al. 1995; Iacono et al. 2015; Balduino et al. 2020). A recent meta-analysis found a significant dose–response association between the level of education and risk of dementia and reported that dementia risk was reduced by 7% for per year increase in education (Xu et al. 2016). The mechanisms that underlie this association are not well understood. One possibility is that highly educated individuals have developed compensatory mechanisms that keep cognition intact for longer by counteracting the effects of the accumulating pathology, and thus truly change the trajectory of functional decline (so-called cognitive reserve). Alternatively, the dramatic delay in dementia onset in those with higher levels of education may simply be due to their higher baseline level of cognitive functioning, and not to the slower rate of decline. Both trends have been described in the literature (Batterham et al. 2011; Muniz-Terrera et al. 2013; Terrera et al. 2014). Additional longitudinal studies relying on precise monitoring of each individual's trajectories of cognitive scores and autopsy endpoints are needed to better understand the mechanisms.

In addition to enhancing cognitive fitness through higher levels of education, there has been much work evaluating the effects on physical fitness and diet on cognitive function and ADNC with age. Late-life physical activity is often associated with resistance and resilience to AD dementia but the underlying mechanisms are unknown (Buchman et al. 2012; Northey et al. 2018). Some studies suggest that, similar to education, exercise may enhance the adaptability of the brain, rendering it better able to cope with ADNC should it develop, thereby conferring resilience (Voss et al. 2010). Other studies show a relationship between reductions in ADNC in association with higher levels of exercise, thereby providing resistance to ADNC (Müller et al. 2018). A healthy diet, specifically consumption of diets rich in antioxidants and anti-inflammatory components can also potentially provide benefits to brain health (Joseph et al. 2009). The Mediterranean diet, which is characterized by a high intake of vegetables, legumes, fruits, nuts, olive oil, and whole grains, and a moderate intake of fish, has been found to have a protective effect in some (Loughrey et al. 2017; Morris et al. 2018; To et al. 2022), but not all, studies (Akbaraly et al. 2019). Caloric restriction (Mouton et al. 2009; Schafer et al. 2015) and intermittent fasting (Anson et al. 2003) have also shown promising results in experimental systems, but comparable studies in humans are insufficiently powered to draw definitive conclusions. Although the current data suggest a trend toward beneficial effect (Ooi et al. 2020; Currenti et al. 2021), the underlying mechanisms are unknown.

Although diet and exercise may play a role in resistance and resilience to ADNC through direct effects on the structure and function of the brain, these modifiers also impart multiple benefits that may result in indirect benefits through promotion of systemic health, including lower body weight, reduced diabetes risk, and improved cardiovascular function. In particular, there is abundant evidence to suggest that maintaining good cardiovascular health, as can be done through healthy diet and exercise, correlates well with successful brain aging, and therefore may play a role in the resistance and resilience to AD (Misiak et al. 2012; Lane et al. 2019). For example, effective management of high blood pressure appears to significantly lower the risk of dementia and midlife weight loss in obese subjects has been shown to improve memory and cognitive scores (Veronese et al. 2017). Despite these correlations, however, little is understood about the underlying mechanisms by which maintaining good peripheral health might lead to resistance or resilience. Indeed, the effects of these systemic changes may derive in part through reduced risk for comorbid pathologies, such as vascular brain injury.

In addition to education, diet, and exercise, social interaction and psychological health also appear to play important roles in the prevention of AD and dementia (James et al. 2011; Hwang et al. 2018; Salinas et al. 2021). Even though a high level of social participation is moderately associated with other health-promoting behaviors, such as physical activity and favorable eating habits (Abe et al. 2022), social engagement alone also seems to have a direct positive impact on cognitive functioning, even after correcting for confounders, such as physical activity and mental health (Cohn-Schwartz 2020). In particular, the development and maintenance of strong social networks has been shown to confer resilience to the presence of ADNC in an aging population (Bennett et al. 2006).

There is much yet to be learned about mechanisms of resistance and resilience from lifestyle habits and dietary or environmental exposures that are associated with an enhanced risk of AD and dementia. Excessive alcohol consumption is known to increase dementia risk, with the effect being most pronounced for early-onset (younger than 65 years of age) dementias (Schwarzinger et al. 2018). However, the dose–response relationship between alcohol use and brain health seems to be complex. Both abstinence and heavy use have been found to be detrimental (Topiwala et al. 2017; Piumatti et al. 2018; Sabia et al. 2018), whereas moderate intake appeared beneficial in some studies (Sabia et al. 2018; Koch et al. 2019). Smoking is associated with increased risk of dementia (Deal et al. 2020; Livingston et al. 2020), and smoking cessation reduces the detrimental effect, even when done at an older age (Choi et al. 2018; Deal et al. 2020). The negative effect of smoking may be mediated through vascular and toxic effects of the inhaled air particulate matter (van der Lee et al. 2018). Similar mechanisms may explain the detrimental effect of air pollution (Peters et al. 2019), an exposure that is associated with a higher incidence of dementia (Chen et al. 2017; Oudin et al. 2018). The history of traumatic brain injury (TBI) is another type of exposure thought to increase the risk of developing dementia (Plassman et al. 2000; Fleminger et al. 2003; Suhanov et al. 2006; Barnes et al. 2014; Gardner et al. 2014; Nordström et al. 2014; Fann et al. 2018). The effect of a single mild concussion appears to be less pronounced compared to severe or multiple impacts, but the extent of trauma sufficient to significantly increase the risk is still not known, and the results are inconsistent across studies (Williams et al. 1991; Launer et al. 1999; Mehta et al. 1999; Helmes et al. 2011; Dams-O'Connor et al. 2013; Crane et al. 2016; Huang et al. 2018). Finally, infections, both local and systemic, and inflammation in general seem to have a detrimental effect on brain health. Neuroinflammation resulting from infections, trauma, or acute vascular events such as stroke or hemorrhage inevitably leads to release of neurotoxic agents and was shown to negatively influence cognition (Pasqualetti et al. 2015). Peripheral chronic inflammatory diseases, such as periodontitis, have also been associated with increased risk of cognitive deficits (Naorungroj et al. 2013). Understanding whether and how these mediators impact the development of ADNC or the brain's ability to cope with it may also provide clues to the mechanisms that underlie resistance and resilience.

Overall, nongenetic factors, including environmental and lifestyle mediators that affect the rate of cognitive decline, can be divided into three broad categories: cognitive stimulation (education and socialization), inflammatory reaction (metabolic and infectious), and toxic influences. Although the underlying mechanisms of action have not been completely elucidated, some may target specific aspects of ADNC pathogenesis, whereas others may impact overall brain health, peripheral health, or aging in general. Each of these mediators provide clues to the pathways that lead to resistance or resilience, and therefore elucidating their mechanisms may uncover novel therapeutic targets.

Potential Therapeutic Approaches

The development of disease-modifying treatments for AD has eluded the field for decades, but recent advances offer the promise of reducing the ADNC and slowing progression of the clinical phenotype (Peng et al. 2023). Additionally, there have been notable symptomatic therapeutic approaches that afford patients some benefits that have been developed (Joe and Ringman 2019; Garcia et al. 2023). Despite these advances, however, the impact of these treatments are relatively minimal and the effective treatment of dementia due to ADNC will most likely require a multipronged approach, targeting several aspects of the pathophysiology (Perry et al. 2015). Here we both summarize the current therapeutic approaches for treating AD dementia and highlight potential novel targets based on our current understanding of resistance and resilience. Although the underlying mechanisms of resistance and resilience are not fully understood, several themes stand out and represent potential therapeutic targets once additional research and clinical studies are completed.

Targeting the Underlying Pathology

The neuropathologic changes that define ADNC (amyloid plaques and tau NFTs) have been a major target of efforts to develop disease-modifying treatments to rid the brain of the underlying pathology along with the downstream effects on neurodegeneration and cognitive function. These approaches have generally focused on reducing the production or accelerating the clearance of these pathologic proteins. With respect to β-amyloid, this has been attempted through a number of different strategies, most resulting in no significant clinical impact. For example, based on the genetic causes of familial AD, inhibitors of the enzymes involved in the processing of the APP have been targeted to prevent the deposition of β-amyloid; unfortunately, secretase inhibitors (α, β, and γ) have largely proven unsuccessful in clinical trials thus far (Kumar et al. 2018; Bazzari and Bazzari 2022; Monteiro et al. 2023). Active and passive immunity against β-amyloid are two additional strategies that have been employed, the latter of which has recently led to the first FDA-approved AD treatments in years (Budd Haeberlein et al. 2022; McDade et al. 2022; Shi et al. 2022; van Dyck et al. 2023; Yadollahikhales and Rojas 2023). These antibody-based therapeutics target soluble and insoluble amyloid β aggregates, ultimately reducing amyloid burden in the brain. There is recent data that not only suggests these strategies are effective in increase β-amyloid clearance, but that they (lecanemab) also can mitigate cognitive decline over time. However, these treatments are not without risk of adverse events, including cerebral edema, and work continues to identify additional approaches to reduce the underlying pathologic burden.

There are several ongoing trials evaluating anti-tau treatments, including those that reduce either tau phosphorylation or aggregation (Medina 2018). Active immunotherapy against tau has been shown to be safe and immunogenic; however, additional studies are necessary to determine the biological and clinical impact of this approach (Novak et al. 2021). Treating comorbid neurodegenerative diseases may promote resilience to ADNC in the brain, because ADNC rarely occurs in the absence of other common comorbid pathologies (Rabinovici et al. 2017). Currently there are no effective disease-modifying treatments for Lewy body pathology or TDP-43 pathology, which are often identified with ADNC, but these are active areas of investigation (Keating et al. 2022; MacDonald et al. 2022). However, treatment of cardiovascular disease risk factors, such as hypertension, hypercholesterolemia, and diabetes, can also help prevent cerebrovascular disease, possibly reducing the severity of cognitive

impairment in the setting of comorbid ADNC (Bergmann and Sano 2006; Wolozin and Bednar 2006; Sabia et al. 2019).

Treating the Effects of Neuron Dysfunction and Loss

In the absence of highly effective disease modifying therapies, much of the current approach for treating AD consists of managing symptoms. Cholinergic neurons in the nucleus basalis of Meynert are thought to be some of the earliest lost in AD, leading to a reduction in acetylcholine production (Hampel et al. 2018). Acetylcholinesterase inhibitors prevent the degradation of acetylcholine, which helps to maintain neuronal activity in the face of cholinergic dysfunction and loss (Lane et al. 2006; Marucci et al. 2021). Another feature seen in AD dementia is an overactive glutamatergic system due to excessive activation of the glutamate receptor subtype, N-methyl-D-aspartate (NMDA) receptor (Wang and Reddy 2017; Liu et al. 2019). NMDA receptor antagonists prevent the overactivation of this receptor, helping to prevent neurotoxicity from excitatory amino acids that contribute to neuron death. These therapeutic approaches help manage some of the consequences of the underlying pathophysiology but can only treat symptoms for a limited time.

Leveraging Approved Therapeutics to Target Pathways of Resilience

Although removing the underlying pathology is one approach to developing novel therapeutics for AD, the study of resistance and resilience has revealed several additional potential targets. Many of these targets already have available therapeutic options that have been used to treat other diseases and therefore have known safety and bioavailability profiles. A number of studies are now evaluating the potential to repurpose mediations developed to treat other conditions for the treatment of AD.

Chronic neuroinflammation has been widely studied in multiple diseases and is thought to be an important driver of AD pathology. Studies identified resilient individuals as having lower inflammation than those with AD pathology and cognitive decline (Barroeta-Espar et al. 2019). Animal models and genetic analysis also suggest brain immune pathways including lower inflammation promote resilience to AD pathology (Neuner et al. 2019; Tesi et al. 2020; Pérez-González et al. 2021). Nonsteroidal anti-inflammatory drugs (NSAIDs) such as COX-2 inhibitors were evaluated for their effect on AD progression with limited success (Aisen 2002; Ho et al. 2006; Jordan et al. 2020) and some risk of increased cardiovascular events. Other ways of targeting inflammation are of interest and currently being pursued. Masitinib is a tyrosine kinase inhibitor and reduces inflammation. A recent report suggests that masitinib was successful at slowing cognitive decline in mild-to-moderate AD patients (Dubois et al. 2023). Mitochondrial dysfunction is another potential driver of AD progression; drugs targeting mitochondrial function are currently under investigation for their effects on cognition (Macdonald et al. 2018). Autophagy is a known driver of aging (Kaushik et al. 2021); preservation of autophagic function was linked to resilience to AD (Tumurbaatar et al. 2023), which suggests that potential gerotherapeutic options like rapamycin may be useful AD therapeutics as well (Kaeberlein and Galvan 2019). Together, these studies provide some promise in repurposing already available therapeutics to target the underlying biology of resilience.

Leveraging the Modifiable Risk Factors

Lifestyle-based approaches to AD management are focused on introducing and supporting lifestyle habits that are considered neuroprotective. They include a combination of nutritious diet, regular exercise, cognitive stimulation, optimization of sleep and social engagement, and a reduction in tobacco and excessive alcohol use.

A diet rich in nutrients with anti-inflammatory, antioxidant, and neuroprotective properties is a well-known factor in maintaining brain health, and its role in the management of AD after onset should not be underestimated. For instance, the Mediterranean diet is considered beneficial for supporting cognitive function

(Féart et al. 2009; Loughrey et al. 2017; Radd-Vagenas et al. 2018; Rainey-Smith et al. 2018) and was shown to improve cognition in aged individuals (Martínez-Lapiscina et al. 2013). Other diets, such as the dietary approaches to stop hypertension (DASH) and the Mediterranean-DASH intervention for neurodegenerative delay (MIND) diet have also shown promising results (Tangney et al. 2014; Berendsen et al. 2017; McEvoy et al. 2017). Further, dietary restrictions, such as intermittent fasting, caloric restriction, and fasting-mimicking diets, promote healthy aging and positively influence the longevity of various species (Fontana and Partridge 2015; Lee and Longo 2016). Therapeutic effects of dietary restrictions on AD pathology, as well as cognitive function, have been demonstrated in transgenic models of AD (Halagappa et al. 2007; Mouton et al. 2009; Parrella et al. 2013).

Maintaining a healthy microbiome is also thought to help prevent dementia due to AD. Alterations in gut microbiota are common in neurodegenerative diseases, including AD, and are thought to contribute to its progression (Fung et al. 2017). Supplementation with probiotics, such as *Bifidobacterium* and *Lactobacterium* species, improves cognitive function in animal models as well as patients with mild cognitive impairment (MCI), possibly through decreasing levels of inflammation and oxidative stress (Kobayashi et al. 2019; Den et al. 2020; Ma et al. 2023).

Sleep disturbances are thought to exacerbate the development of ADNC and cognitive impairment, and improvement in sleep quantity and quality is expected to be beneficial for slowing the disease progression. There is a relative paucity of studies of sleep interventions in AD and MCI, but some positive outcomes have been associated with successful management of obstructive sleep apnea (Cooke et al. 2009), psychotherapy (Cassidy-Eagle et al. 2018), and melatonin treatment (Cruz-Aguilar et al. 2018, 2021).

Both physical and social activities are thought to be protective against dementia. There is evidence that physical inactivity is a risk factor for developing dementia (Livingston et al. 2020), and regular exercise has been shown to improve cognition and quality of life in older adults and patients with AD (Heyn et al. 2004; Erickson et al. 2011; Garuffi et al. 2013; Hoffmann et al. 2016). Similarly, social isolation and the absence of cognitively stimulating activities are associated with increased risk of developing dementia (Penninkilampi et al. 2018; Saito et al. 2018; Livingston et al. 2020), and several studies have reported a positive effect of psychosocial interventions and cognitive stimulation on cognition (Clare et al. 2010; Mortimer et al. 2012; Lin et al. 2018).

CONCLUSION

AD is a major public health crisis and there is an urgent need to identify novel therapeutic targets for the treatment and prevention of the underlying pathologic processes that contribute to the development of AD pathology, the impact of that pathology on brain function, or a combination of the two. Prevention of ADNC occurs naturally in a small but important subset of individuals referred to as resistant to AD. A better understanding of what factors led to the successful aging of these individuals and their ability to resist ADNC may identify critical pathways that can be targeted and manipulated through lifestyle, pharmaceutical, or molecular interventions in individuals who do not naturally possess those defenses, ultimately providing a preventative treatment for AD. Alternatively, the ability to cope with the presence of significant burden of ADNC in the brain is observed in an even smaller group of individuals referred to as resilient to AD. Identifying the relevant pathways that permit an individual to maintain normal levels of cognitive functioning despite harboring high levels of AD pathology in the brain could lead to interventional treatments to prevent dementia in individuals who do develop ADNC.

There has been progress toward a better understanding of the mechanisms of resistance and resilience. The focus on genes and pathways that together confer either an increased or decreased risk of AD could ultimately identify relevant biological pathways that can be further tested in model systems and probed for potential therapeutic targets. Similarly, studies on the modifiable mediators of AD risk, including diet, exercise, education, and other lifestyle or environmental exposures, show correlations between certain behaviors and healthy brain aging. Much work remains to be done to take these genetic, lifestyle, and environmental modifiers and pinpoint specific mechanisms and targetable pathways that prevent or mitigate the effects of AD pathology. To this end, focusing on resistant and resilient individuals using ever improving definitions of resistance and resilience, combined with a growing understanding of the underlying pathophysiology of AD, holds great potential.

REFERENCES

Abe T, Seino S, Tomine Y, Nishi M, Hata T, Shinkai S, Fujiwara Y, Kitamura A. 2022. Identifying the specific associations between participation in social activities and healthy lifestyle behaviours in older adults. *Maturitas* **155:** 24–31. doi:10.1016/j.maturitas.2021.10.003

Aisen PS. 2002. Evaluation of selective COX-2 inhibitors for the treatment of Alzheimer's disease. *J Pain Symptom Manage* **23:** S35–S40. doi:10.1016/s0885-3924(02)00374-3

Akbaraly TN, Singh-Manoux A, Dugravot A, Brunner EJ, Kivimäki M, Sabia S. 2019. Association of midlife diet with subsequent risk for dementia. *J Am Med Assoc* **321:** 957–968. doi:10.1001/jama.2019.1432

Alzheimer's Association. 2020. 2020 Alzheimer's disease facts and figures. *Alzheimers Dement* **16:** 391–460. doi:10.1002/alz.12068

Anson RM, Guo Z, de Cabo R, Iyun T, Rios M, Hagepanos A, Ingram DK, Lane MA, Mattson MP. 2003. Intermittent fasting dissociates beneficial effects of dietary restriction on glucose metabolism and neuronal resistance to injury from calorie intake. *Proc Natl Acad Sci* **100:** 6216–6220. doi:10.1073/pnas.1035720100

Arenaza-Urquijo EM, Vemuri P. 2018. Resistance vs resilience to Alzheimer disease: clarifying terminology for preclinical studies. *Neurology* **90:** 695–703. doi:10.1212/WNL.0000000000005303

Balduino E, de Melo BAR, de Sousa Mota da Silva L, Martinelli JE, Cecato JF. 2020. The "SuperAgers" construct in clinical practice: neuropsychological assessment of illiterate and educated elderly. *Int Psychogeriatr* **32:** 191–198. doi:10.1017/S1041610219001364

Barnes DE, Kaup A, Kirby KA, Byers AL, Diaz-Arrastia R, Yaffe K. 2014. Traumatic brain injury and risk of dementia in older veterans. *Neurology* **83:** 312–319. doi:10.1212/WNL.0000000000000616

Barroeta-Espar I, Weinstock LD, Perez-Nievas BG, Meltzer AC, Siao Tick Chong M, Amaral AC, Murray ME, Moulder KL, Morris JC, Cairns NJ, et al. 2019. Distinct cytokine profiles in human brains resilient to Alzheimer's pathology. *Neurobiol Dis* **121:** 327–337. doi:10.1016/j.nbd.2018.10.009

Batterham PJ, Mackinnon AJ, Christensen H. 2011. The effect of education on the onset and rate of terminal decline. *Psychol Aging* **26:** 339–350. doi:10.1037/a0021845

Bazzari FH, Bazzari AH. 2022. BACE1 inhibitors for Alzheimer's disease: the past, present and any future? *Molecules* **27:** 8823. doi:10.3390/molecules27248823

Bellenguez C, Küçükali F, Jansen IE, Kleineidam L, Moreno-Grau S, Amin N, Naj AC, Campos-Martin R, Grenier-Boley B, Andrade V, et al. 2022. New insights into the genetic etiology of Alzheimer's disease and related dementias. *Nat Genet* **54:** 412–436. doi:10.1038/s41588-022-01024-z

Bennett DA, Schneider JA, Tang Y, Arnold SE, Wilson RS. 2006. The effect of social networks on the relation between Alzheimer's disease pathology and level of cognitive function in old people: a longitudinal cohort study. *Lancet Neurol* **5:** 406–412. doi:10.1016/S1474-4422(06)70417-3

Berendsen AAM, Kang JH, van de Rest O, Feskens EJM, de Groot LCPGM, Grodstein F. 2017. The dietary approaches to stop hypertension diet, cognitive function, and cognitive decline in American older women. *J Am Med Dir Assoc* **18:** 427–432. doi:10.1016/j.jamda.2016.11.026

Bergmann C, Sano M. 2006. Cardiac risk factors and potential treatments in Alzheimer's disease. *Neurol Res* **28:** 595–604. doi:10.1179/016164106X130498

Bertram L, Tanzi RE. 2012. The genetics of Alzheimer's disease. *Prog Mol Biol Transl Sci* **107:** 79–100. doi:10.1016/B978-0-12-385883-2.00008-4

Bird TD. 1993. Early-Onset familial Alzheimer disease—retired chapter, for historical reference only. In *GeneReviews* (ed. Adam MP, Ardinger HH, Pagon RA, et al.). University of Washington, Seattle.

Boros BD, Greathouse KM, Gentry EG, Curtis KA, Birchall EL, Gearing M, Herskowitz JH. 2017. Dendritic spines provide cognitive resilience against Alzheimer's disease. *Ann Neurol* **82:** 602–614. doi:10.1002/ana.25049

Braak H, Braak E. 1991. Neuropathological stageing of Alzheimer-related changes. *Acta Neuropathol* **82:** 239–259. doi:10.1007/BF00308809

Braak H, Alafuzoff I, Arzberger T, Kretzschmar H, Del Tredici K. 2006. Staging of Alzheimer disease-associated neurofibrillary pathology using paraffin sections and immunocytochemistry. *Acta Neuropathol* **112:** 389–404. doi:10.1007/s00401-006-0127-z

Braak H, Thal DR, Ghebremedhin E, Del Tredici K. 2011. Stages of the pathologic process in Alzheimer disease: age categories from 1 to 100 years. *J Neuropathol Exp Neurol* **70:** 960–969. doi:10.1097/NEN.0b013e318232a379

Brettschneider J, Del Tredici K, Lee VMY, Trojanowski JQ. 2015. Spreading of pathology in neurodegenerative diseases: a focus on human studies. *Nat Rev Neurosci* **16:** 109–120. doi:10.1038/nrn3887

Buchman AS, Boyle PA, Yu L, Shah RC, Wilson RS, Bennett DA. 2012. Total daily physical activity and the risk of AD and cognitive decline in older adults. *Neurology* **78:** 1323–1329. doi:10.1212/WNL.0b013e3182535d35

Budd Haeberlein S, Aisen PS, Barkhof F, Chalkias S, Chen T, Cohen S, Dent G, Hansson O, Harrison K, von Hehn C, et al. 2022. Two randomized phase 3 studies of aducanumab in early Alzheimer's disease. *J Prev Alzheimers Dis* **9:** 197–210. doi:10.14283/jpad.2022.30

Cassidy-Eagle E, Siebern A, Unti L, Glassman J, O'Hara R. 2018. Neuropsychological functioning in older adults with mild cognitive impairment and insomnia randomized to CBT-I or control group. *Clin Gerontol* **41:** 136–144. doi:10.1080/07317115.2017.1384777

Chen H, Kwong JC, Copes R, Tu K, Villeneuve PJ, van Donkelaar A, Hystad P, Martin RV, Murray BJ, Jessiman B, et al. 2017. Living near major roads and the incidence of dementia, Parkinson's disease, and multiple sclerosis: a population-based cohort study. *Lancet* **389:** 718–726. doi:10.1016/S0140-6736(16)32399-6

Chen ST, Volle D, Jalil J, Wu P, Small GW. 2019. Health-promoting strategies for the aging brain. *Am J Geriatr Psychiatry* **27:** 213–236. doi:10.1016/j.jagp.2018.12.016

Choi D, Choi S, Park SM. 2018. Effect of smoking cessation on the risk of dementia: a longitudinal study. *Ann Clin Transl Neurol* **5:** 1192–1199. doi:10.1002/acn3.633

Clare L, Linden DEJ, Woods RT, Whitaker R, Evans SJ, Parkinson CH, van Paasschen J, Nelis SM, Hoare Z, Yuen KSL, et al. 2010. Goal-oriented cognitive rehabilitation for people with early-stage Alzheimer disease: a single-blind randomized controlled trial of clinical efficacy. *Am J Geriatr Psychiatry* **18:** 928–939. doi:10.1097/JGP.0b013e3181d5792a

Cohn-Schwartz E. 2020. Pathways from social activities to cognitive functioning: the role of physical activity and mental health. *Innov Aging* **4:** igaa015. doi:10.1093/geroni/igaa015

Cooke JR, Ancoli-Israel S, Liu L, Loredo JS, Natarajan L, Palmer BS, He F, Corey-Bloom J. 2009. Continuous positive airway pressure deepens sleep in patients with Alzheimer's disease and obstructive sleep apnea. *Sleep Med* **10:** 1101–1106. doi:10.1016/j.sleep.2008.12.016

Corrada MM, Berlau DJ, Kawas CH. 2012. A population-based clinicopathological study in the oldest-old: the 90+ study. *Curr Alzheimer Res* **9:** 709–717. doi:10.2174/156720512801322537

Crane PK, Gibbons LE, Dams-O'Connor K, Trittschuh E, Leverenz JB, Keene CD, Sonnen J, Montine TJ, Bennett DA, Leurgans S, et al. 2016. Association of traumatic brain injury with late-life neurodegenerative conditions and neuropathologic findings. *JAMA Neurol* **73:** 1062–1069. doi:10.1001/jamaneurol.2016.1948

Cruz-Aguilar MA, Ramírez-Salado I, Guevara MA, Hernández-González M, Benitez-King G. 2018. Melatonin effects on EEG activity during sleep onset in mild-to-moderate Alzheimer's disease: a pilot study. *J Alzheimers Dis Rep* **2:** 55–65. doi:10.3233/ADR-170019

Cruz-Aguilar MA, Ramírez-Salado I, Hernández-González M, Guevara MA, Del Río JM. 2021. Melatonin effects on EEG activity during non-rapid eye movement sleep in mild-to-moderate Alzheimer's disease: a pilot study. *Int J Neurosci* **131:** 580–590. doi:10.1080/00207454.2020.1750392

Crystal H, Dickson D, Fuld P, Masur D, Scott R, Mehler M, Masdeu J, Kawas C, Aronson M, Wolfson L. 1988. Clinico-pathologic studies in dementia: nondemented subjects with pathologically confirmed Alzheimer's disease. *Neurology* **38:** 1682–1687. doi:10.1212/WNL.38.11.1682

Currenti W, Godos J, Castellano S, Caruso G, Ferri R, Caraci F, Grosso G, Galvano F. 2021. Association between time restricted feeding and cognitive status in older Italian adults. *Nutrients* **13**: 191. doi:10.3390/nu13010191

Dams-O'Connor K, Gibbons LE, Bowen JD, McCurry SM, Larson EB, Crane PK. 2013. Risk for late-life re-injury, dementia and death among individuals with traumatic brain injury: a population-based study. *J Neurol Neurosurg Psychiatry* **84**: 177–182. doi:10.1136/jnnp-2012-303938

Deal JA, Power MC, Palta P, Alonso A, Schneider ALC, Perryman K, Bandeen-Roche K, Sharrett AR. 2020. Relationship of cigarette smoking and time of quitting with incident dementia and cognitive decline. *J Am Geriatr Soc* **68**: 337–345. doi:10.1111/jgs.16228

Den H, Dong X, Chen M, Zou Z. 2020. Efficacy of probiotics on cognition, and biomarkers of inflammation and oxidative stress in adults with Alzheimer's disease or mild cognitive impairment—a meta-analysis of randomized controlled trials. *Aging* **12**: 4010–4039. doi:10.18632/aging.102810

Dickson DW, Crystal HA, Mattiace LA, Masur DM, Blau AD, Davies P, Yen SH, Aronson MK. 1992. Identification of normal and pathological aging in prospectively studied nondemented elderly humans. *Neurobiol Aging* **13**: 179–189. doi:10.1016/0197-4580(92)90027-u

Dubois B, López-Arrieta J, Lipschitz S, Doskas T, Spiru L, Moroz S, Venger O, Vermersch P, Moussy A, Mansfield CD, et al. 2023. Masitinib for mild-to-moderate Alzheimer's disease: results from a randomized, placebo-controlled, phase 3, clinical trial. *Alzheimers Res Ther* **15**: 39. doi:10.1186/s13195-023-01169-x

Erickson KI, Voss MW, Prakash RS, Basak C, Szabo A, Chaddock L, Kim JS, Heo S, Alves H, White SM, et al. 2011. Exercise training increases size of hippocampus and improves memory. *Proc Natl Acad Sci* **108**: 3017–3022. doi:10.1073/pnas.1015950108

Escott-Price V, Sims R, Bannister C, Harold D, Vronskaya M, Majounie E, Badarinarayan N, Morgan K, Passmore P, Holmes C, et al. 2015. Common polygenic variation enhances risk prediction for Alzheimer's disease. *Brain* **138**: 3673–3684. doi:10.1093/brain/awv268

Fann JR, Ribe AR, Pedersen HS, Fenger-Grøn M, Christensen J, Benros ME, Vestergaard M. 2018. Long-term risk of dementia among people with traumatic brain injury in Denmark: a population-based observational cohort study. *Lancet Psychiatry* **5**: 424–431. doi:10.1016/S2215-0366(18)30065-8

Féart C, Samieri C, Rondeau V, Amieva H, Portet F, Dartigues JF, Scarmeas N, Barberger-Gateau P. 2009. Adherence to a Mediterranean diet, cognitive decline, and risk of dementia. *J Am Med Assoc* **302**: 638–648. doi:10.1001/jama.2009.1146

Fleminger S, Oliver DL, Lovestone S, Rabe-Hesketh S, Giora A. 2003. Head injury as a risk factor for Alzheimer's disease: the evidence 10 years on; a partial replication. *J Neurol Neurosurg Psychiatry* **74**: 857–862. doi:10.1136/jnnp.74.7.857

Fontana L, Partridge L. 2015. Promoting health and longevity through diet: from model organisms to humans. *Cell* **161**: 106–118. doi:10.1016/j.cell.2015.02.020

Fung TC, Olson CA, Hsiao EY. 2017. Interactions between the microbiota, immune and nervous systems in health and disease. *Nat Neurosci* **20**: 145–155. doi:10.1038/nn.4476

Garcia MJ, Leadley R, Lang S, Ross J, Vinand E, Ballard C, Gsteiger S. 2023. Real-world use of symptomatic treatments in early Alzheimer's disease. *J Alzheimers Dis* **91**: 151–167. doi:10.3233/JAD-220471

Gardner RC, Burke JF, Nettiksimmons J, Kaup A, Barnes DE, Yaffe K. 2014. Dementia risk after traumatic brain injury vs nonbrain trauma: the role of age and severity. *JAMA Neurol* **71**: 1490–1497. doi:10.1001/jamaneurol.2014.2668

Garuffi M, Costa JLR, Hernández SSS, Vital TM, Stein AM, dos Santos JG, Stella F. 2013. Effects of resistance training on the performance of activities of daily living in patients with Alzheimer's disease. *Geriatr Gerontol Int* **13**: 322–328. doi:10.1111/j.1447-0594.2012.00899.x

Halagappa VKM, Guo Z, Pearson M, Matsuoka Y, Cutler RG, Laferla FM, Mattson MP. 2007. Intermittent fasting and caloric restriction ameliorate age-related behavioral deficits in the triple-transgenic mouse model of Alzheimer's disease. *Neurobiol Dis* **26**: 212–220. doi:10.1016/j.nbd.2006.12.019

Hampel H, Mesulam MM, Cuello AC, Farlow MR, Giacobini E, Grossberg GT, Khachaturian AS, Vergallo A, Cavedo E, Snyder PJ, et al. 2018. The cholinergic system in the pathophysiology and treatment of Alzheimer's disease. *Brain* **141**: 1917–1933. doi:10.1093/brain/awy132

Helmes E, Østbye T, Steenhuis RE. 2011. Incremental contribution of reported previous head injury to the prediction of diagnosis and cognitive functioning in older adults. *Brain Inj* **25**: 338–347. doi:10.3109/02699052.2011.556104

Heyn P, Abreu BC, Ottenbacher KJ. 2004. The effects of exercise training on elderly persons with cognitive impairment and dementia: a meta-analysis. *Arch Phys Med Rehabil* **85**: 1694–1704. doi:10.1016/j.apmr.2004.03.019

Ho L, Qin W, Stetka BS, Pasinetti GM. 2006. Is there a future for cyclo-oxygenase inhibitors in Alzheimer's disease? *CNS Drugs* **20**: 85–98. doi:10.2165/00023210-200620020-00001

Hoffmann K, Sobol NA, Frederiksen KS, Beyer N, Vogel A, Vestergaard K, Brændgaard H, Gottrup H, Lolk A, Wermuth L, et al. 2016. Moderate-to-high intensity physical exercise in patients with Alzheimer's disease: a randomized controlled trial. *J Alzheimers Dis* **50**: 443–453. doi:10.3233/JAD-150817

Hohman TJ, Dumitrescu L, Cox NJ, Jefferson AL, Alzheimer's Neuroimaging Initiative. 2017. Genetic resilience to amyloid related cognitive decline. *Brain Imaging Behav* **11**: 401–409. doi:10.1007/s11682-016-9615-5

Hollingworth P, Harold D, Sims R, Gerrish A, Lambert JC, Carrasquillo MM, Abraham R, Hamshere ML, Pahwa JS, Moskvina V, et al. 2011. Common variants at ABCA7, MS4A6A/MS4A4E, EPHA1, CD33 and CD2AP are associated with Alzheimer's disease. *Nat Genet* **43**: 429–435. doi:10.1038/ng.803

Huang CH, Lin CW, Lee YC, Huang CY, Huang RY, Tai YC, Wang KW, Yang SN, Sun YT, Wang HK. 2018. Is traumatic brain injury a risk factor for neurodegeneration? A meta-analysis of population-based studies. *BMC Neurol* **18**: 184. doi:10.1186/s12883-018-1187-0

Huq AJ, Fulton-Howard B, Riaz M, Laws S, Sebra R, Ryan J, Renton AE, Goate AM, Masters CL, Storey E, et al. 2021. Polygenic score modifies risk for Alzheimer's disease in *APOE* ε4 homozygotes at phenotypic extremes. *Alzheimers Dement* 13: e12226. doi:10.1002/dad2.12226

Hwang J, Park S, Kim S. 2018. Effects of participation in social activities on cognitive function among middle-aged and older adults in Korea. *Int J Environ Res Public Health* 15: 2315. doi:10.3390/ijerph15102315

Hyman BT, Phelps CH, Beach TG, Bigio EH, Cairns NJ, Carrillo MC, Dickson DW, Duyckaerts C, Frosch MP, Masliah E, et al. 2012. National Institute on Aging-Alzheimer's Association guidelines for the neuropathologic assessment of Alzheimer's disease. *Alzheimers Dement* 8: 1–13. doi:10.1016/j.jalz.2011.10.007

Iacono D, Zandi P, Gross M, Markesbery WR, Pletnikova O, Rudow G, Troncoso JC. 2015. APOEε2 and education in cognitively normal older subjects with high levels of AD pathology at autopsy: findings from the Nun Study. *Oncotarget* 6: 14082–14091. doi:10.18632/oncotarget.4118

James BD, Wilson RS, Barnes LL, Bennett DA. 2011. Late-life social activity and cognitive decline in old age. *J Int Neuropsychol Soc* 17: 998–1005. doi:10.1017/S1355617711000531

Joe E, Ringman JM. 2019. Cognitive symptoms of Alzheimer's disease: clinical management and prevention. *BMJ* 367: l6217. doi:10.1136/bmj.l6217

Jordan F, Quinn TJ, McGuinness B, Passmore P, Kelly JP, Tudur Smith C, Murphy K, Devane D. 2020. Aspirin and other non-steroidal anti-inflammatory drugs for the prevention of dementia. *Cochrane Database Syst Rev* 4: CD011459. doi:10.1002/14651858.CD011459.pub2

Joseph J, Cole G, Head E, Ingram D. 2009. Nutrition, brain aging, and neurodegeneration. *J Neurosci* 29: 12795–12801. doi:10.1523/JNEUROSCI.3520-09.2009

Kaeberlein M, Galvan V. 2019. Rapamycin and Alzheimer's disease: time for a clinical trial? *Sci Transl Med* 11: eaar4289. doi:10.1126/scitranslmed.aar4289

Katzman R, Terry R, DeTeresa R, Brown T, Davies P, Fuld P, Renbing X, Peck A. 1988. Clinical, pathological, and neurochemical changes in dementia: a subgroup with preserved mental status and numerous neocortical plaques. *Ann Neurol* 23: 138–144. doi:10.1002/ana.410230206

Kaushik S, Tasset I, Arias E, Pampliega O, Wong E, Martinez-Vicente M, Cuervo AM. 2021. Autophagy and the hallmarks of aging. *Ageing Res Rev* 72: 101468. doi:10.1016/j.arr.2021.101468

Keating SS, San Gil R, Swanson MEV, Scotter EL, Walker AK. 2022. TDP-43 pathology: from noxious assembly to therapeutic removal. *Prog Neurobiol* 211: 102229. doi:10.1016/j.pneurobio.2022.102229

Knopman DS, DeKosky ST, Cummings JL, Chui H, Corey-Bloom J, Relkin N, Small GW, Miller B, Stevens JC. 2001. Practice parameter: diagnosis of dementia (an evidence-based review). Report of the Quality Standards Subcommittee of the American Academy of Neurology. *Neurology* 56: 1143–1153. doi:10.1212/wnl.56.9.1143

Kobayashi Y, Kinoshita T, Matsumoto A, Yoshino K, Saito I, Xiao JZ. 2019. Bifidobacterium breve A1 supplementation improved cognitive decline in older adults with mild cognitive impairment: an open-label, single-arm study. *J Prev Alzheimers Dis* 6: 70–75. doi:10.14283/jpad.2018.32

Koch M, Fitzpatrick AL, Rapp SR, Nahin RL, Williamson JD, Lopez OL, DeKosky ST, Kuller LH, Mackey RH, Mukamal KJ, et al. 2019. Alcohol consumption and risk of dementia and cognitive decline among older adults with or without mild cognitive impairment. *JAMA Netw Open* 2: e1910319. doi:10.1001/jamanetworkopen.2019.10319

Kumar D, Ganeshpurkar A, Kumar D, Modi G, Gupta SK, Singh SK. 2018. Secretase inhibitors for the treatment of Alzheimer's disease: long road ahead. *Eur J Med Chem* 148: 436–452. doi:10.1016/j.ejmech.2018.02.035

Lambert JC, Heath S, Even G, Campion D, Sleegers K, Hiltunen M, Combarros O, Zelenika D, Bullido MJ, Tavernier B, et al. 2009. Genome-wide association study identifies variants at CLU and CR1 associated with Alzheimer's disease. *Nat Genet* 41: 1094–1099. doi:10.1038/ng.439

Lambert JC, Ibrahim-Verbaas CA, Harold D, Naj AC, Sims R, Bellenguez C, Jun G, DeStefano AL, Bis JC, Beecham GW, et al. 2013. Meta-analysis of 74,046 individuals identifies 11 new susceptibility loci for Alzheimer's disease. *Nat Genet* 45: 1452–1458. doi:10.1038/ng.2802

Lane RM, Potkin SG, Enz A. 2006. Targeting acetylcholinesterase and butyrylcholinesterase in dementia. *Int J Neuropsychopharmacol* 9: 101–124. doi:10.1017/S1461145705005833

Lane CA, Barnes J, Nicholas JM, Sudre CH, Cash DM, Parker TD, Malone IB, Lu K, James SN, Keshavan A, et al. 2019. Associations between blood pressure across adulthood and late-life brain structure and pathology in the neuroscience substudy of the 1946 British birth cohort (insight 46): an epidemiological study. *Lancet Neurol* 18: 942–952. doi:10.1016/S1474-4422(19)30228-5

Latimer CS, Burke BT, Liachko NF, Currey HN, Kilgore MD, Gibbons LE, Henriksen J, Darvas M, Domoto-Reilly K, Jayadev S, et al. 2019. Resistance and resilience to Alzheimer's disease pathology are associated with reduced cortical pTau and absence of limbic-predominant age-related TDP-43 encephalopathy in a community-based cohort. *Acta Neuropathol Commun* 7: 91. doi:10.1186/s40478-019-0743-1

Launer LJ, Andersen K, Dewey ME, Letenneur L, Ott A, Amaducci LA, Brayne C, Copeland JR, Dartigues JF, Kragh-Sorensen P, et al. 1999. Rates and risk factors for dementia and Alzheimer's disease: results from EURODEM pooled analyses. EURODEM incidence research group and work groups. European studies of dementia. *Neurology* 52: 78–84. doi:10.1212/wnl.52.1.78

Lee C, Longo V. 2016. Dietary restriction with and without caloric restriction for healthy aging. *F1000Res* 5: F1000 Faculty Rev-117. doi:10.12688/f1000research.7136.1

Lin HC, Yang YP, Cheng WY, Wang JJ. 2018. Distinctive effects between cognitive stimulation and reminiscence therapy on cognitive function and quality of life for different types of behavioural problems in dementia. *Scand J Caring Sci* 32: 594–602. doi:10.1111/scs.12484

Liu J, Chang L, Song Y, Li H, Wu Y. 2019. The role of NMDA receptors in Alzheimer's disease. *Front Neurosci* 13: 43. doi:10.3389/fnins.2019.00043

Livingston G, Huntley J, Sommerlad A, Ames D, Ballard C, Banerjee S, Brayne C, Burns A, Cohen-Mansfield J, Cooper C, et al. 2020. Dementia prevention, intervention, and care: 2020 report of the Lancet Commission. *Lancet* **396:** 413–446. doi:10.1016/S0140-6736(20)30367-6

Loughrey DG, Lavecchia S, Brennan S, Lawlor BA, Kelly ME. 2017. The impact of the Mediterranean diet on the cognitive functioning of healthy older adults: a systematic review and meta-analysis. *Adv Nutr* **8:** 571–586. doi:10.3945/an.117.015495

Lu T, Aron L, Zullo J, Pan Y, Kim H, Chen Y, Yang TH, Kim HM, Drake D, Liu XS, et al. 2014. REST and stress resistance in ageing and Alzheimer's disease. *Nature* **507:** 448–454. doi:10.1038/nature13163

Ma X, Kim JK, Shin YJ, Son YH, Lee DY, Park HS, Kim DH. 2023. Alleviation of cognitive impairment-like behaviors, neuroinflammation, colitis, and gut dysbiosis in 5xFAD transgenic and aged mice by lactobacillus mucosae and bifidobacterium longum. *Nutrients* **15:** 3381. doi:10.3390/nu15153381

Macdonald R, Barnes K, Hastings C, Mortiboys H. 2018. Mitochondrial abnormalities in Parkinson's disease and Alzheimer's disease: can mitochondria be targeted therapeutically? *Biochem Soc Trans* **46:** 891–909. doi:10.1042/BST20170501

MacDonald S, Shah AS, Tousi B. 2022. Current therapies and drug development pipeline in lewy body dementia: an update. *Drugs Aging* **39:** 505–522. doi:10.1007/s40266-022-00939-w

Martínez-Lapiscina EH, Clavero P, Toledo E, Estruch R, Salas-Salvadó J, San Julián B, Sanchez-Tainta A, Ros E, Valls-Pedret C, Martinez-Gonzalez MÁ. 2013. Mediterranean diet improves cognition: the PREDIMED-NAVARRA randomised trial. *J Neurol Neurosurg Psychiatry* **84:** 1318–1325. doi:10.1136/jnnp-2012-304792

Marucci G, Buccioni M, Ben DD, Lambertucci C, Volpini R, Amenta F. 2021. Efficacy of acetylcholinesterase inhibitors in Alzheimer's disease. *Neuropharmacology* **190:** 108352. doi:10.1016/j.neuropharm.2020.108352

Maurer K, Volk S, Gerbaldo H. 1997. Auguste D and Alzheimer's disease. *Lancet* **349:** 1546–1549. doi:10.1016/S0140-6736(96)10203-8

McDade E, Cummings JL, Dhadda S, Swanson CJ, Reyderman L, Kanekiyo M, Koyama A, Irizarry M, Kramer LD, Bateman RJ. 2022. Lecanemab in patients with early Alzheimer's disease: detailed results on biomarker, cognitive, and clinical effects from the randomized and open-label extension of the phase 2 proof-of-concept study. *Alzheimers Res Ther* **14:** 191. doi:10.1186/s13195-022-01124-2

McEvoy CT, Guyer H, Langa KM, Yaffe K. 2017. Neuroprotective diets are associated with better cognitive function: the health and retirement study. *J Am Geriatr Soc* **65:** 1857–1862. doi:10.1111/jgs.14922

McKhann G, Drachman D, Folstein M, Katzman R, Price D, Stadlan EM. 1984. Clinical diagnosis of Alzheimer's disease: report of the NINCDS-ADRDA Work Group under the auspices of Department of Health and Human Services Task Force on Alzheimer's disease. *Neurology* **34:** 939–944. doi:10.1212/wnl.34.7.939

McKhann GM, Knopman DS, Chertkow H, Hyman BT, Jack CR J, Kawas CH, Klunk WE, Koroshetz WJ, Manly JJ, Mayeux R, et al. 2011. The diagnosis of dementia due to Alzheimer's disease: recommendations from the National

Institute on Aging-Alzheimer's Association workgroups on diagnostic guidelines for Alzheimer's disease. *Alzheimers Dement* **7:** 263–269. doi:10.1016/j.jalz.2011.03.005

Medina M. 2018. An overview on the clinical development of tau-based therapeutics. *Int J Mol Sci* **19:** 1160. doi:10.3390/ijms19041160

Medway C, Morgan K. 2014. Review: the genetics of Alzheimer's disease; putting flesh on the bones. *Neuropathol Appl Neurobiol* **40:** 97–105. doi:10.1111/nan.12101

Mehta KM, Ott A, Kalmijn S, Slooter AJ, van Duijn CM, Hofman A, Breteler MM. 1999. Head trauma and risk of dementia and Alzheimer's disease: the Rotterdam study. *Neurology* **53:** 1959–1962. doi:10.1212/wnl.53.9.1959

Mirra SS. 1997. The CERAD neuropathology protocol and consensus recommendations for the postmortem diagnosis of Alzheimer's disease: a commentary. *Neurobiol Aging* **18:** S91–S94. doi:10.1016/s0197-4580(97)00058-4

Mirra SS, Heyman A, McKeel D, Sumi SM, Crain BJ, Brownlee LM, Vogel FS, Hughes JP, van Belle G, Berg L. 1991. The consortium to establish a registry for Alzheimer's disease (CERAD). Part II: Standardization of the neuropathologic assessment of Alzheimer's disease. *Neurology* **41:** 479–486. doi:10.1212/wnl.41.4.479

Misiak B, Leszek J, Kiejna A. 2012. Metabolic syndrome, mild cognitive impairment and Alzheimer's disease—the emerging role of systemic low-grade inflammation and adiposity. *Brain Res Bull* **89:** 144–149. doi:10.1016/j.brainresbull.2012.08.003

Monteiro KLC, Dos Santos Alcântara MG, Freire NML, Brandão EM, do Nascimento VL, Dos Santos Viana LM, de Aquino TM, da Silva-Júnior EF. 2023. BACE-1 inhibitors targeting Alzheimer's disease. *Curr Alzheimer Res* **20:** 131–148. doi:10.2174/1567205020666230612155953

Montine TJ, Phelps CH, Beach TG, Bigio EH, Cairns NJ, Dickson DW, Duyckaerts C, Frosch MP, Masliah E, Mirra SS, et al. 2012. National Institute on Aging–Alzheimer's Association guidelines for the neuropathologic assessment of Alzheimer's disease: a practical approach. *Acta Neuropathol* **123:** 1–11. doi:10.1007/s00401-011-0910-3

Montine TJ, Monsell SE, Beach TG, Bigio EH, Bu Y, Cairns NJ, Frosch M, Henriksen J, Kofler J, Kukull WA, et al. 2016. Multisite assessment of NIA-AA guidelines for the neuropathologic evaluation of Alzheimer's disease. *Alzheimers Dement* **12:** 164–169. doi:10.1016/j.jalz.2015.07.492

Montine TJ, Cholerton BA, Corrada MM, Edland SD, Flanagan ME, Hemmy LS, Kawas CH, White LR. 2019. Concepts for brain aging: resistance, resilience, reserve, and compensation. *Alzheimers Res Ther* **11:** 22. doi:10.1186/s13195-019-0479-y

Morris MC, Wang Y, Barnes LL, Bennett DA, Dawson-Hughes B, Booth SL. 2018. Nutrients and bioactives in green leafy vegetables and cognitive decline: prospective study. *Neurology* **90:** e214–e222. doi:10.1212/WNL.0000000000004815

Mortimer JA, Snowdon DA, Markesbery WR. 2003. Head circumference, education and risk of dementia: findings from the Nun Study. *J Clin Exp Neuropsychol* **25:** 671–679. doi:10.1076/jcen.25.5.671.14584

Mortimer JA, Ding D, Borenstein AR, DeCarli C, Guo Q, Wu Y, Zhao Q, Chu S. 2012. Changes in brain volume and cognition in a randomized trial of exercise and social interaction in a community-based sample of non-demented Chinese elders. *J Alzheimers Dis* **30**: 757–766. doi:10.3233/JAD-2012-120079

Mouton PR, Chachich ME, Quigley C, Spangler E, Ingram DK. 2009. Caloric restriction attenuates amyloid deposition in middle-aged dtg APP/PS1 mice. *Neurosci Lett* **464**: 184–187. doi:10.1016/j.neulet.2009.08.038

Mukherjee S, Kim S, Gibbons LE, Nho K, Risacher SL, Glymour MM, Habeck C, Lee GJ, Mormino E, Ertekin-Taner N, et al. 2012. Genetic architecture of resilience of executive functioning. *Brain Imaging Behav* **6**: 621–633. doi:10.1007/s11682-012-9184-1

Müller S, Preische O, Sohrabi HR, Gräber S, Jucker M, Ringman JM, Martins RN, McDade E, Schofield PR, Ghetti B, et al. 2018. Relationship between physical activity, cognition, and Alzheimer pathology in autosomal dominant Alzheimer's disease. *Alzheimers Dement* **14**: 1427–1437. doi:10.1016/j.jalz.2018.06.3059

Muniz-Terrera G, van den Hout A, Piccinin AM, Matthews FE, Hofer SM. 2013. Investigating terminal decline: results from a UK population-based study of aging. *Psychol Aging* **28**: 377–385. doi:10.1037/a0031000

Naj AC, Jun G, Beecham GW, Wang L-S, Vardarajan BN, Buros J, Gallins PJ, Buxbaum JD, Jarvik GP, Crane PK, et al. 2011. Common variants at MS4A4/MS4A6E, CD2AP, CD33 and EPHA1 are associated with late-onset Alzheimer's disease. *Nat Genet* **43**: 436–441. doi:10.1038/ng.801

Naorungroj S, Slade GD, Beck JD, Mosley TH, Gottesman RF, Alonso A, Heiss G. 2013. Cognitive decline and oral health in middle-aged adults in the ARIC study. *J Dent Res* **92**: 795–801. doi:10.1177/0022034513497960

Nelson PT, Alafuzoff I, Bigio EH, Bouras C, Braak H, Cairns NJ, Castellani RJ, Crain BJ, Davies P, Del Tredici K, et al. 2012. Correlation of Alzheimer disease neuropathologic changes with cognitive status: a review of the literature. *J Neuropathol Exp Neurol* **71**: 362–381. doi:10.1097/NEN.0b013e31825018f7

Neuner SM, Heuer SE, Zhang JG, Philip VM, Kaczorowski CC. 2019. Identification of pre-symptomatic gene signatures that predict resilience to cognitive decline in the genetically diverse AD-BXD model. *Front Genet* **10**: 35. doi:10.3389/fgene.2019.00035

Nordström P, Michaëlsson K, Gustafson Y, Nordström A. 2014. Traumatic brain injury and young onset dementia: a nationwide cohort study. *Ann Neurol* **75**: 374–381. doi:10.1002/ana.24101

Northey JM, Cherbuin N, Pumpa KL, Smee DJ, Rattray B. 2018. Exercise interventions for cognitive function in adults older than 50: a systematic review with meta-analysis. *Br J Sports Med* **52**: 154–160. doi:10.1136/bjsports-2016-096587

Novak P, Kovacech B, Katina S, Schmidt R, Scheltens P, Kontsekova E, Ropele S, Fialova L, Kramberger M, Paulenka-Ivanovova N, et al. 2021. ADAMANT: a placebo-controlled randomized phase 2 study of AADvac1, an active immunotherapy against pathological tau in Alzheimer's disease. *Nat Aging* **1**: 521–534. doi:10.1038/s43587-021-00070-2

Nyberg L, Lövdén M, Riklund K, Lindenberger U, Bäckman L. 2012. Memory aging and brain maintenance. *Trends Cogn Sci* **16**: 292–305. doi:10.1016/j.tics.2012.04.005

Ooi TC, Meramat A, Rajab NF, Shahar S, Ismail IS, Azam AA, Sharif R. 2020. Intermittent fasting enhanced the cognitive function in older adults with mild cognitive impairment by inducing biochemical and metabolic changes: a 3-year progressive study. *Nutrients* **12**: 2644. doi:10.3390/nu12092644

Ott A, Breteler MM, van Harskamp F, Claus JJ, van der Cammen TJ, Grobbee DE, Hofman A. 1995. Prevalence of Alzheimer's disease and vascular dementia: association with education. The Rotterdam study. *BMJ* **310**: 970–973. doi:10.1136/bmj.310.6985.970

Oudin A, Segersson D, Adolfsson R, Forsberg B. 2018. Association between air pollution from residential wood burning and dementia incidence in a longitudinal study in northern Sweden. *PLoS ONE* **13**: e0198283. doi:10.1371/journal.pone.0198283

Parrella E, Maxim T, Maialetti F, Zhang L, Wan J, Wei M, Cohen P, Fontana L, Longo VD. 2013. Protein restriction cycles reduce IGF-1 and phosphorylated tau, and improve behavioral performance in an Alzheimer's disease mouse model. *Aging Cell* **12**: 257–268. doi:10.1111/acel.12049

Pasqualetti G, Brooks DJ, Edison P. 2015. The role of neuroinflammation in dementias. *Curr Neurol Neurosci Rep* **15**: 17. doi:10.1007/s11910-015-0531-7

Peng Y, Jin H, Xue YH, Chen Q, Yao SY, Du MQ, Liu S. 2023. Current and future therapeutic strategies for Alzheimer's disease: an overview of drug development bottlenecks. *Front Aging Neurosci* **15**: 1206572. doi:10.3389/fnagi.2023.1206572

Penninkilampi R, Casey AN, Singh MF, Brodaty H. 2018. The association between social engagement, loneliness, and risk of dementia: a systematic review and meta-analysis. *J Alzheimers Dis* **66**: 1619–1633. doi:10.3233/JAD-180439

Pérez-González M, Badesso S, Lorenzo E, Guruceaga E, Pérez-Mediavilla A, García-Osta A, Cuadrado-Tejedor M. 2021. Identifying the main functional pathways associated with cognitive resilience to Alzheimer's disease. *Int J Mol Sci* **22**: 9120. doi:10.3390/ijms22179120

Perez-Nievas BG, Stein TD, Tai HC, Dols-Icardo O, Scotton TC, Barroeta-Espar I, Fernandez-Carballo L, de Munain EL, Perez J, Marquie M, et al. 2013. Dissecting phenotypic traits linked to human resilience to Alzheimer's pathology. *Brain* **136**: 2510–2526. doi:10.1093/brain/awt171

Perry D, Sperling R, Katz R, Berry D, Dilts D, Hanna D, Salloway S, Trojanowski JQ, Bountra C, Krams M, et al. 2015. Building a roadmap for developing combination therapies for Alzheimer's disease. *Expert Rev Neurother* **15**: 327–333. doi:10.1586/14737175.2015.996551

Peters R, Ee N, Peters J, Booth A, Mudway I, Anstey KJ. 2019. Air pollution and dementia: a systematic review. *J Alzheimers Dis* **70**: S145–S163. doi:10.3233/JAD-180631

Piumatti G, Moore SC, Berridge DM, Sarkar C, Gallacher J. 2018. The relationship between alcohol use and long-term cognitive decline in middle and late life: a longitudinal analysis using UK Biobank. *J Public Health* **40**: 304–311. doi:10.1093/pubmed/fdx186

Plassman BL, Havlik RJ, Steffens DC, Helms MJ, Newman TN, Drosdick D, Phillips C, Gau BA, Welsh-Bohmer KA,

Burke JR, et al. 2000. Documented head injury in early adulthood and risk of Alzheimer's disease and other dementias. *Neurology* **55:** 1158–1166. doi:10.1212/wnl.55.8.1158

Rabinovici GD, Carrillo MC, Forman M, DeSanti S, Miller DS, Kozauer N, Petersen RC, Randolph C, Knopman DS, Smith EE, et al. 2017. Multiple comorbid neuropathologies in the setting of Alzheimer's disease neuropathology and implications for drug development. *Alzheimers Dement* **3:** 83–91. doi:10.1016/j.trci.2016.09.002

Radd-Vagenas S, Duffy SL, Naismith SL, Brew BJ, Flood VM, Fiatarone Singh MA. 2018. Effect of the Mediterranean diet on cognition and brain morphology and function: a systematic review of randomized controlled trials. *Am J Clin Nutr* **107:** 389–404. doi:10.1093/ajcn/nqx070

Rainey-Smith SR, Gu Y, Gardener SL, Doecke JD, Villemagne VL, Brown BM, Taddei K, Laws SM, Sohrabi HR, Weinborn M, et al. 2018. Mediterranean diet adherence and rate of cerebral Aβ-amyloid accumulation: data from the Australian imaging, biomarkers and lifestyle study of ageing. *Transl Psychiatry* **8:** 238. doi:10.1038/s41398-018-0293-5

Ramanan VK, Lesnick TG, Przybelski SA, Heckman MG, Knopman DS, Graff-Radford J, Lowe VJ, Machulda MM, Mielke MM, Jack CR, et al. 2021. Coping with brain amyloid: genetic heterogeneity and cognitive resilience to Alzheimer's pathophysiology. *Acta Neuropathol Commun* **9:** 48. doi:10.1186/s40478-021-01154-1

Riley KP, Snowdon DA, Desrosiers MF, Markesbery WR. 2005. Early life linguistic ability, late life cognitive function, and neuropathology: findings from the Nun Study. *Neurobiol Aging* **26:** 341–347. doi:10.1016/j.neurobiolaging.2004.06.019

Sabia S, Fayosse A, Dumurgier J, Dugravot A, Akbaraly T, Britton A, Kivimäki M, Singh-Manoux A. 2018. Alcohol consumption and risk of dementia: 23 year follow-up of Whitehall II cohort study. *BMJ* **362:** k2927. doi:10.1136/bmj.k2927

Sabia S, Fayosse A, Dumurgier J, Schnitzler A, Empana JP, Ebmeier KP, Dugravot A, Kivimäki M, Singh-Manoux A. 2019. Association of ideal cardiovascular health at age 50 with incidence of dementia: 25 year follow-up of Whitehall II cohort study. *BMJ* **366:** l4414. doi:10.1136/bmj.l4414

Saito T, Murata C, Saito M, Takeda T, Kondo K. 2018. Influence of social relationship domains and their combinations on incident dementia: a prospective cohort study. *J Epidemiol Community Health* **72:** 7–12. doi:10.1136/jech-2017-209811

Salinas J, O'Donnell A, Kojis DJ, Pase MP, DeCarli C, Rentz DM, Berkman LF, Beiser A, Seshadri S. 2021. Association of social support with brain volume and cognition. *JAMA Netw Open* **4:** e2121122. doi:10.1001/jamanetworkopen.2021.21122

Schafer MJ, Alldred MJ, Lee SH, Calhoun ME, Petkova E, Mathews PM, Ginsberg SD. 2015. Reduction of β-amyloid and γ-secretase by calorie restriction in female Tg2576 mice. *Neurobiol Aging* **36:** 1293–1302. doi:10.1016/j.neurobiolaging.2014.10.043

Schneider JA, Aggarwal NT, Barnes L, Boyle P, Bennett DA. 2009. The neuropathology of older persons with and without dementia from community versus clinic cohorts. *J Alzheimers Dis* **18:** 691–701. doi:10.3233/JAD-2009-1227

Schwarzinger M, Pollock BG, Hasan OSM, Dufouil C, Rehm J, QalyDays Study Group. 2018. Contribution of alcohol use disorders to the burden of dementia in France 2008-13: a nationwide retrospective cohort study. *Lancet Public Health* **3:** e124–e132. doi:10.1016/S2468-2667(18)30022-7

Serrano-Pozo A, Das S, Hyman BT. 2021. APOE and Alzheimer's disease: advances in genetics, pathophysiology, and therapeutic approaches. *Lancet Neurol* **20:** 68–80. doi:10.1016/S1474-4422(20)30412-9

Seshadri S, Fitzpatrick AL, Ikram MA, DeStefano AL, Gudnason V, Boada M, Bis JC, Smith AV, Carrasquillo MM, Lambert JC. 2010. Genome-wide analysis of genetic loci associated with Alzheimer disease. *J Am Med Assoc* **303:** 1832–1840. doi:10.1001/jama.2010.574

Shi M, Chu F, Zhu F, Zhu J. 2022. Impact of anti-amyloid-β monoclonal antibodies on the pathology and clinical profile of Alzheimer's disease: a focus on aducanumab and lecanemab. *Front Aging Neurosci* **14:** 870517. doi:10.3389/fnagi.2022.870517

Stern Y. 2002. What is cognitive reserve? theory and research application of the reserve concept. *J Int Neuropsychol Soc* **8:** 448–460. doi:10.1017/S1355617702813248

Stern Y. 2009. Cognitive reserve. *Neuropsychologia* **47:** 2015–2028. doi:10.1016/j.neuropsychologia.2009.03.004

Suhanov AV, Pilipenko PI, Korczyn AD, Hofman A, Voevoda MI, Shishkin SV, Simonova GI, Nikitin YP, Feigin VL. 2006. Risk factors for Alzheimer's disease in Russia: a case-control study. *Eur J Neurol* **13:** 990–995. doi:10.1111/j.1468-1331.2006.01391.x

Tangney CC, Li H, Wang Y, Barnes L, Schneider JA, Bennett DA, Morris MC. 2014. Relation of DASH- and Mediterranean-like dietary patterns to cognitive decline in older persons. *Neurology* **83:** 1410–1416. doi:10.1212/WNL.0000000000000884

Terrera GM, Minett T, Brayne C, Matthews FE. 2014. Education associated with a delayed onset of terminal decline. *Age Ageing* **43:** 26–31. doi:10.1093/ageing/aft150

Tesi N, van der Lee SJ, Hulsman M, Jansen IE, Stringa N, van Schoor NM, Scheltens P, van der Flier WM, Huisman M, Reinders MJT, et al. 2020. Immune response and endocytosis pathways are associated with the resilience against Alzheimer's disease. *Transl Psychiatry* **10:** 332. doi:10.1038/s41398-020-01018-7

Thal DR, Rüb U, Orantes M, Braak H. 2002. Phases of Aβ-deposition in the human brain and its relevance for the development of AD. *Neurology* **58:** 1791–1800. doi:10.1212/wnl.58.12.1791

To J, Shao ZY, Gandawidjaja M, Tabibi T, Grysman N, Grossberg GT. 2022. Comparison of the impact of the Mediterranean diet, anti-inflammatory diet, Seventh-day Adventist diet, and ketogenic diet relative to cognition and cognitive decline. *Curr Nutr Rep* **11:** 161–171. doi:10.1007/s13668-022-00407-2

Tomlinson BE, Blessed G, Roth M. 1968. Observations on the brains of non-demented old people. *J Neurol Sci* **7:** 331–356. doi:10.1016/0022-510x(68)90154-8

Topiwala A, Allan CL, Valkanova V, Zsoldos E, Filippini N, Sexton C, Mahmood A, Fooks P, Singh-Manoux A, Mackay CE, et al. 2017. Moderate alcohol consumption as risk factor for adverse brain outcomes and cognitive decline: longitudinal cohort study. *BMJ* **357:** j2353. doi:10 .1136/bmj.j2353

Tumurbaatar B, Fracassi A, Scaduto P, Guptarak J, Woltjer R, Jupiter D, Taglialatela G. 2023. Preserved autophagy in cognitively intact non-demented individuals with Alzheimer's neuropathology. *Alzheimers Dement* doi:10 .1002/alz.13074

van der Lee SJ, Teunissen CE, Pool R, Shipley MJ, Teumer A, Chouraki V, van Lent DM, Tynkkynen J, Fischer K, Hernesniemi J, et al. 2018. Circulating metabolites and general cognitive ability and dementia: evidence from 11 cohort studies. *Alzheimers Dement* **14:** 707–722. doi:10 .1016/j.jalz.2017.11.012

van Dyck CH, Swanson CJ, Aisen P, Bateman RJ, Chen C, Gee M, Kanekiyo M, Li D, Reyderman L, Cohen S, et al. 2023. Lecanemab in early Alzheimer's disease. *N Engl J Med* **388:** 9–21. doi:10.1056/NEJMoa2212948

Veronese N, Facchini S, Stubbs B, Luchini C, Solmi M, Manzato E, Sergi G, Maggi S, Cosco T, Fontana L. 2017. Weight loss is associated with improvements in cognitive function among overweight and obese people: a systematic review and meta-analysis. *Neurosci Biobehav Rev* **72:** 87–94. doi:10.1016/j.neubiorev.2016.11.017

Voss M, Prakash R, Erickson K, Basak C, Chaddock L, Kim J, Alves H, Heo S, Szabo A, White S, et al. 2010. Plasticity of brain networks in a randomized intervention trial of exercise training in older adults. *Front Aging Neurosci* **2:** 32. doi:10.3389/fnagi.2010.00032

Walker JM, Kazempour Dehkordi S, Fracassi A, Vanschoiack A, Pavenko A, Taglialatela G, Woltjer R, Richardson TE, Zare H, Orr ME. 2022. Differential protein expression in the hippocampi of resilient individuals identified by digital spatial profiling. *Acta Neuropathol Commun* **10:** 23. doi:10.1186/s40478-022-01324-9

Wang R, Reddy PH. 2017. Role of glutamate and NMDA receptors in Alzheimer's disease. *J Alzheimers Dis* **57:** 1041–1048. doi:10.3233/JAD-160763

Wang Y, Du Y, Li J, Qiu C. 2019. Lifespan intellectual factors, genetic susceptibility, and cognitive phenotypes in aging: implications for interventions. *Front Aging Neurosci* **11:** 129. doi:10.3389/fnagi.2019.00129

Williams DB, Annegers JF, Kokmen E, O'Brien PC, Kurland LT. 1991. Brain injury and neurologic sequelae: a cohort study of dementia, parkinsonism, and amyotrophic lateral sclerosis. *Neurology* **41:** 1554–1557. doi:10.1212/wnl.41 .10.1554

Wolozin B, Bednar MM. 2006. Interventions for heart disease and their effects on Alzheimer's disease. *Neurol Res* **28:** 630–636. doi:10.1179/016164106X130515

World Health Organization. 2019. *Risk reduction of cognitive decline and dementia: WHO guidelines.* World Health Organization, Geneva. https://www.who.int/publications /i/item/9789241550543

Xu W, Tan L, Wang HF, Tan MS, Tan L, Li JQ, Zhao QF, Yu JT. 2016. Education and risk of dementia: dose-response meta-analysis of prospective cohort studies. *Mol Neurobiol* **53:** 3113–3123. doi:10.1007/s12035-015-9211-5

Yadollahikhales G, Rojas JC. 2023. Anti-amyloid immunotherapies for Alzheimer's disease: a 2023 clinical update. *Neurotherapeutics* **20:** 914–931. doi:10.1007/s13311-023-01405-0

Zhang MY, Katzman R, Salmon D, Jin H, Cai GJ, Wang ZY, Qu GY, Grant I, Yu E, Levy P. 1990. The prevalence of dementia and Alzheimer's disease in Shanghai, China: impact of age, gender, and education. *Ann Neurol* **27:** 428–437. doi:10.1002/ana.410270412

International Gains to Achieving Healthy Longevity

Andrew Scott,[1] Julian Ashwin,[2] Martin Ellison,[3] and David Sinclair[4]

[1]London Business School and Research Fellow, Centre for Economic Policy Research, Regent's Park, London NW1 4SA, United Kingdom

[2]London Business School, Regent's Park, London NW1 4SA, United Kingdom

[3]University of Oxford, Nuffield College, NuCamp, CEPR, Oxford OX1 1NF, United Kingdom

[4]Department of Genetics, Blavatnik Institute, Boston, Massachusetts 02115, USA

Correspondence: ascott@london.edu

Utilizing economic tools, we evaluate the gains from improving the relationship between biological and chronological age in dollar terms. We show that the gains to individuals are substantial because targeting aging exploits synergies between health and life expectancy and the complementarities across different diseases. Gains are boosted by improvements in life expectancy and a rising number of older people. We compute the value of slowing aging in a range of countries and estimate that increasing life expectancy by 1 year has an annual benefit of ~4%–5% of gross domestic product (GDP). Augmenting GDP with these measures of health gains reveals the growing importance of achieving healthy longevity as a means of boosting welfare, with the need being particularly acute in the United States.

The advent of the global pandemic in 2020 led to massive disruption for the world economy, with actions taken by individuals and governments to minimize the health impact of the pandemic leading to dramatic falls in gross domestic product (GDP) (Bonadio et al. 2020). Many lessons will be drawn from Covid-19, but central among them should be just how much we value our health.

While attention has been focused on the Covid-19 pandemic, a greater threat to the world's health and economic future in the coming decades is the rising incidence of age-related diseases. With life expectancy gains increasingly driven by mortality improvements at older ages (Vaupel et al. 2021), more years are spent by individuals in the "red zone" characterized by high levels of frailty and poorer health (Olshansky and Carnes 2019). These trends are producing an increase in global deaths from noncommunicable diseases (expected to rise by 66% between 2016 and 2040 [Foreman et al. 2018]) and more years spent in poor health, lower productivity, and placing an increased burden on society.

Given these two facts, how much we value health and the rising burden of age-related diseases, it is no surprise that the benefits of achieving healthy longevity are estimated to be substantial. Using different economic methodologies, both Goldman et al. (2013) and Scott et al. (2021) calculate multi-trillion-dollar benefits from improvements in slowing the rate at which we age.

Applying economic tools to evaluate longevity gains provides insights over and above simply arriving at a dollar value. As shown in this paper, these tools reveal the relative importance of extending life expectancy versus compressing morbidity (Fries 1980), the relative merits of tackling single diseases versus the aging process itself, as well as revealing an important interplay between the dynamics of health and life expectancy. The tools also point to a virtuous circle whereby the longer and healthier we live, the more we value additional gains in healthy longevity. This leads to the conclusion that not only is targeting aging a key research priority today, but we are entering a new epidemiological transition (Olshansky and Ault 1986) where improvements in how we age lead to greater interest in further gains.

The paper begins by outlining the economic tools used to evaluate health gains and applying them to issues of healthy longevity and the benefits of increased longevity versus compressing morbidity. It then shows why focusing on aging itself is important relative to targeting single diseases and evaluates the relative benefits of reversing rather than slowing aging. An explanation is provided as to why the importance of targeting aging has only recently emerged as a priority. The focus then shifts from the individual to the aggregate level by calculating the total value of improvements in aging for a number of high-income countries. This analysis places a dollar value on improvements in healthy longevity. When the measures are used in combination with GDP data to consider the welfare performance of a range of countries over recent decades, it shows how extending the healthy period of life and compressing morbidity is becoming ever more important and relevant.

EVALUATING GAINS TO HEALTH AND LONGEVITY

There are three broad approaches to assigning a dollar value to the gains arising from healthy longevity. The first is to calculate the impact in terms of current and future GDP growth, as longer, healthier lives lead to an increase in education, employment, and productivity, and have the potential to generate an economic longevity dividend (Scott 2021). The second is to estimate savings in terms of lower health costs and expenditures that arise from reductions in age-related diseases (Fries et al. 1993). The third places a monetary estimate (Viscusi 2018) on how much individuals value health gains, independently of any impact on their income or expenditure.

Each of these approaches is important and provides an insight into a different question. The GDP calculations have appeal to Ministries of Finance, but they require economic models that incorporate shifts in healthy longevity and the various mechanisms through which this influences economic growth (e.g., delayed retirement, greater investments in health and education, influences on innovation, and so on). Successful application of this approach requires the development of a canonical model for the economics of longevity, which is currently absent (Scott 2021).

The magnitude of potential health cost savings arising from extending healthy life span are clearly attractive to Ministries of Health. However, this focus on cost savings is restrictive from a welfare point of view as it rules out potentially highly valuable treatments. That is important given that both individuals and society are likely willing to spend more on reducing the incidence of age-related diseases than they are on dealing with their implications. As stressed by Hall and Jones (2007) given how valuable health improvements are, the consequence of rising prosperity is an ever-higher proportion of income on health outcomes. With age-related diseases increasingly the most important health challenge, this points to rising medical costs as being acceptable to achieve healthy longevity.

This focus on measuring the welfare gains from health improvements is the basis of the third approach and is the one used in this paper. That is, to use the value of statistical life (VSL) framework (Viscusi 2004) to derive a willingness to pay (WTP) measure for improvements in healthy longevity. These WTP measures place a dollar value on gains to health or life expectancy. Importantly, they are not based solely on considerations of how the gains impact the economy or an individual's earning potential, but instead capture the broad value individuals and society place on health. As Covid-19 shows, this is considerable. According to Greenstone and Nigam (2020), the VSL for the United States currently stands at $11.5 million, based on updated Environmental Protection Agency (EPA) figures for inflation and economic growth.

The VSL approach is related to attempts to measure the cost effectiveness of health expenditures by considering the cost in terms of quality-adjusted life years (QALY) of different treatments. For example, in the United Kingdom, the National Institute for Health and Care Excellence (NICE) considers treatments that cost <£30,000 per QALY saved to be good value. With UK life expectancy currently being 83 years, the value of saving a life at birth becomes 83 × £30,000, or ~£2.5 million.

Murphy and Topel (2006) developed a VSL model based on an economic analysis of the life cycle. Given expectations about health and life expectancy, interest rates, and wages, individuals decide how to structure their lives in terms of work and leisure, consumption, and savings. Changes in any of these variables lead to changes in lifetime economic decisions. For instance, the economic model shows how individuals respond to an increase in life expectancy by increasing labor supply and changing consumption and savings at different ages to support their longer lives.

These responses matter as they lead to changes in the VSL, and it is these changes that enable calculation of an individual's WTP for health improvements. The shifts in behavior are also important in enabling a dynamic analysis of how the WTP adjusts in response to changes in health and life expectancy, which is key for understanding future trends around the value of healthy longevity.

The VSL depends on two features—the *quantity* and *quality* of life. The quantity of life is captured by life expectancy in the form of a survival function showing the probability of surviving to a given age. The quality of life is cap-

tured by three variables—health, consumption, and leisure. As health and life expectancy change, individuals reevaluate and adjust their life plans in terms of consumption, savings, and work to finance longer lives and benefit from health changes. These changes contribute to shifts in the VSL.

This VSL framework can be used to evaluate the relative merits of living longer or achieving a compression of morbidity. In Scott et al. (2021), this is done by considering two scenarios—Struldbrugg and Dorian Gray. In the Struldbrugg scenario, life expectancy is increased by improvements in the survival function that lead to higher survival probabilities at each age. However, the assumption is that the relationship between health and age is unchanged, as with the life of the Struldbruggs on the island of Luggnagg in Jonathan Swift's *Gulliver's Travels* who live forever but in ever-declining health.

The Dorian Gray scenario is the opposite. In Oscar Wilde's novel *The Portrait of Dorian Gray*, Gray strikes a bargain so that his portrait ages but his body does not, allowing him to remain youthful in appearance until he dies. This is the case where health improves at each age, but life expectancy remains unchanged (mortality is the same). In the limit, healthy life expectancy becomes the same as life expectancy and there is a full compression of morbidity.

Using these two scenarios, Scott et al. (2021) arrive at the following conclusions:

- Gains to life expectancy are valuable under the Struldbrugg scenario, despite no improvements in health. A rise in life expectancy at birth from the current U.S. level of 78.9 to 79.9 years is estimated to be worth $118,000 to an individual at birth.

- Increasing life expectancy without changing health suffers from diminishing returns, due to declining health and the extra work required to finance longer lives. The result is that a rise in life expectancy from 88.9 to 89.9 years is worth only $81,800.

- More valuable is to raise healthy life expectancy, even in the absence of gains to life expectancy. Raising U.S. healthy life expectancy at birth from its current value of 68.9 to 69.9 years is worth an estimated $242,000.

- Gains from compressing morbidity diminish but remain high. In the United States, it is currently more beneficial to achieve a full compression of morbidity than to increase life expectancy.

- The gains to healthy longevity are largest at older ages because the older you are the more likely you are to benefit from health gains at older ages, the gains happen sooner for older people and so are discounted less, and better health in later life leads to a relative reallocation of consumption toward those years.

The logic behind these results can be seen in Figure 1. Figure 1A shows the value at birth of achieving a 1-year increase in life expectancy by reducing mortality, evaluated at different initial levels of life expectancy and healthy life expectancy (HLE). Figure 1B does the same but for 1 year increases in HLE achieved by improving health. These show that increases in HLE are more valuable than increases in life expectancy at every point in the grid. They also show that there are diminishing returns to improvements that only affect either health or mortality. Above all, Figure 1 shows the complementarity between health and longevity. For any given level of life expectancy, the higher the HLE, the greater the gains from improvements in mortality. Similarly for any given level of HLE, the greater the longevity, the greater the value of improvements in health. The complementarity between health and longevity is an important part of the value of targeting aging.

TARGETING BIOLOGICAL AGE

Both the Struldbrugg and Dorian Gray scenarios are based on changes in how we age. In Struldbrugg, the relationship between mortality rates and chronological age is improved, while in Dorian Gray, it is the relationship between health and chronological age that changes.

A more profound possibility exists if mortality and morbidity are jointly related to an underlying concept of biological age. For example, it has been shown that broad measures of health such as frailty indices (Mitnitski et al. 2002) capture health and mortality risks better than chronological age (Rockwood et al. 2017). If frailty is driven by biological aging, then improvements in how we age could simultaneously shift both the survival and health functions. Doing so would boost life expectancy and healthy life expectancy in tandem, triggering the complementarities detailed above. Indeed, for laboratory animals or humans, gains in overall health due to the slowing of aging are almost always associated with an increase in life span (Campisi et al. 2019; Olshansky et al. 2019).

Scott et al. (2021) refer to the slowing down of biological age as the *Peter Pan* scenario, based on J.M. Barrie's play about a boy who never grows up. In the extreme case, where biological age is constant regardless of chronological age, no aging occurs. The Peter Pan scenario leads to more valuable outcomes than either Dorian Gray or Struldbrugg because it exploits the complementarities shown in Figure 1.

The Peter Pan scenario illustrates two mechanisms through which targeting biological aging leads to more valuable outcomes than treatments focused on single specific diseases. The first is a simple *aggregation* effect. If biological age is the driver of multiple age-related diseases then targeting aging will lead to more valuable outcomes simply because it aggregates across numerous diseases. The second is through the elimination of *competing risks*. Reducing the incidence of, say, cancer, leads to improvements in life expectancy and health, but the gains are limited by the existence of other age-specific diseases such as dementia, chronic obstructive pulmonary disease (COPD), etc. The complementarity between health and life expectancy means the gains from eliminating cancer are greater if these other age-related diseases are also absent. The result (Scott et al. 2021) is that reducing the joint incidence of age-related diseases is more valuable (by ~20%–30%) than the sum of reducing the incidence of each disease separately.

The Peter Pan scenario involves slowing down biological aging. Another possibility that can be considered in our simulations is reversing

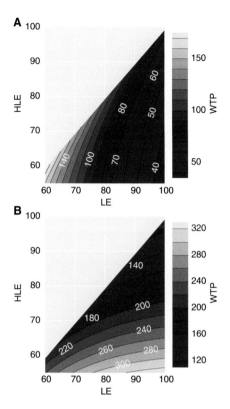

Figure 1. (*A*) Willingness to pay (WTP) in thousand U.S. dollars for one extra year of life expectancy (LE) by improving mortality. Increases in LE are more valued for higher healthy life expectancy (HLE). (*B*) WTP in thousand U.S. dollars for one extra year of healthy life expectancy by improving health. Increases in HLE are more valued for higher LE.

the biological aging process. Recent discoveries point to aging being a result, at least in part, of a loss of information at the epigenetic (gene regulation) level, and to the existence of a back-up copy of this information that can be accessed when certain embryonic genes are turned on in adult tissues (Zhang et al. 2020). Scott et al. (2021) refer to this as the Wolverine scenario, based on the Marvel character of the same name who has the capacity to regenerate limbs and organs. Scott et al. (2021) compare the case of Peter Pan (a permanent slowdown in the rate of biological aging) to a one-time Wolverine treatment at age 50 years. Conditional on achieving the same improvement in life expectancy, they show that the gains are broadly similar,

although Peter Pan is slightly preferred to Wolverine.

Figure 2 shows why the Peter Pan and Wolverine scenarios are similar despite their different biological foundations. The impact of Peter Pan is to reduce the rate at which health declines with age (here assumed to start from age 30), hence the health function is higher at all ages relative to the baseline. By contrast, under Wolverine, there is a reset of health to an earlier level (here assumed to occur at age 50). Peter Pan therefore leads to higher health for all ages past 30, while Wolverine only has a benefit for those aged 50 and above. Furthermore, Peter Pan is eventually higher than Wolverine at higher ages because Wolverine resets rather than slows the rate of aging. The net effect of these relative shifts is that the WTP for Peter Pan and Wolverine are broadly alike.

This logic though is based on the assumption that Wolverine is a one-time intervention. Imagine instead if a Wolverine reset can be performed every year, indefinitely, and without loss of efficacy. While this may seem a radical extension, it is again worth stressing the similarities with Peter Pan. In fact, repeated Wolverine is isomorphic to Peter Pan. Consider the case where Wolverine is repeated every 12 months and produces a reversal in biological age of 3 months. That is exactly equivalent to Peter Pan where the rate of aging is slowed down by 25% (i.e., every 12 months biological age only increases by 9 months).[5] At least within our framework, Peter Pan and repeated Wolverine are the same and their merits then depend on the relative biological feasibility and costs.

Table 1 shows the WTP for repeated annual applications of Wolverine treatments in which biological age is reversed by 3, 6, 9, or 12 months each year, starting at age 30, 50, or 70. The WTP for these interventions is substantial because

---

[5]Oeppen and Vaupel (2002) document a historical 2- to 3-year improvement in best practice life expectancy every decade. This is akin to a 25% reset of biological age each year in terms of its impact on mortality (i.e., biological age in terms of impact on mortality rises only 9 months each calendar year).

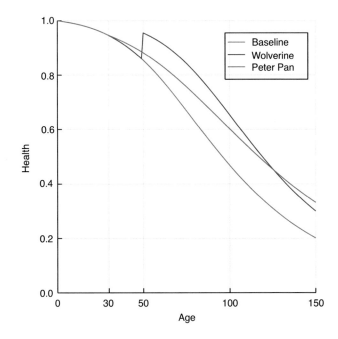

Figure 2. Comparing health effects of Peter Pan and Wolverine. In both cases, life expectancy at birth is increased to 100 years, driven by slower biological aging from age 30 for Peter Pan and a one-off reversal in biological age at 50 for Wolverine.

they lead to major increases in both life expectancy and healthy life expectancy.[6]

Consider the extreme case of repeated annual Wolverine treatments that starts at age 50 and each reverse aging by 12 months. The impact of this is that every year after age 50 is characterized by the same mortality rate and health as at age 50, regardless of advancing chronological age. Not surprisingly, the WTP at birth for such an intervention is enormous ($4.425 mn).

The WTP is higher if the reset locks in the mortality and health of a 30-year-old ($7.16 mn), and lower if the lock-in occurs at the mortality and health of a 70-year-old ($1 mn). It is worth noting the very extreme life expectancy

that locking in at the mortality of a 30-year-old produces. At this level of life expectancy, our economic model is being pushed into uncomfortable terrain where its applicability is questionable even allowing the extreme scientific assumptions underpinning the scenario.

A NEW EPIDEMIOLOGICAL TRANSITION

The above analysis shows treatments that slow down biological aging are very valuable, as doing so exploits a number of complementarities between health and life expectancy. However, the importance of exploiting these synergies has not always been so great. That is changing for two reasons.

The first is relatively simple. The benefits of targeting aging depend on the probability of experiencing age-related diseases. In 1933, a newborn in the United States had a 21% chance of reaching 80 years of age. Assuming no changes in future mortality, a newborn in 2019 had a 59% chance of doing so. This shift in probability leads to a significant increase in the WTP for

---

[6]Our results are based on a fixed schedule for wages that declines with age, calibrated to the empirical evidence in Casanova (2012). Given the large changes in life expectancy in Table 1, it is likely that changes in lifelong learning, health, and career decisions would lead to significant variations in wages especially at older ages, all of which would lead to substantial changes in the WTP (and probably much higher estimates).

Table 1. Effects of repeated Wolverine (reversing aging)

Starting age	Annual reset	Life expectancy	Healthy life expectancy	WTP at birth ($000s)
Baseline		78.9	68.7	
30	3 mo	91	79	1290
30	6 mo	113	98	2996
30	9 mo	167.9	146.4	5205
30	12 mo	1782.6	1686.9	7161
50	3 mo	85	73.5	564
50	6 mo	95.3	81.7	1362
50	9 mo	118.1	100.5	2585
50	12 mo	307.3	267.5	4425
70	3 mo	80.5	69.8	117
70	6 mo	82.9	71.5	281
70	9 mo	87	74.5	532
70	12 mo	99.3	83.9	999

tackling aging. That is because the gains from reducing age-related diseases depend on the probability of experiencing them.

The value of improvements in how we age has therefore increased as life expectancy has increased. This is shown in Fig. 3A, which plots the WTP at birth for a 10% "Dorian Gray" slowdown in the rate of biological aging (assumed only to impact health and not mortality, and starting at age 50) but evaluated using mortality rates in the United States in each year between 1933 and 2020. The increased probability since 1933 of the young becoming old leads to a substantial increase in the WTP for improvements in aging. Since 1941, the value has doubled, and has increased by 13% even compared with 20 years ago.

The second reason why the WTP for healthy longevity gains increases is due to changes in population size and structure. Improvements in mortality mean fewer people dying and a larger population, which directly increases the gains to society of any health improvements. In addition, improvements in longevity mean not just more people but more older people. As the old value gains from increased longevity more than the young, this compositional effect boosts the social gains from targeting aging. This is shown in Fig. 3B, which uses the population age structure between 1933 and 2020 and the WTP at different ages to construct an estimate of the social gains from healthy aging. These have increased as the proportion of the population aged over 50 has increased.

These two factors (longer lives, more old people) together lead to a rising value for targeting aging and point to the emergence of a new epidemiological transition (Olshansky and Ault 1986) focused on tackling age-related diseases.

INTERNATIONAL GAINS

Scott et al. (2021) use calculations of individual WTP for improvements in healthy longevity and population projections for the United States to calculate aggregate WTP numbers of economic value at a national level. In this section, we extend the analysis to a range of other high-income countries.[7] To do so, we follow Viscusi and Masterman (2017) and calculate the VSL for country i using the following equation (and for 2020 GDP)[8]:

$$VSL_i = VSL_{US}\left(\frac{Y_i}{Y_{US}}\right)^{\eta},$$

where η is the elasticity of the VSL with respect to income, which, following Viscusi and Master-

---

[7]While we can in theory perform the same calculations for low- and middle-income countries, a number of assumptions and calibrations of our model suggest restricting our focus in this way.

[8]The numbers for the United States are based on the most recent data and a different population series, so are not directly comparable with Scott et al. (2021).

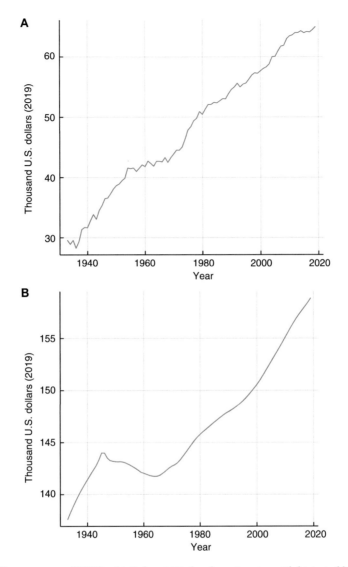

Figure 3. (*A*) Willingness to pay (WTP) at birth for a 10% slowdown in aging with historical life expectancy and survival rates. (*B*) Average individual WTP for a 10% slowdown in aging with historical population structure.

man (2017), is set equal to 1. We also need to calibrate our survival and health functions for different countries. We do this by adjusting the life span in our mortality functions so that the survival curve matches the life expectancy for each country and the health function matches healthy life expectancy. We then use the latest United Nations (UN) (2019) data on the size and age structure of the population to calculate the aggregate value of a slowdown in aging (as in Peter Pan) that leads to a 1-year increase in life expectancy from its current base (phased in over a 10-year period).

The aggregate WTP for all countries (shown in Table 2) is sizeable and between 4% and 5% of GDP on an annual basis (assuming 2% interest rates). The precise value varies across countries depending upon GDP per capita (the higher the GDP, the higher the VSL), the size and structure of the population (the more people and the more older people the higher the aggregate WTP), and also the starting level of life expectancy and

Table 2. International gains to targeting aging

	Life expectancy	Healthy life expectancy	Population (mn)	GDP per capita ($000s)	WTP current ($trn)	WTP future generations ($trn)	WTP total ($trn)
Australia	83	70.9	25.5	47	2.2	0.7	2.9
Canada	82.2	71.3	37.74	43.4	3.1	0.9	4
France	82.5	72.1	65.27	40.9	5	1.2	6.2
Germany	81.7	70.9	83.78	47.1	7.6	1.6	9.2
Israel	82.6	72.4	8.66	38.6	0.6	0.3	0.9
Italy	83	71.9	60.46	35.1	4.1	0.6	4.7
Japan	84.3	74.1	126.48	40.4	9.5	1.3	10.8
Netherlands	81.8	71.4	17.13	52.4	1.7	0.4	2.1
New Zealand	82	70.2	4.82	40.6	0.4	0.1	0.5
Spain	83.2	72.1	46.75	34.2	3.1	0.5	3.6
Sweden	82.4	71.9	10.1	50	1	0.3	1.3
UK	81.4	70.1	67.89	39.1	5.1	1.4	6.5
USA	78.5	66.1	331	58.2	38.4	12.5	50.9

healthy life expectancy (the lower either is, the more valuable are gains to healthy life expectancy). The same results that Scott et al. (2021) found for the United States hold here—the value of slowing aging and supporting healthy longevity is enormous. Health matters and the most important health issues for aging populations relate to age-related diseases.

ASSESSING PERFORMANCE

The VSL methodology can be used not just to construct dollar estimates for hypothetical gains in healthy longevity but also to value actual gains achieved in the past (Table 3; see Murphy and Topel 2006). Combining the dollar value of these health gains with the income generated by the economy (in other words GDP) gives a broad measure of welfare.

Table 3 shows the performance of this broad measure of welfare for various countries since 1990, in terms of the separate contributions of GDP per capita and the dollar value of health improvements and a combined aggregate measure.[9]

GDP per capita has generally increased for all countries, although the rate of increase

slowed in the wake of the Global Financial Crisis (2007–2009). An even more marked slowdown is apparent in the aggregate WTP for health and longevity gains. For every country except Israel, the monetary value of health gains achieved over the most recent period are the lowest since 1990. The performance of the United States is especially striking, with the aggregate WTP being *negative*. In other words, there has been an overall deterioration in health and life expectancy that has lowered welfare. The United States ranks first in 1990 and second in 2018 among these 13 countries in terms of GDP but based on the combined index the United States sees its ranking fall to 11th. While the United States is a dramatic example, Table 3 shows that there has been a substantial reduction in the value of health gains achieved in high-income countries in recent years.

Given that health challenges in these nations increasingly concern age-related diseases, the combined index is another way of understanding the main conclusion of this paper: there are substantial welfare gains to improving how we age. According to Table 3, the welfare gains from current health improvements are slowing, both in absolute terms and also relative to the size of the economy. While there is much focus on the negative impact to countries from slower GDP growth and secular stagnation, Table 3 points to the equal if not overriding importance of im-

---

[9]Data on health and mortality is taken from Global Burden of Disease data, with health measured using the proportion of years lost to disease in each age bracket.

Table 3. Economic value of gains to GDP and health 1990–2018

	Australia	Canada	France	Germany	Israel	Italy	Japan	Netherlands	New Zealand	Spain	Sweden	United Kingdom	United States
GDP per capita													
1990–1999	39.7	32.3	30.3	31.5	25.7	29.2	29.5	34.1	27.7	20.4	35.0	33.5	41.9
2000–2009	50.4	38.5	35.6	35.8	28.6	32.9	31.9	42.6	34.8	25.5	44.9	41.6	51.6
2010–2018	57.8	44.0	37.6	40.4	34.8	30.9	34.2	45.8	40.1	26.0	50.7	44.5	56.4
WTP per capita													
1990–1999	25.4	5.7	14.9	22.0	6.6	19.8	17.0	8.7	22.2	12.1	16.4	16.1	14.3
2000–2009	26.2	19.2	21.8	17.9	19.2	21.8	15.7	30.1	24.5	15.8	20.6	29.6	16.8
2010–2018	10.4	0.8	11.1	4.0	10.6	7.6	12.1	3.3	2.1	5.6	11.6	1.7	−14.2
GDP + WTP per capita													
1990–1999	65.2	38.0	45.2	53.5	32.4	49.0	46.4	42.8	50.0	32.6	51.4	49.7	56.1
2000–2009	76.6	57.7	57.5	53.7	47.8	54.6	47.6	72.7	59.3	41.3	65.5	71.2	68.4
2010–2018	68.2	44.7	48.7	44.4	45.4	38.5	46.2	49.1	42.3	31.6	62.2	46.2	42.2
Share of health capital: WTP/(WTP + GDP)													
1990–1999	0.39	0.15	0.33	0.41	0.20	0.40	0.37	0.20	0.44	0.37	0.32	0.33	0.25
2000–2009	0.34	0.33	0.38	0.33	0.40	0.40	0.33	0.41	0.41	0.38	0.31	0.42	0.25
2010–2018	0.15	0.02	0.23	0.09	0.23	0.20	0.26	0.07	0.05	0.18	0.19	0.04	−0.34

Cite this article as *Cold Spring Harb Perspect Med* doi: 10.1101/cshperspect.a041202

proving health and life expectancy. Given current population structures and survival curves, there must be a focus on targeting aging itself.

CONCLUDING REMARKS

There are few things that matter to society as much as health. Given increases in life expectancy and shifts in the age structure of the population, it is now a priority to guarantee that we age well, on both an individual and national level. Evaluations with economic tools show that the dollar value of improvements in healthy longevity run into multiple trillions of dollars at a country and global level. Despite the importance of achieving such healthy longevity, current approaches to increasing health and longevity are not working. Our estimates point to deteriorating performance in generating health gains in high-income countries, both in absolute terms and relative to the size of economic gains. As populations age, governments need to set health and life expectancy as a policy goal and search for instruments that achieve healthy longevity gains. As part of this approach, a relative shift in focus in medical research and drug development toward targeting the aging process rather than specific single diseases seems warranted given the potential value and current diminishing success in achieving healthy longevity.

ACKNOWLEDGMENTS

A.S. and J.A. are grateful for support from ESRC Grant T002204. David is grateful for support from NIH Grants R01AG019719 and the Dalio Foundation. David's activities outside of Harvard Medical School are at sinclair.hms.harvard.edu/david-sinclairs-affiliations.

APPENDIX

Model

The life-cycle model used is based on that of Murphy and Topel (2006), with parameters calibrated as in Scott et al. (2021). Both mortality and health are based on frailty that increases with age a:

$$F(a) = e^{\delta a - T}.$$

Mortality is defined as a Gompertz function:

$$\mu(a) = M_1 F(a)^\gamma.$$

The survival rate $S(a, t)$ then gives the probability of an individual of age a surviving to time t. Health is based on the ratio of disability at birth to current disability:

$$H(a) = \left(\frac{D_0 + D_1 F(0)^\psi}{D_0 + D_1 F(a)^\psi} \right)^\alpha.$$

Agents choose their consumption and leisure over the life cycle to maximize utility subject to a standard budget constraint.

$$\int_a^\infty H(t) u(c(t), \; l(t)) S(a, t) e^{-\rho(t-a)},$$

where instantaneous utility u has a constant elasticity of substitution (CES) form.

$$u(z) = \frac{z^{1-1/\sigma} - z_0^{1-1/\sigma}}{1 - 1/\sigma},$$

$$z = \left(\phi c^{1-\frac{1}{\eta}} + (1 - \phi) l^{1-\frac{1}{\eta}} \right)^{\eta/(\eta-1)}.$$

Parameters are calibrated to match the U.S. economy as in Scott et al. (2021).

We use analytic expressions based on Murphy and Topel (2006) to calculate WTP for hypothetical changes in health and survival rates:

$$WTP(a) = \int_a^\infty v(t) \Delta S(a, t) dt$$

$$+ \frac{\Delta H(t)}{H(t)} \frac{u(c(t), \; l(t))}{u_c(c(t), \; l(t))} dt,$$

where $v(t)$ is the value of a life year at age t. Social WTP is then found by weighting the WTP at each age a by the total population in that age bracket.

The extra year of life expectancy from improving mortality in Fig. 1A is generated by changing M_1 in the mortality function. The extra year of healthy life expectancy from improving health in Fig. 1B is generated by changing D_1 in the health equation. The Peter Pan exercises work through changing δ and the Wolverine exercises through resetting a to a previous level of health and mortality.

Data

Historical mortality and population structure data for the United States used in Fig. 3 are taken from the Human Mortality Database (www.mortality.org). In Fig. 3A, we use historical survival rates but otherwise use the baseline calibrations, and evaluate WTP at birth for a 10% slowdown in aging with respect to health starting at age 50. In Fig. 3B, we use the calculated WTP for the same change using the baseline calibration and compute the average WTP across society using the historical population structures.

For the international comparison of social WTP shown in Table 2, we use our baseline model but calibrate T to set life expectancy and α to set healthy life expectancy according to data from the World Health Organization (apps.who.int/gho/data). We then scale the wage distribution to set the VSL according to GDP data from the World Bank (data.worldbank.org/indicator/NY.GDP.MKTP.CD). Finally, we use current population data and future fertility projections from the UN World Population Prospects 2019 (population.un.org/wpp/Download/Standard/Population). We compute the WTP for an extra year of life expectancy by slowing down aging through the δ parameter, phased in linearly over 10 years.

To assess international performance, we use mortality rates and years lost to disease from the Global Burden of Disease data set (ghdx.healthdata.org/gbd-2019) to compute survival and health curves for each country over time. The VSL for each country is calculated using the

World Bank GDP data mentioned above, and the wage distribution is scaled accordingly. In each year, we calculate the WTP for the health and survival curves of the following year.

REFERENCES

Bonadio B, Huo Z, Levchenko AA, Pandalai-Nayar N. 2020. Global supply chains in the pandemic. NBER Working Paper 27224, National Bureau of Economic Research, Cambridge, MA.

Campisi J, Kapahi P, Lithgow GJ, Melov S, Newman JC, Verdin E. 2019. From discoveries in ageing research to therapeutics for healthy ageing. Nature 571: 183–192. doi:10.1038/s41586-019-1365-2

Casanova M. 2012. Wage and earnings profiles at older ages. University of Chicago, Chicago.

Foreman KJ, Marquez N, Dolgert A, Fukutaki K, Fullman N, McGaughey M, Pletcher MA, Smith AE, Tang K, Yuan CW, et al. 2018. Forecasting life expectancy, years of life lost, and all-cause and cause-specific mortality for 250 causes of death: reference and alternative scenarios for 2016–40 for 195 countries and territories. Lancet 392: 2052–2090. doi:10.1016/S0140-6736(18)31694-5

Fries JF. 1980. Aging, natural death, and the compression of morbidity. N Engl J Med 303: 130–135. doi:10.1056/NEJM198007173030304

Fries JF, Everett Koop C, Beadle CE, Cooper PP, England MJ, Greaves RF, Sokolov JJ, Wright D; Health Project Consortium. 1993. Reducing health care costs by reducing the need and demand for medical services. N Engl J Med 329: 321–325. doi:10.1056/NEJM199307293290506

Goldman DP, Cutler D, Rowe JW, Michaud PC, Sullivan J, Peneva D, Olshansky SJ. 2013. Substantial health and economic returns from delayed aging may warrant a new focus for medical research. Health Aff 32: 1698–1705. doi:10.1377/hlthaff.2013.0052

Greenstone M, Nigam V. 2020. Does social distancing matter? COVID Econ 1: 1–22.

Hall RE, Jones CI. 2007. The value of life and the rise in health spending. Q J Econ 122: 39–72. doi:10.1162/qjec.122.1.39

Mitnitski AB, Mogilner AJ, MacKnight C, Rockwood K. 2002. The accumulation of deficits with age and possible invariants of aging. ScientificWorldJournal 2: 1816–1822. doi:10.1100/tsw.2002.861

Murphy KM, Topel RH. 2006. The value of health and longevity. J Polit Econ 114: 871–904. doi:10.1086/508033

Oeppen J, Vaupel JW. 2002. Broken limits to life expectancy. Science 296: 1029–1031. doi:10.1126/science.1069655

Olshansky SJ, Ault AB. 1986. The fourth stage of the epidemiologic transition: the age of delayed degenerative diseases. Milbank Q 64: 355–391. doi:10.2307/3350025

Olshansky SJ, Carnes BA. 2019. Inconvenient truths about human longevity. J Gerontol A Biol Sci Med Sci 74: S7–S12. doi:10.1093/gerona/glz098

Olshansky SJ, Perry D, Miller RA, Butler RN. 2019. The longevity dividend. In Encyclopedia of gerontology and population aging. Springer, Berlin.

Rockwood K, Blodgett JM, Theou O, Sun MH, Feridooni HA, Mitnitski A, Rose RA, Godin J, Gregson E, Howlett SE. 2017. A frailty index based on deficit accumulation quantifies mortality risk in humans and in mice. *Sci Rep* **7:** 43068. doi:10.1038/srep43068

Scott AJ. 2021. Achieving a three-dimensional longevity dividend. *Nat Aging* **1:** 500–505. doi:10.1038/s43587-021-00074-y

Scott AJ, Ellison M, Sinclair DA. 2021. The economic value of targeting aging. *Nat Aging* **1:** 616–623. doi:10.1038/s43587-021-00080-0

Vaupel JW, Villavicencio F, Bergeron-Boucher MP. 2021. Demographic perspectives on the rise of longevity. *Proc Natl Acad Sci* **118:** e2019536118. doi:10.1073/pnas.2019536118

Viscusi WK. 2004. The value of risks to life and health. *J Econ Lit* **31:** 1912–1946.

Viscusi WK. 2018. *Pricing lives: guideposts for a safer society.* Princeton University Press, Princeton, NJ.

Viscusi WK, Masterman CJ. 2017. Income elasticities and global values of a statistical life. *J Benefit Cost Anal* **8:** 226–250. doi:10.1017/bca.2017.12

Zhang W, Qu J, Liu GH, Belmonte JCI. 2020. The ageing epigenome and its rejuvenation. *Nat Rev Mol Cell Biol* **21:** 137–150. doi:10.1038/s41580-019-0204-5

Discovering Biological Mechanisms of Exceptional Human Health Span and Life Span

Sofiya Milman and Nir Barzilai

Institute for Aging Research, Department of Medicine, Divisions of Endocrinology and Geriatrics, Department of Genetics, Albert Einstein College of Medicine, Bronx, New York 10461, USA

Correspondence: Sofiya.milman@einsteinmed.edu

Humans age at different rates and families with exceptional longevity provide an opportunity to understand why some people age slower than others. Unique features exhibited by centenarians include a family history of extended life span, compression of morbidity with resultant extension of health span, and longevity-associated biomarker profiles. These biomarkers, including low-circulating insulin-like growth factor 1 (IGF-1) and elevated high-density lipoprotein (HDL) cholesterol levels, are associated with functional genotypes that are enriched in centenarians, suggesting that they may be causative for longevity. While not all genetic discoveries from centenarians have been validated, in part due to exceptional life span being a rare phenotype in the general population, the APOE2 and FOXO3a genotypes have been confirmed in a number of populations with exceptional longevity. However, life span is now recognized as a complex trait and genetic research methods to study longevity are rapidly extending beyond classical Mendelian genetics to polygenic inheritance methodologies. Moreover, newer approaches are suggesting that pathways that have been recognized for decades to control life span in animals may also regulate life span in humans. These discoveries led to strategic development of therapeutics that may delay aging and prolong health span.

RATIONALE FOR STUDYING HUMAN EXCEPTIONAL LONGEVITY

The U.S. Centers for Disease Control and Prevention (CDC) publishes an annual report on the rate of death from individual diseases, stratified by age groups (CDC 2023). What is striking about these reports is that the rate of death increases logarithmically with advancing age for all diseases that typically affect older adults, including heart disease, cancer, stroke, diabetes mellitus type 2 (T2DM), and Alzheimer's disease. The incidence of these diseases parallels the death rate, a pattern that has been confirmed in different populations, including from the United Kingdom (Fig. 1; Zenin et al. 2019). To put these statistics in perspective: an elevated low-density lipoprotein (LDL) cholesterol level, one of the best known and aggressively treated risk factors for coronary disease, is associated with a fourfold increase in the risk for heart disease (Gordon et al. 1977); on the other hand, advancing from age 40 yr to 70 yr raises the risk of coronary heart disease by as

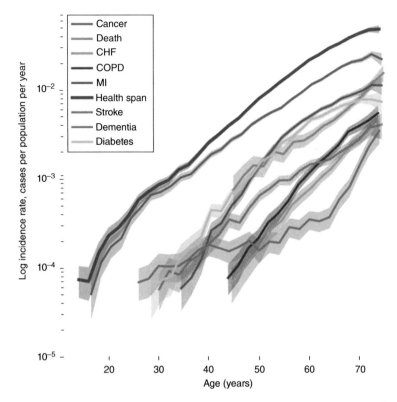

Figure 1. Log incidence rate of disease, cases per population per year. (CHF) Congestive heart failure, (COPD) chronic obstructive pulmonary disease, (MI) myocardial infarction. (Image reprinted from Zenin et al. 2019 under a Creative Commons Attribution 4.0 International License, http://creativecommons.org/licenses/by/4.0.)

much as 100-fold. Notably, the lines depicting disease-specific incidence and mortality are nearly parallel for all age-related diseases, suggesting that these diseases may share a common biological mechanism: the biology of aging. This demonstrates that aging is a major risk factor that all these age-related diseases have in common. If we accept the notion that aging is the common and major risk factor for all age-related diseases, then we conclude that unless aging itself is delayed, our best attempts at preventing each disease individually will result in exchanging one disease for another. The return for curing individual diseases is small. For example, statistical models project that delaying cancer would increase the population of older adults by only 0.8% over a 50-yr period, whereas delaying aging would result in an ~7% increase, with most of these individuals remaining free of disability (Goldman et al. 2013). Furthermore, de-

laying aging and extending life span even by 1 yr is expected to yield ~$38 trillion in economic value, with changes in retirement age and participation in leisurely activities contributing to the gains (Scott et al. 2021).

When thinking about aging, it is important to recognize that chronological and biological age are not the same. It is well recognized that some individuals appear younger than their chronological age, whereas others appear older. This observation highlights an opportunity for scientific discovery that until recently has been missed: to understand the biologic underpinnings of why some people age faster while others age slower. At one extreme of the rate-of-aging spectrum are progeroid syndromes, such as Hutchinson–Gilford progeria and Werner syndromes, rare diseases that manifest clinically as accelerated aging, and that have been traditionally studied to advance our understanding of the aging process (Martin 2005). More recently, scientists have become interested in studying people with exceptional longevity, who represent the other end of the rate-of-aging spectrum, in an effort to discover the genetic and biological determinants of delayed aging.

Centenarians are a unique group of individuals who exemplify delayed aging. The delay in aging manifests as an extension of disease-free survival, which has been repeatedly observed in centenarians. Analyses from the New England Centenarian Study (Andersen et al. 2012), the Long Life Family Study (Sebastiani et al. 2013), and the Longevity Genes Project (LGP) (Ismail et al. 2014) have all demonstrated that individuals with exceptional longevity manifest compression of morbidity, characterized by a smaller proportion of time spent living with chronic illness; as a result, their health span approximates their life span. These studies reveal that individuals with exceptional longevity were significantly delayed in the ages of onset for most age-related diseases, including hypertension, cardiovascular disease, cancer, T2DM, stroke, osteoporosis, and Alzheimer's disease. Thus, not only do centenarians live longer, they live healthier. Although a large proportion of centenarians delay or escape from age-related diseases altogether (Evans et al. 2014), a number of individuals achieve exceptional longevity despite having developed one or several of these diseases (Andersen et al. 2012; Ailshire et al. 2015). This suggests that these people likely possess protective factors that allow them to be resilient and survive in spite of health ailments.

The inherent differences between chronological and biological age, and between the diverse rates of aging, offer scientists opportunities to study the variations in biology and genetics among these different groups. As exemplified in other work in the literature, in a variety of animal models, several mechanisms have already been identified that can delay aging. Investigating whether these same mechanisms apply to humans with exceptional longevity serves to validate these discoveries as important for human aging. Furthermore, studies are underway for the discovery of age-delaying mechanisms that are specific to humans by using centenarian populations. The rationale for studying centenarians is that they are the "poster children" for what we are ultimately aiming to achieve: extension of health span and not merely life span.

EVIDENCE FOR HERITABILITY OF EXCEPTIONAL LONGEVITY

Demographers and epidemiologists have attributed ~15%–30% of the variation in life span to heritable factors (McGue et al. 1993; Herskind et al. 1996; Mitchell et al. 2001). Several studies have found positive correlations between the life spans of parents and their biological offspring (Atzmon et al. 2004; Schoenmaker et al. 2006; Westendorp et al. 2009). However, the advances of modern medicine, including preventive measures and treatments, have extended the life spans of the contemporary generations beyond what would have been predicted based on their inheritance. Thus, offspring whose parents died from cardiovascular disease resulting from hereditary hyperlipidemia can now enjoy an extension of their life span aided by treatment with cholesterol-lowering medications and interventions such as coronary artery bypass graft surgery or revascularization of coronary arteries with angioplasty. Despite these significant medical advances, achievement of exceptional longevity remains a rare occurrence, with individuals age 95 and older accounting for only 0.14% of the U.S. population in 2010 (Howden and Meyer 2011). Yet, in spite of its rarity, exceptional longevity clusters in families, pointing to a strong relationship between genetics and longevity.

Data suggests that offspring of parents who achieved a life span of at least 70 yr have a much greater probability of living longer compared to offspring of parents with shorter life spans, with this association becoming stronger as the parental life span lengthens (Gavrilov et al. 2001). This relationship is even more pronounced in families with exceptional longevity. Siblings of centenarians have been shown to be approximately 4–5 times more likely to achieve longevity, with male siblings being 17 times more likely to become centenarians themselves (Perls et al. 1998, 2002). The parents of centenarians were found to be seven times more likely to have survived to age 90 and beyond, compared to parents of those with usual life span (Atzmon et al. 2004). Even if genetics account for smaller differences in the rate of aging, identification of these genes is important for devising strategies that can delay the aging process. Furthermore, since exceptional longevity is heritable, studying the families of centenarians to identify genetic determinants of exceptional longevity offers tremendous promise for discovery.

Familial longevity is likely mediated through protection from age-related disease, which is inherited by the offspring from their parents. Centenarians and their offspring have a lower prevalence and later age-of-onset of heart disease, stroke, hypertension, T2DM, Alzheimer's disease, and cancer (Anderson et al. 1991; Atzmon et al. 2004; Adams et al. 2008; Lipton et al. 2010; Altmann-Schneider et al. 2013). This heritable protection from disease has also been demonstrated in several large studies. A prospective population-based study with >23 yr of follow-up found that the incidence of Alzheimer's disease was 43% lower in offspring of parents with exceptional longevity compared to offspring of parents with a usual life span (Lipton et al. 2010). A similar association was observed in a cohort whose parents achieved more modest longevity. In a secondary analysis of the Diabetes Prevention Program (DPP), a large clinical trial designed to compare strategies for prevention of T2DM in individuals at high risk for T2DM, parental longevity was associated with a delay in the incidence of T2DM among the offspring, with the children of parents with longest life spans experiencing the greatest delay in disease onset (Florez et al. 2011). The effect of parental life span on diabetes prevention was found to be just as strong as the effect of metformin, a drug used in the study to prevent T2DM (Florez et al. 2011). These results demonstrate that extended parental life span is strongly associated with better health outcomes in the offspring, even in populations who achieve less extreme degrees of longevity.

Although environmental influences may have a significant effect on health and life span in the general population, this does not appear to be the case in centenarians. A study that compared individuals with exceptional longevity to their contemporaries who did not achieve longevity found that centenarians were as likely as their shorter-lived peers to have been overweight or obese (Rajpathak et al. 2011). Furthermore, the proportion of centenarians who smoked, consumed alcohol daily, had not participated in regular physical activity, or had not followed a low-calorie diet throughout their middle age was similar to that among their peers from the same birth cohort. In fact, as many as 60% of male and 30% of female centenarians had been smokers (Rajpathak et al. 2011). Thus, the centenarians had not engaged in a healthier lifestyle compared to their peers. Furthermore, a recent study that compared the lifestyle habits and cardiovascular disease prevalence in adults aged 65 yr and older, who either had at least one parent with exceptional longevity or no parent with exceptional longevity, demonstrated analogous findings. Despite having similar lifestyle habits and dietary intake, inclusive of various nutrient components, individuals with a history of parental longevity had a 35% lower prevalence of cardiovascular disease compared to those without parental longevity (Gubbi et al. 2017). These findings support the notion that genes contribute to the observed dissociation between environmental risk factors and health outcomes in individuals with genetic predisposition to longevity, with these genes likely serving a protective role.

GENETICS OF EXCEPTIONAL LONGEVITY

For over two decades, centenarian populations of diverse Americans, as well as ethnically homogeneous populations of Mormons, Ashkenazi Jews (AJs), Icelandics, Okinawan Japanese, Italians, Irish, and Dutch, among others, have contributed to studies that aimed to identify the genetic underpinnings of longevity. One prevailing hypothesis of longevity had been that centenarians lacked genetic variants linked to increased risk for cardiovascular disease, Alzheimer's disease, T2DM, and other age-related diseases; thus, this hypothesis proposed that centenarians had a "perfect genome." However, it has become clear from a number of studies that centenarians harbor many disease-associated genotypes. A whole genome-sequencing analysis of 44 centenarians revealed that this group carried a total of 227 autosomal and seven X-chromosome-coding, single-nucleotide variants (SNVs) that are likely to cause disease according to the ClinVar database (Freudenberg-Hua et al. 2014). Among these SNVs were variants associated with Parkinson's, Alzheimer's, neurodegenerative, neoplastic, and cardiac diseases. Yet, despite over 95 yr of exposure to these risky genotypes, the centenarians did not exhibit any of the diseases for which they were genetic carriers. Similarly, recent whole-exome sequencing studies that compared the number of disease-associated gene variants between individuals with longevity and those without familial longevity did not find significant differences (Gutman et al. 2020a; Lin et al. 2021). Although some studies did find that individuals with exceptional longevity had lower polygenic risk scores (PRSs) for several age-related diseases compared to younger population controls, their genomes were not devoid of risk-associated variants (Gunn et al. 2022; Torres et al. 2022). These observations led to the conclusion that there are longevity-associated protective genotypes in centenarians that delay aging or specifically protect against the manifestations of age-related diseases. Subsequently, many studies have been undertaken to identify longevity-associated genes. The earlier studies mostly relied on candidate gene and genome-wide association study (GWAS) approaches, whereas more recently, polygenic approaches have been explored.

A number of longevity-associated genes have been discovered through the application of the candidate gene approach. These genes of interest were selected for investigation because they were previously implicated in aging or health span and single-nucleotide polymorphisms (SNPs) within these genes were linked with longevity. These included *PON1* (Bonafè et al. 2002; Rea et al. 2004; Franceschi et al. 2005; Marchegiani et al. 2006; Tan et al. 2006), *IGF-1* (Bonafè et al. 2003; Kojima et al. 2004; van Heemst et al. 2005), *PAPR-1*, cytokine genes, genes that code for enzymatic antioxidants such as superoxide dismutases (Andersen et al. 1998; Mecocci et al. 2000), *ADIPOQ* (Atzmon

et al. 2008), genes regulating telomere length (Atzmon et al. 2010), and components of lipid metabolism, with several examples described below (Barzilai et al. 2003; Vergani et al. 2006). Other genes that have been implicated in human aging, and not only longevity, are updated on genomics.senescence.info/genes.

The cholesteryl ester transfer protein (*CETP*) longevity-associated variant was identified in AJ centenarians. The *CETP* codon 405 isoleucine to valine variant was associated with low levels of plasma CETP, high levels of high-density lipoprotein (HDL) cholesterol, and large lipoprotein particle size (Barzilai et al. 2003). This genotype was also shown to be protective against cognitive decline and Alzheimer's disease in an independent diverse population (Sanders et al. 2010). This same genotype was validated by another research group in an Italian population (Vergani et al. 2006). Additional genotype in the *CETP* gene was also found to be significantly associated with higher HDL cholesterol in the Long Life Family Study (LLFS) (Feitosa et al. 2014). Although not all studies have confirmed these findings, it is important to keep in mind that a particular SNP may not exhibit a similar phenotype in all populations. Therefore, the biological phenotype itself (in the example above, the HDL cholesterol level) should be tested for association with longevity rather than a particular SNP that may have differential expression in varying populations.

Another lipid-related genotype, homozygosity for the apolipoprotein C-3 (*APOC-3*)-641C allele was also associated with exceptional longevity in AJs (Atzmon et al. 2006). It too exhibited a unique lipid phenotype and low levels of plasma APOC-3. In a striking example of validation, carriers of a different *APOC3* genotype in a homogenous Pennsylvania Amish population also exhibited low APOC-3 levels, favorable lipid phenotype, better arterial health score, and longevity (Pollin et al. 2008). These findings demonstrate the power of discovery in selected genetically homogeneous populations. *APOC-3* genotype was also identified to be related to exceptional longevity in the LLFS (Feitosa et al. 2014) but the phenotype associated with this SNP has not been defined yet.

One of the strengths of GWAS compared to the candidate gene approach is that these studies are unbiased and their results could provide insights into novel mechanisms that at the outset may not have been predicted to have a role in longevity. Several research groups have conducted GWASs for longevity (Beekman et al. 2010; Sebastiani et al. 2012), yet most earlier studies have either not yielded significant results or identified few loci on chromosome 19 that included the *APOE* gene (Deelen et al. 2011; Nebel et al. 2011; Sebastiani et al. 2012; Lu et al. 2014; Zeng et al. 2016). There are several explanations for these disappointing results. First, relying on common genetic variants that occur at frequencies >5% in the general population to study the uncommon event of exceptional longevity that occurs at a rate of <1% in the population is likely to miss the rare longevity-associated genotypes (Howden and Meyer 2011). Therefore, exome or whole-genome sequencing are expected to contribute to the identification of longevity-associated rare variants. Second, to conduct an effective GWAS in a genetically diverse population requires a very large study cohort to overcome the challenges of genetic diversity and identify rare genetic variants at sufficient proportions; yet, studies to date lack adequate power for these discoveries. Thus, it is of paramount importance to establish very large centenarian cohort studies to advance the discovery of genetics of longevity.

Several approaches have been established to overcome the limitations outlined above. For example, meta-analyses of longevity-associated GWASs increased the cohort size and thereby the power for discovery of longevity variants. This approach resulted in the confirmation of variants in *FOXO3*, as well as variants previously associated with human longevity in a locus on chromosome 19 that included genes *PVLR2*, *TOMM40*, *APOE*, and *APOC1* (Deelen et al. 2014; Broer et al. 2015; Sebastiani et al. 2017), although the association with *FOXO3* did not persist when only exceptional longevity was considered (Bae et al. 2018). On the other hand, in a follow-up study, *APOE* was confirmed to be associated with exceptional longevity. In an analysis of 28,297 participants from seven longevity cohorts from around the world, the ε2ε2 and ε2ε3 genotypes compared to the ε3ε3 genotype were identified as significantly associated with increased odds of reaching extreme longevity (Sebastiani et al. 2019). Additionally, meta-analyses contributed to the discovery of new variants related to longevity in genes *USP42* and *TMTC2*, and in GPR78 locus (Sebastiani et al. 2017; Deelen et al. 2019).

Another approach focused on genetically homogeneous populations. Given our understanding of genetic research challenges, it is not surprising that many important genetic discoveries were made in relatively genetically homogeneous populations. One such example is the Icelandic population that originated from a small number of founders and expanded to ~500,000 people. Others include the Amish (Pollin et al. 2008) and AJs, a larger population (Barzilai et al. 2003; Atzmon et al. 2008, 2009b, 2010; Suh et al. 2008). The advantage of studying a genetically homogeneous population was demonstrated by a finding that an addition of each AJ subject contributed 20 times more genetic variability to the cohort as compared to the addition of a European subject to a cohort of European ancestry of identical sample size (Carmi et al. 2014). One of the ways in which genetically similar populations contribute to genetic discovery is that these populations accumulate rare variants at higher frequencies than diverse populations. Gene variants that are rare in the general population may occur at higher frequencies in homogenous populations due to the founder effect, as is the case with mutations in the *BRCA* and *HEXA* genes that cause breast and/or ovarian cancer and Tay–Sachs disease, respectively, at higher frequencies among AJs. Accumulation of rare longevity-associated genetic variants in founder populations will increase the power of GWAS to withstand the rigorous statistical analysis that is applied to genome-wide data.

Lessons learned from genetic research conducted over the past several decades led to the recognition that longevity is a complex trait; therefore, the classical Mendelian approach previously employed in genetic research must be extended to include multiple genotypes, genes, and pathways. For example, many SNPs that fall below the threshold for GWAS significance may still be relevant for longevity in aggregate. Indeed, Sebastiani et al. have identified 281 SNPs that can distinguish centenarians from individuals without familial longevity (Sebastiani et al. 2012). In line with this changed approach, a recent analysis used whole-exome sequence data from a large cohort of centenarians and controls to examine enrichment of pathways for rare longevity-associated variants. This analysis revealed that conserved longevity-associated pathways, including insulin/insulin-like growth factor 1, AMPK, and mammalian target of rapamycin (mTOR) signaling pathways, were enriched in rare coding variants among centenarians compared to controls (Lin et al. 2021). These same pathways have been consistently associated with extension of life span in numerous experimental models (Kenyon et al. 1993; Brown-Borg et al. 1996). Thus, confirming the relevance of these pathways in human aging strengthens the evidence for their role in human life span and health span. Additionally, newer approaches allow for identification of gene–gene interactions between disease-associated genes and longevity-associated genes that protect from disease. For example, the study above also identified rare coding variants in the Wnt signaling pathway that exhibited a pro-longevity effect in individuals with *APOE4* risk alleles (Lin et al. 2021).

FROM MODEL ORGANISMS TO HUMANS: TRANSLATING THE BIOLOGY OF AGING

The LGP and LonGenity are studies that include families of AJs with exceptional longevity. Since longevity carries a substantial genetic component, these studies conduct genetic and detailed phenotypic analyses in the families with exceptional longevity in an effort to determine the functions of genes of interest. Using the candidate gene approach in this AJ cohort, several favorable genotypes were identified in multiple genes, which were associated with unique biological phenotypes.

Longevity-associated genotypes and phenotypes that have influenced clinical recommendations are related to thyroid-stimulating hormone (TSH) and its receptor (TSHR) (Atzmon et al.

2009a,b). The metabolic rate theory of aging suggests that there exists an inverse relationship between basal metabolic rate and aging, with several hypothyroid mammalian models exhibiting longer life span. Centenarians have higher plasma TSH levels, although they are not hypothyroid, and their offspring also exhibit this phenotype with significant heritability (Atzmon et al. 2009a; Rozing et al. 2010). These clinical features have been supported by a National Health and Nutrition Examination Survey (NHANES III) conducted across the United States and led to the recommendation to not supplement older adults with mild elevations in TSH and normal thyroxine levels with thyroid hormone (Tabatabaie and Surks 2013).

Among various naturally occurring examples and experimental models, disruption of the growth hormone/insulin-like growth factor 1 (GH/IGF-1) action results in extension of life span and health span. These disruptions, which are associated with a small body size (dwarfism) across species, result in numerous biological indices of delayed aging, including enhanced stress resistance and a major increase in life span (Kenyon et al. 1993; Brown-Borg et al. 1996). One naturally occurring example in humans that highlights the importance of GH/IGF-1 signaling in extended health span comes from a population of individuals with Laron syndrome, who are carriers of a rare mutation in the GH receptor (*GHR*) gene that results in GHR deficiency. A group with this genotype was studied in Ecuador and appears to have a negligible prevalence of T2DM and cancer (Guevara-Aguirre et al. 2011). Although they do not exhibit exceptional longevity, they are protected from major age-related diseases.

Studies of individuals with exceptional longevity, have identified and validated several SNPs in genes within the insulin/IGF-1 signaling pathway to be associated with exceptional longevity, but for the most part no specific phenotype related to these SNPs has been identified (Pawlikowska et al. 2009). An exception to this has been the identification of a functional IGF-1 receptor (*IGF1R*) gene mutation discovered by sequencing the *IGF1* and *IGF1R* genes of centenarians (Suh et al. 2008). Heterozygous mutations in the *IGF1R* gene have been overrepresented among centenarians compared to the controls without familial longevity and have been associated with high serum IGF-1 levels in the setting of reduced activity of the IGF1R, as measured in transformed lymphocytes (Suh et al. 2008). Partial IGF-1 resistance conferred by these longevity-associated *IGF1R* genotypes was confirmed in a study conducted on wild-type cells transformed with the mutant genes (Tazearslan et al. 2011). A particular *IGF1R* genotype was also associated with longevity in the LLFS; however, its associated phenotype has not yet been defined.

Additional evidence from epidemiologic studies links reduced GH/IGF-1 signaling with exceptional longevity and extended health span. Nonagenarians and centenarians with lower circulating IGF-1 levels or IGF-1/IGBP-3 ratios demonstrated extended survival and preserved functional status (Milman et al. 2014; van der Spoel et al. 2015). Furthermore, females with exceptional longevity and IGF-1 levels in the first tertile had 61% lower odds of being cognitively impaired compared to females with IGF-1 levels in the upper two tertiles (Perice et al. 2016). Even though this finding was not observed in males with exceptional longevity, the association between lower IGF-1 levels and survival was noted among both males and females who achieved longevity despite having had cancer (Milman et al. 2014). Although, lower IGF-1 levels predicted life expectancy in exceptionally long-lived individuals, supporting the role of the GH/IGF-1 pathway in exceptional longevity, previous studies in middle-aged and younger individuals have not consistently demonstrated associations between IGF-1 and life span or health span (Milman et al. 2016). However, the largest to-date IGF-1 study conducted in the UK Biobank cohort found an interaction between age and circulating IGF-1 level. The study demonstrated that higher baseline IGF-1 levels were associated with greater hazard for mortality and age-related morbidity, including dementia, vascular disease, diabetes, and cancer, with advancing age (Fig. 2; Zhang et al. 2021). This finding supports the theory of antagonistic pleiotropy and may explain why prior studies that have not accounted for age-IGF-1 interactions have reached inconsistent conclusions on the role of GH/IGF-1 in aging.

A recent study identified two linked rare genetic variants (N308K/A313S) in *SIRT6* gene-encoding sirtuin 6, a protein deacylase and mono-ADP-ribosylase enzyme, to be enriched among AJ centenarians (Simon et al. 2022). Functional characterization of these alleles demonstrated that they enhance genome maintenance through suppression of LINE1 retrotransposons, augmentation of DNA double-strand break repair, and improved interaction with Lamin A/C (LMNA) (Simon et al. 2022). These results provided additional evidence for the role of *SIRT6* in human longevity, which has been previously implicated in regulation of life span in model organisms (Tian et al. 2019).

Other genomic mechanisms, no doubt, also contribute to aging, including epigenomic mechanisms. Methylation patterns have been noted to change with aging and may affect the transcribed DNA. Initial studies have shown significant differences in methylation patterns between centenarians and younger controls, with several groups currently pursuing this line of research (Gutman et al. 2020b; Daunay et al. 2022; Gensous et al. 2022). Finally, longevity-associated microRNAs have been identified (Gombar et al. 2012), with a number of microRNAs linked to frailty resilience (Inglés et al. 2022).

EXCEPTIONAL LONGEVITY RESEARCH GUIDES DEVELOPMENT OF AGE-DELAYING DRUGS

The goal of longevity research is to identify pathways that are relevant to human aging and to develop therapeutics that will delay aging by targeting these pathways. Longevity and extension of healthy life span have been achieved in model organisms via a variety of genetic manipulations, drugs, and environmental influences, thereby providing the preclinical foundation needed to proceed to drug development.

The pharmaceutical industry has relied on genetic discoveries made in longevity studies, as well as other studies, to identify individuals who have naturally occurring genetic variants or mutations that confer desirable phenotypes. The goal for pharmaceutical development is to formulate drugs that mimic the actions of favorable

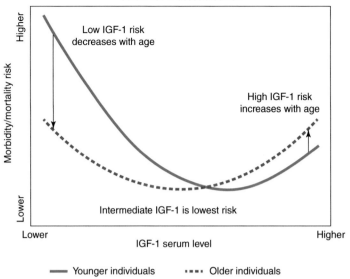

Figure 2. The antagonistic pleiotropy of insulin-like growth factor 1 (IGF-1). (Figure created based on data in Zhang et al. 2021.)

genetic variants. Observing the carriers of these genetic variants for any detrimental health effects informs drug makers of any potential side effects that may arise from a drug that targets the desired pathway. For example, the observation that centenarians are enriched with a unique *CETP* genotype that exposes them to a lifetime of lower CETP levels that is also associated with high HDL levels and large lipoprotein particle size, suggests that decreased CETP function is safe (Barzilai et al. 2003). In fact, a number of CETP inhibitors were developed and tested in clinical trials, including anacetrapib, which demonstrated reduction of major coronary events (The HPS3/TIMI55–REVEAL Collaborative Group et al. 2017). Similar observations were made about the APOC-3 protein and, after demonstrated efficacy in phase 2 trials (Lee et al. 2013; Tardif et al. 2022), APOC-3 inhibitors are now being tested in phase 3 trials.

Another group of therapeutic agents that may be effective against aging, based on prior knowledge gained through longevity research, is monoclonal antibodies directed against the IGF-1 receptor. These were initially developed by several pharmaceutical industries as antineoplastic therapies; however, they were not successful at treating cancer due to significant mutagenesis within cancer cells that resulted in eventual resistance to these drugs. Nonetheless, these compounds are available for preclinical testing in aging research and a recent study demonstrated that administration of anti-IGF1R monoclonal antibodies to middle-aged rodents resulted in median life extension and health-span improvement in female mice (Mao et al. 2018). Similarly, the GH/IGF-1 pathway, which may be important for human aging, can be targeted by the GH receptor antagonist that is currently in clinical use for the treatment of acromegaly, a condition of GH excess (Kopchick 2003). Although to the best of our knowledge, the above-mentioned therapeutics are presently not being developed for extension of human life span and health span, these drugs may be tested in the future for the indication of delaying aging and age-associated diseases.

Other compounds may target aging more directly, even though they are in clinical use for other indications. One example is a class of drugs that inhibit the mTOR enzyme. These drugs are primarily used as immune modulators post organ transplantation, but, recently, also have been shown to improve the immune response to vaccinations in older adults (Mannick et al. 2014), thereby demonstrating their potential utility in the treatment of health conditions associated with aging.

Metformin, a medication currently recommended as the first-line treatment for T2DM, is another drug of interest for the treatment of aging. Several research groups tested the effect of metformin on aging and demonstrated that it caused extension in life span and health span in a number of rodent models (Anisimov et al. 2008, 2010, 2011; Smith et al. 2010; Martin-Montalvo et al. 2013). Metformin also extended the life span of nematodes (Cabreiro et al. 2013), suggesting that its action is mediated via an evolutionarily conserved mechanism. Numerous investigators looked at the potential anti-aging effects of this drug in populations treated with metformin for T2DM. The large United Kingdom Prospective Diabetes Study (UKPDS) demonstrated that metformin reduced the incidence of cardiovascular disease (Holman et al. 2008; Anfossi et al. 2010). This finding has been validated and reproduced by other studies and meta-analysis (Johnson et al. 2005; Lamanna et al. 2011; Roumie et al. 2012; Hong et al. 2013; Whittington et al. 2013). In addition, a number of investigations suggested that metformin use is associated with a decreased incidence of cancer (Libby et al. 2009; Landman et al. 2010; Lee et al. 2011; Monami et al. 2011; Tseng 2012), with many animal and cell models demonstrating the inhibitory effects of metformin on tumorigenesis (Seibel et al. 2008; Tosca et al. 2010; Liu et al. 2011; Salani et al. 2012; Anisimov and Bartke 2013; Karnevi et al. 2013; Quinn et al. 2013). Metformin likely inhibits complex IV in the mitochondria and initiates a biological cascade that targets many hallmarks of aging (LaMoia et al. 2022).

In the future, other compounds discovered to be important for longevity may be developed into drugs. For example, the level of humanin, a mitochondrial-derived peptide, decreases with aging but has been shown to be up to threefold higher in the offspring of centenarians (Muzumdar et al. 2009), thus making it an attractive candidate for drug development.

A major obstacle to the development of therapeutic agents for the treatment of aging is the fact that the FDA does not recognize aging as a preventable condition. The pharmaceutical industry is not incentivized to develop drugs that are not covered by health insurance companies. The same was true for medications that treat hypertension, until studies demonstrated that lowering blood pressure prevented cardiovascular disease and stroke. As additional evidence demonstrates the benefits of targeting biological aging to delay age-related diseases and disability, the tide may turn for gerotherapeutics as well.

CONCLUDING REMARKS

This review demonstrates that biological and genetic experimental methods can help scientists uncover why some people age more slowly than others. Although such discoveries in humans have the advantage of being directly relevant to human longevity, many longevity-associated genes and pathways first identified in animal models subsequently have been confirmed in centenarian cohorts, demonstrating that both experimental and clinical models are beneficial for advancing aging research. Nonetheless, drug targets that have support from human genetic studies are at least twice as likely to be successful in clinical trials and to result in eventual FDA approval (King et al. 2019). Therefore, pharmaceutical developers who are interested in drug targets that have the potential to delay aging are looking for supporting information in the genomes of centenarians. Thus, it is of utmost importance to increase the number of centenarians in research to strengthen the power for genetic discovery and validation of biological pathways that regulate healthy longevity. Such an effort is underway with the recent launch of the Super-Agers Family Study that aims to enroll 10,000 families with exceptional longevity. Development of drugs based on genetics of centenarians will result in unique therapeutics that target not only specific diseases but the biology of aging itself. One barrier for the development of drugs that target aging is that, at present, the FDA does not recognize aging as an indication for treatment. However, efforts are ongoing to test metformin for its effectiveness to delay aging in a placebo-controlled clinical trial, Taming Aging with Metformin (TAME), which will establish a new paradigm for testing pharmaceutical compounds for the indication of delaying multiple age-related diseases (Barzilai et al. 2016). The need is urgent to change this paradigm to accelerate drug development and realize the longevity dividend.

ACKNOWLEDGMENTS

S.M. is supported by grants from the National Institutes of Health (R01AG061155, P30AG03 8072, UH3AG064704, U19AG073172, R56AG0 44829) and the American Federation for Aging Research. N.B. is supported by grants from the National Institutes of Health (P01AG021654), The Nathan Shock Center of Excellence for the Biology of Aging (P30AG038072), and the Glenn Center for the Biology of Human Aging (Paul Glenn Foundation for Medical Research). The content is solely the responsibility of the authors and does not necessarily represent the official views of the National Institutes of Health.

REFERENCES

Adams ER, Nolan VG, Andersen SL, Perls TT, Terry DF. 2008. Centenarian offspring: start healthier and stay healthier. *J Am Geriatr Soc* **56:** 2089–2092. doi:10.1111/j .1532-5415.2008.01949.x

Ailshire JA, Beltran-Sanchez H, Crimmins EM. 2015. Becoming centenarians: disease and functioning trajectories of older U.S. adults as they survive to 100. *J Gerontol A Biol Sci Med Sci* **70:** 193–201. doi:10.1093/gerona/glu124

Altmann-Schneider I, van der Grond J, Slagboom PE, Westendorp RG, Maier AB, van Buchem MA, de Craen AJ. 2013. Lower susceptibility to cerebral small vessel disease in human familial longevity: the Leiden Longevity Study. *Stroke* **44:** 9–14. doi:10.1161/STROKEAHA.112.671438

Andersen HR, Jeune B, Nybo H, Nielsen JB, Andersen-Ranberg K, Grandjean P. 1998. Low activity of superoxide dismutase and high activity of glutathione reductase in erythrocytes from centenarians. *Age Ageing* **27:** 643–648. doi:10.1093/ageing/27.5.643

Andersen SL, Sebastiani P, Dworkis DA, Feldman L, Perls TT. 2012. Health span approximates life span among many supercentenarians: compression of morbidity at the approximate limit of life span. *J Gerontol A Biol Sci Med Sci* **67A:** 395–405. doi:10.1093/gerona/glr223

Anderson KM, Odell PM, Wilson PW, Kannel WB. 1991. Cardiovascular disease risk profiles. *Am Heart J* **121:** 293–298. doi:10.1016/0002-8703(91)90861-B

Anfossi G, Russo I, Bonomo K, Trovati M. 2010. The cardiovascular effects of metformin: further reasons to consider an old drug as a cornerstone in the therapy of type 2 diabetes mellitus. *Curr Vasc Pharmacol* **8:** 327–337. doi:10.2174/157016110791112359

Anisimov VN, Bartke A. 2013. The key role of growth hormone-insulin-IGF-1 signaling in aging and cancer. *Crit Rev Oncol Hematol* **87:** 201–223. doi:10.1016/j.critrevonc .2013.01.005

Anisimov VN, Berstein LM, Egormin PA, Piskunova TS, Popovich IG, Zabezhinski MA, Tyndyk ML, Yurova MV, Kovalenko IG, Poroshina TE, et al. 2008. Metformin slows down aging and extends life span of female SHR mice. *Cell Cycle* **7:** 2769–2773. doi:10.4161/cc.7.17.6625

Anisimov VN, Egormin PA, Piskunova TS, Popovich IG, Tyndyk ML, Yurova MN, Zabezhinski MA, Anikin IV, Karkach AS, Romanyukha AA. 2010. Metformin extends life span of HER-2/neu transgenic mice and in combination with melatonin inhibits growth of transplantable tumors in vivo. *Cell Cycle* **9:** 188–197. doi:10.4161/cc.9.1 .10407

Anisimov VN, Berstein LM, Popovich IG, Zabezhinski MA, Egormin PA, Piskunova TS, Semenchenko AV, Tyndyk ML, Yurova MN, Kovalenko IG, et al. 2011. If started early in life, metformin treatment increases life span and postpones tumors in female SHR mice. *Aging (Albany NY)* **3:** 148–157. doi:10.18632/aging.100273

Atzmon G, Schechter C, Greiner W, Davidson D, Rennert G, Barzilai N. 2004. Clinical phenotype of families with longevity. *J Am Geriatr Soc* **52:** 274–277. doi:10.1111/j.1532-5415.2004.52068.x

Atzmon G, Rincon M, Schechter CB, Shuldiner AR, Lipton RB, Bergman A, Barzilai N. 2006. Lipoprotein genotype and conserved pathway for exceptional longevity in humans. *PLoS Biol* **4:** e113. doi:10.1371/journal.pbio.004 0113

Atzmon G, Pollin TI, Crandall J, Tanner K, Schechter CB, Scherer PE, Rincon M, Siegel G, Katz M, Lipton RB, et al. 2008. Adiponectin levels and genotype: a potential regulator of life span in humans. *J Gerontol A Biol Sci Med Sci* **63:** 447–453. doi:10.1093/gerona/63.5.447

Atzmon G, Barzilai N, Hollowell JG, Surks MI, Gabriely I. 2009a. Extreme longevity is associated with increased serum thyrotropin. *J Clin Endocrinol Metab* **94:** 1251–1254. doi:10.1210/jc.2008-2325

Atzmon G, Barzilai N, Surks MI, Gabriely I. 2009b. Genetic predisposition to elevated serum thyrotropin is associated with exceptional longevity. *J Clin Endocrinol Metab* **94:** 4768–4775. doi:10.1210/jc.2009-0808

Atzmon G, Cho M, Cawthon RM, Budagov T, Katz M, Yang X, Siegel G, Bergman A, Huffman DM, Schechter CB, et al. 2010. Evolution in health and medicine Sackler colloquium: genetic variation in human telomerase is associated with telomere length in Ashkenazi centenarians. *Proc Natl Acad Sci* **107**(Suppl 1): 1710–1717. doi:10.1073/pnas .0906191106

Bae H, Gurinovich A, Malovini A, Atzmon G, Andersen SL, Villa F, Barzilai N, Puca A, Perls TT, Sebastiani P. 2018. Effects of FOXO3 polymorphisms on survival to extreme longevity in four centenarian studies. *J Gerontol A Biol Sci Med Sci* **73:** 1439–1447. doi:10.1093/gerona/glx124

Barzilai N, Atzmon G, Schechter C, Schaefer EJ, Cupples AL, Lipton R, Cheng S, Shuldiner AR. 2003. Unique lipoprotein phenotype and genotype associated with exceptional longevity. *JAMA* **290:** 2030–2040. doi:10.1001/jama.290 .15.2030

Barzilai N, Crandall JP, Kritchevsky SB, Espeland MA. 2016. Metformin as a tool to target aging. *Cell Metab* **23:** 1060–1065. doi:10.1016/j.cmet.2016.05.011

Beekman M, Nederstigt C, Suchiman HE, Kremer D, van der Breggen R, Lakenberg N, Alemayehu WG, de Craen AJ, Westendorp RG, Boomsma DI, et al. 2010. Genome-wide association study (GWAS)-identified disease risk alleles do not compromise human longevity. *Proc Natl Acad Sci* **107:** 18046–18049. doi:10.1073/pnas.1003540107

Bonafè M, Marchegiani F, Cardelli M, Olivieri F, Cavallone L, Giovagnetti S, Pieri C, Marra M, Antonicelli R, Troiano L, et al. 2002. Genetic analysis of Paraoxonase (PON1) locus reveals an increased frequency of Arg192 allele in centenarians. *Eur J Hum Genet* **10:** 292–296. doi:10.1038/sj.ejhg.5200806

Bonafè M, Barbieri M, Marchegiani F, Olivieri F, Ragno E, Giampieri C, Mugianesi E, Centurelli M, Franceschi C, Paolisso G. 2003. Polymorphic variants of insulin-like growth factor I (IGF-I) receptor and phosphoinositide 3-kinase genes affect IGF-I plasma levels and human longevity: cues for an evolutionarily conserved mechanism of life span control. *J Clin Endocrinol Metab* **88:** 3299–3304. doi:10.1210/jc.2002-021810

Broer L, Buchman AS, Deelen J, Evans DS, Faul JD, Lunetta KL, Sebastiani P, Smith JA, Smith AV, Tanaka T, et al. 2015. GWAS of longevity in CHARGE consortium confirms APOE and FOXO3 candidacy. *J Gerontol A Biol Sci Med Sci* **70:** 110–118. doi:10.1093/gerona/glu166

Brown-Borg HM, Borg KE, Meliska CJ, Bartke A. 1996. Dwarf mice and the ageing process. *Nature* **384:** 33. doi:10.1038/384033a0

Cabreiro F, Au C, Leung KY, Vergara-Irigaray N, Cochemé HM, Noori T, Weinkove D, Schuster E, Greene ND, Gems D. 2013. Metformin retards aging in *C. elegans* by altering microbial folate and methionine metabolism. *Cell* **153:** 228–239. doi:10.1016/j.cell.2013.02.035

Carmi S, Hui KY, Kochav E, Liu X, Xue J, Grady F, Guha S, Upadhyay K, Ben-Avraham D, Mukherjee S, et al. 2014. Sequencing an Ashkenazi reference panel supports population-targeted personal genomics and illuminates Jewish and European origins. *Nat Commun* **5:** 4835. doi:10.1038/ncomms5835

CDC. 2023. Leading causes of death and injury. Centers for Disease Control and Prevention, Atlanta. http://www.cdc.gov/nchs/hus.htm

Daunay A, Hardy LM, Bouyacoub Y, Sahbatou M, Touvier M, Blanché H, Deleuze JF, How-Kit A. 2022. Centenarians consistently present a younger epigenetic age than their chronological age with four epigenetic clocks based on a small number of CpG sites. *Aging (Albany NY)* **14:** 7718–7733. doi:10.18632/aging.204316

Deelen J, Beekman M, Uh HW, Helmer Q, Kuningas M, Christiansen L, Kremer D, van der Breggen R, Suchiman HE, Lakenberg N, et al. 2011. Genome-wide association study identifies a single major locus contributing to survival into old age; the APOE locus revisited. *Aging Cell* **10:** 686–698. doi:10.1111/j.1474-9726.2011.00705.x

Deelen J, Beekman M, Uh HW, Broer L, Ayers KL, Tan Q, Kamatani Y, Bennet AM, Tamm R, Trompet S, et al. 2014. Genome-wide association meta-analysis of human lon-gevity identifies a novel locus conferring survival beyond 90 years of age. *Hum Mol Genet* **23:** 4420–4432. doi:10.1093/hmg/ddu139

Deelen J, Evans DS, Arking DE, Tesi N, Nygaard M, Liu X, Wojczynski MK, Biggs ML, van der Spek A, Atzmon G, et al. 2019. A meta-analysis of genome-wide association studies identifies multiple longevity genes. *Nat Commun* **10:** 3669. doi:10.1038/s41467-019-11558-2

Evans CJ, Ho Y, Daveson BA, Hall S, Higginson IJ, Gao W. 2014. Place and cause of death in centenarians: a population-based observational study in England, 2001 to 2010. *PLoS Med* **11:** e1001653. doi:10.1371/journal.pmed.1001653

Feitosa MF, Wojczynski MK, Straka R, Kammerer CM, Lee JH, Kraja AT, Christensen K, Newman AB, Province MA, Borecki IB. 2014. Genetic analysis of long-lived families reveals novel variants influencing high density-lipoprotein cholesterol. *Front Genet* **5:** 159. doi:10.3389/fgene.2014.00159

Florez H, Ma Y, Crandall JP, Perreault L, Marcovina SM, Bray GA, Saudek CD, Barrett-Connor E, Knowler WC. 2011. Parental longevity and diabetes risk in the Diabetes Prevention Program. *J Gerontol A Biol Sci Med Sci* **66A:** 1211–1217. doi:10.1093/gerona/glr114

Franceschi C, Olivieri F, Marchegiani F, Cardelli M, Cavallone L, Capri M, Salvioli S, Valensin S, De Benedictis G, Di Iorio A, et al. 2005. Genes involved in immune response/inflammation, IGF1/insulin pathway and response to oxidative stress play a major role in the genetics of human longevity: the lesson of centenarians. *Mech Ageing Dev* **126:** 351–361. doi:10.1016/j.mad.2004.08.028

Freudenberg-Hua Y, Freudenberg J, Vacic V, Abhyankar A, Emde AK, Ben-Avraham D, Barzilai N, Oschwald D, Christen E, Koppel J, et al. 2014. Disease variants in genomes of 44 centenarians. *Mol Genet Genomic Med* **2:** 438–450. doi:10.1002/mgg3.86

Gavrilov L, Gavrilova N, Semyonova V, Evdokushkina G. 2001. Parental age effects on human longevity. In *Annual Meeting of the Gerontological Society of America*. Chicago, November 15–18.

Gensous N, Sala C, Pirazzini C, Ravaioli F, Milazzo M, Kwiatkowska KM, Marasco E, De Fanti S, Giuliani C, Pellegrini C, et al. 2022. A targeted epigenetic clock for the prediction of biological age. *Cells* **11:** 4044. doi:10.3390/cells11244044

Goldman DP, Cutler D, Rowe JW, Michaud PC, Sullivan J, Peneva D, Olshansky SJ. 2013. Substantial health and economic returns from delayed aging may warrant a new focus for medical research. *Health Aff (Millwood)* **32:** 1698–1705. doi:10.1377/hlthaff.2013.0052

Gombar S, Jung HJ, Dong F, Calder B, Atzmon G, Barzilai N, Tian XL, Pothof J, Hoeijmakers JH, Campisi J, et al. 2012. Comprehensive microRNA profiling in B-cells of human centenarians by massively parallel sequencing. *BMC Genomics* **13:** 353. doi:10.1186/1471-2164-13-353

Gordon T, Castelli WP, Hjortland MC, Kannel WB, Dawber TR. 1977. High density lipoprotein as a protective factor against coronary heart disease. the Framingham Study. *Am J Med* **62:** 707–714. doi:10.1016/0002-9343(77)90874-9

Gubbi S, Schwartz E, Crandall J, Verghese J, Holtzer R, Atzmon G, Braunstein R, Barzilai N, Milman S. 2017. Effect of exceptional parental longevity and lifestyle factors on prevalence of cardiovascular disease in offspring. *Am J Cardiol* **120:** 2170–2175. doi:10.1016/j.amjcard.2017.08.040

Guevara-Aguirre J, Balasubramanian P, Guevara-Aguirre M, Wei M, Madia F, Cheng CW, Hwang D, Martin-Montalvo A, Saavedra J, Ingles S, et al. 2011. Growth hormone receptor deficiency is associated with a major reduction in pro-aging signaling, cancer, and diabetes in humans. *Sci Transl Med* **3:** 70ra13. doi:10.1126/scitranslmed.3001845

Gunn S, Wainberg M, Song Z, Andersen S, Boudreau R, Feitosa MF, Tan Q, Montasser ME, O'Connell JR, Stitziel N, et al. 2022. Distribution of 54 polygenic risk scores for common diseases in long lived individuals and their offspring. *Geroscience* **44:** 719–729. doi:10.1007/s11357-022-00518-2

Gutman D, Lidzbarsky G, Milman S, Gao T, Sin-Chan P, Gonzaga-Jauregui C, Regeneron Genetics C, Deelen J, Shuldiner AR, Barzilai N, et al. 2020a. Similar burden of pathogenic coding variants in exceptionally long-lived individuals and individuals without exceptional longevity. *Aging Cell* **19:** e13216. doi:10.1111/acel.13216

Gutman D, Rivkin E, Fadida A, Sharvit L, Hermush V, Rubin E, Kirshner D, Sabin I, Dwolatzky T, Atzmon G. 2020b. Exceptionally long-lived individuals (ELLI) demonstrate slower aging rate calculated by DNA methylation clocks as possible modulators for healthy longevity. *Int J Mol Sci* **21:** 615. doi:10.3390/ijms21020615

Herskind AM, McGue M, Holm NV, Sørensen TI, Harvald B, Vaupel JW. 1996. The heritability of human longevity: a population-based study of 2872 Danish twin pairs born 1870–1900. *Hum Genet* **97:** 319–323. doi:10.1007/BF02185763

Holman RR, Paul SK, Bethel MA, Matthews DR, Neil HA. 2008. 10-year follow-up of intensive glucose control in type 2 diabetes. *N Engl J Med* **359:** 1577–1589. doi:10.1056/NEJMoa0806470

Hong J, Zhang Y, Lai S, Lv A, Su Q, Dong Y, Zhou Z, Tang W, Zhao J, Cui L, et al. 2013. Effects of metformin versus glipizide on cardiovascular outcomes in patients with type 2 diabetes and coronary artery disease. *Diabetes Care* **36:** 1304–1311. doi:10.2337/dc12-0719

Howden LM, Meyer JA. 2011. Age and sex composition: 2010, 2010 census briefs. Available at http://www.census.gov/prod/cen2010/briefs/c2010br-03.pdf

Inglés M, Belenguer-Varea A, Serna E, Mas-Bargues C, Tarazona-Santabalbina FJ, Borrás C, Vina J. 2022. Functional transcriptomic analysis of centenarians' offspring reveals a specific genetic footprint that may explain that they are less frail than age-matched noncentenarians' offspring. *J Gerontol A Biol Sci Med Sci* **77:** 1931–1938. doi:10.1093/gerona/glac119

Ismail K NL, Sebastiani P, Milman S, Perls TT, Barzilai N. 2014. Individuals with exceptional longevity exhibit increased health span and delayed onset of age-related diseases. In *Presidential Poster Session of the American Geriatrics Society Annual Meeting*, Orlando, FL.

Johnson JA, Simpson SH, Toth EL, Majumdar SR. 2005. Reduced cardiovascular morbidity and mortality associated with metformin use in subjects with type 2 diabetes. *Diabet Med* **22:** 497–502. doi:10.1111/j.1464-5491.2005.01448.x

Karnevi E, Said K, Andersson R, Rosendahl AH. 2013. Metformin-mediated growth inhibition involves suppression of the IGF-I receptor signalling pathway in human pancreatic cancer cells. *BMC Cancer* **13:** 235. doi:10.1186/1471-2407-13-235

Kenyon C, Chang J, Gensch E, Rudner A, Tabtiang R. 1993. A *C. elegans* mutant that lives twice as long as wild type. *Nature* **366:** 461–464. doi:10.1038/366461a0

King EA, Davis JW, Degner JF. 2019. Are drug targets with genetic support twice as likely to be approved? Revised estimates of the impact of genetic support for drug mechanisms on the probability of drug approval. *PLoS Genet* **15:** e1008489. doi:10.1371/journal.pgen.1008489

Kojima T, Kamei H, Aizu T, Arai Y, Takayama M, Nakazawa S, Ebihara Y, Inagaki H, Masui Y, Gondo Y, et al. 2004. Association analysis between longevity in the Japanese population and polymorphic variants of genes involved in insulin and insulin-like growth factor 1 signaling pathways. *Exp Gerontol* **39:** 1595–1598. doi:10.1016/j.exger.2004.05.007

Kopchick JJ. 2003. Discovery and mechanism of action of pegvisomant. *Eur J Endocrinol* **148**(Suppl 2): S21–S25. doi:10.1530/eje.0.148s021

Lamanna C, Monami M, Marchionni N, Mannucci E. 2011. Effect of metformin on cardiovascular events and mortality: a meta-analysis of randomized clinical trials. *Diabetes Obes Metab* **13:** 221–228. doi:10.1111/j.1463-1326.2010.01349.x

LaMoia TE, Butrico GM, Kalpage HA, Goedeke L, Hubbard BT, Vatner DF, Gaspar RC, Zhang XM, Cline GW, Nakahara K, et al. 2022. Metformin, phenformin, and galegine inhibit complex IV activity and reduce glycerol-derived gluconeogenesis. *Proc Natl Acad Sci* **119:** e2122287119. doi:10.1073/pnas.2122287119

Landman GW, Kleefstra N, van Hateren KJ, Groenier KH, Gans RO, Bilo HJ. 2010. Metformin associated with lower cancer mortality in type 2 diabetes: ZODIAC-16. *Diabetes Care* **33:** 322–326. doi:10.2337/dc09-1380

Lee MS, Hsu CC, Wahlqvist ML, Tsai HN, Chang YH, Huang YC. 2011. Type 2 diabetes increases and metformin reduces total, colorectal, liver and pancreatic cancer incidences in Taiwanese: a representative population prospective cohort study of 800,000 individuals. *BMC Cancer* **11:** 20. doi:10.1186/1471-2407-11-20

Lee RG, Crosby J, Baker BF, Graham MJ, Crooke RM. 2013. Antisense technology: an emerging platform for cardiovascular disease therapeutics. *J Cardiovasc Transl Res* **6:** 969–980. doi:10.1007/s12265-013-9495-7

Libby G, Donnelly LA, Donnan PT, Alessi DR, Morris AD, Evans JM. 2009. New users of metformin are at low risk of incident cancer: a cohort study among people with type 2 diabetes. *Diabetes Care* **32:** 1620–1625. doi:10.2337/dc08-2175

Lin J-R, Sin-Chan P, Napolioni V, Torres GG, Mitra J, Zhang Q, Jabalameli MR, Wang Z, Nguyen N, Gao T, et al. 2021. Rare genetic coding variants associated with human longevity and protection against age-related diseases. *Nature Aging* **1:** 783–794. doi:10.1038/s43587-021-00108-5

Lipton RB, Hirsch J, Katz MJ, Wang C, Sanders AE, Verghese J, Barzilai N, Derby CA. 2010. Exceptional parental longevity associated with lower risk of Alzheimer's disease and memory decline. *J Am Geriatr Soc* **58**: 1043–1049. doi:10.1111/j.1532-5415.2010.02868.x

Liu B, Fan Z, Edgerton SM, Yang X, Lind SE, Thor AD. 2011. Potent anti-proliferative effects of metformin on trastuzumab-resistant breast cancer cells via inhibition of erbB2/IGF-1 receptor interactions. *Cell Cycle* **10**: 2959–2966. doi:10.4161/cc.10.17.16359

Lu F, Guan H, Gong B, Liu X, Zhu R, Wang Y, Qian J, Zhou T, Lan X, Wang P, et al. 2014. Genetic variants in PVRL2-TOMM40-APOE region are associated with human longevity in a Han Chinese population. *PLoS ONE* **9**: e99580. doi:10.1371/journal.pone.0099580

Mannick JB, Del Giudice G, Lattanzi M, Valiante NM, Praestgaard J, Huang B, Lonetto MA, Maecker HT, Kovarik J, Carson S, et al. 2014. mTOR inhibition improves immune function in the elderly. *Sci Transl Med* **6**: 268ra179. doi:10.1126/scitranslmed.3009892

Mao K, Quipildor GF, Tabrizian T, Novaj A, Guan F, Walters RO, Delahaye F, Hubbard GB, Ikeno Y, Ejima K, et al. 2018. Late-life targeting of the IGF-1 receptor improves healthspan and lifespan in female mice. *Nat Commun* **9**: 2394. doi:10.1038/s41467-018-04805-5

Marchegiani F, Marra M, Spazzafumo L, James RW, Boemi M, Olivieri F, Cardelli M, Cavallone L, Bonfigli AR, Franceschi C. 2006. Paraoxonase activity and genotype predispose to successful aging. *J Gerontol A Biol Sci Med Sci* **61**: 541–546. doi:10.1093/gerona/61.6.541

Martin GM. 2005. Genetic modulation of senescent phenotypes in *Homo sapiens*. *Cell* **120**: 523–532. doi:10.1016/j.cell.2005.01.031

Martin-Montalvo A, Mercken EM, Mitchell SJ, Palacios HH, Mote PL, Scheibye-Knudsen M, Gomes AP, Ward TM, Minor RK, Blouin MJ, et al. 2013. Metformin improves healthspan and lifespan in mice. *Nat Commun* **4**: 2192. doi:10.1038/ncomms3192

McGue M, Vaupel JW, Holm N, Harvald B. 1993. Longevity is moderately heritable in a sample of Danish twins born 1870-1880. *J Gerontol* **48**: B237–B244. doi:10.1093/geronj/48.6.B237

Mecocci P, Polidori MC, Troiano L, Cherubini A, Cecchetti R, Pini G, Straatman M, Monti D, Stahl W, Sies H, et al. 2000. Plasma antioxidants and longevity: a study on healthy centenarians. *Free Radic Biol Med* **28**: 1243–1248. doi:10.1016/S0891-5849(00)00246-X

Milman S, Atzmon G, Huffman DM, Wan J, Crandall JP, Cohen P, Barzilai N. 2014. Low insulin-like growth factor-1 level predicts survival in humans with exceptional longevity. *Aging Cell* **13**: 769–771. doi:10.1111/acel.12213

Milman S, Huffman DM, Barzilai N. 2016. The somatotropic axis in human aging: framework for the current state of knowledge and future research. *Cell Metab* **23**: 980–989. doi:10.1016/j.cmet.2016.05.014

Mitchell BD, Hsueh WC, King TM, Pollin TI, Sorkin J, Agarwala R, Schaffer AA, Shuldiner AR. 2001. Heritability of life span in the Old Order Amish. *Am J Med Genet* **102**: 346–352. doi:10.1002/ajmg.1483

Monami M, Colombi C, Balzi D, Dicembrini I, Giannini S, Melani C, Vitale V, Romano D, Barchielli A, Marchionni N, et al. 2011. Metformin and cancer occurrence in insulin-treated type 2 diabetic patients. *Diabetes Care* **34**: 129–131. doi:10.2337/dc10-1287

Muzumdar RH, Huffman DM, Atzmon G, Buettner C, Cobb LJ, Fishman S, Budagov T, Cui L, Einstein FH, Poduval A, et al. 2009. Humanin: a novel central regulator of peripheral insulin action. *PLoS ONE* **4**: e6334. doi:10.1371/journal.pone.0006334

Nebel A, Kleindorp R, Caliebe A, Nothnagel M, Blanché H, Junge O, Wittig M, Ellinghaus D, Flachsbart F, Wichmann HE, et al. 2011. A genome-wide association study confirms APOE as the major gene influencing survival in long-lived individuals. *Mech Ageing Dev* **132**: 324–330. doi:10.1016/j.mad.2011.06.008

Pawlikowska L, Hu D, Huntsman S, Sung A, Chu C, Chen J, Joyner AH, Schork NJ, Hsueh WC, Reiner AP, et al. 2009. Association of common genetic variation in the insulin/IGF1 signaling pathway with human longevity. *Aging Cell* **8**: 460–472. doi:10.1111/j.1474-9726.2009.00493.x

Perice L, Barzilai N, Verghese J, Weiss EF, Holtzer R, Cohen P, Milman S. 2016. Lower circulating insulin-like growth factor-I is associated with better cognition in females with exceptional longevity without compromise to muscle mass and function. *Aging (Albany NY)* **8**: 2414–2424. doi:10.18632/aging.101063

Perls TT, Bubrick E, Wager CG, Vijg J, Kruglyak L. 1998. Siblings of centenarians live longer. *Lancet* **351**: 1560. doi:10.1016/S0140-6736(05)61126-9

Perls TT, Wilmoth J, Levenson R, Drinkwater M, Cohen M, Bogan H, Joyce E, Brewster S, Kunkel L, Puca A. 2002. Life-long sustained mortality advantage of siblings of centenarians. *Proc Natl Acad Sci* **99**: 8442–8447. doi:10.1073/pnas.122587599

Pollin TI, Damcott CM, Shen H, Ott SH, Shelton J, Horenstein RB, Post W, McLenithan JC, Bielak LF, Peyser PA, et al. 2008. A null mutation in human *APOC3* confers a favorable plasma lipid profile and apparent cardioprotection. *Science* **322**: 1702–1705. doi:10.1126/science.1161524

Quinn BJ, Dallos M, Kitagawa H, Kunnumakkara AB, Memmott RM, Hollander MC, Gills JJ, Dennis PA. 2013. Inhibition of lung tumorigenesis by metformin is associated with decreased plasma IGF-I and diminished receptor tyrosine kinase signaling. *Cancer Prev Res (Phila)* **6**: 801–810. doi:10.1158/1940-6207.CAPR-13-0058-T

Rajpathak SN, Liu Y, Ben-David O, Reddy S, Atzmon G, Crandall J, Barzilai N. 2011. Lifestyle factors of people with exceptional longevity. *J Am Geriatr Soc* **59**: 1509–1512. doi:10.1111/j.1532-5415.2011.03498.x

Rea IM, McKeown PP, McMaster D, Young IS, Patterson C, Savage MJ, Belton C, Marchegiani F, Olivieri F, Bonafe M, et al. 2004. Paraoxonase polymorphisms PON1 192 and 55 and longevity in Italian centenarians and Irish nonagenarians. A pooled analysis. *Exp Gerontol* **39**: 629–635. doi:10.1016/j.exger.2003.11.019

Roumie CL, Hung AM, Greevy RA, Grijalva CG, Liu X, Murff HJ, Elasy TA, Griffin MR. 2012. Comparative effectiveness of sulfonylurea and metformin monotherapy on cardiovascular events in type 2 diabetes mellitus: a cohort study. *Ann Intern Med* **157**: 601–610. doi:10.7326/0003-4819-157-9-201211060-00003

Rozing MP, Houwing-Duistermaat JJ, Slagboom PE, Beekman M, Frölich M, de Craen AJ, Westendorp RG, van Heemst D. 2010. Familial longevity is associated with decreased thyroid function. *J Clin Endocrinol Metab* **95:** 4979–4984. doi:10.1210/jc.2010-0875

Salani B, Maffioli S, Hamoudane M, Parodi A, Ravera S, Passalacqua M, Alama A, Nhiri M, Cordera R, Maggi D. 2012. Caveolin-1 is essential for metformin inhibitory effect on IGF1 action in non-small-cell lung cancer cells. *FASEB J* **26:** 788–798. doi:10.1096/fj.11-192088

Sanders AE, Wang C, Katz M, Derby CA, Barzilai N, Ozelius L, Lipton RB. 2010. Association of a functional polymorphism in the cholesteryl ester transfer protein (*CETP*) gene with memory decline and incidence of dementia. *JAMA* **303:** 150–158. doi:10.1001/jama.2009.1988

Schoenmaker M, de Craen AJ, de Meijer PH, Beekman M, Blauw GJ, Slagboom PE, Westendorp RG. 2006. Evidence of genetic enrichment for exceptional survival using a family approach: the Leiden Longevity Study. *Eur J Hum Genet* **14:** 79–84. doi:10.1038/sj.ejhg.5201508

Scott AJ, Ellison M, Sinclair DA. 2021. The economic value of targeting aging. *Nature Aging* **1:** 616–623. doi:10.1038/s43587-021-00080-0

Sebastiani P, Solovieff N, Dewan AT, Walsh KM, Puca A, Hartley SW, Melista E, Andersen S, Dworkis DA, Wilk JB, et al. 2012. Genetic signatures of exceptional longevity in humans. *PLoS ONE* **7:** e29848. doi:10.1371/journal.pone.0029848

Sebastiani P, Sun FX, Andersen SL, Lee JH, Wojczynski MK, Sanders JL, Yashin A, Newman AB, Perls TT. 2013. Families enriched for exceptional longevity also have increased health-span: findings from the Long Life Family Study. *Front Public Health* **1:** 38. doi:10.3389/fpubh.2013.00038

Sebastiani P, Gurinovich A, Bae H, Andersen S, Malovini A, Atzmon G, Villa F, Kraja AT, Ben-Avraham D, Barzilai N, et al. 2017. Four genome-wide association studies identify new extreme longevity variants. *J Gerontol A Biol Sci Med Sci* **72:** 1453–1464. doi:10.1093/gerona/glx027

Sebastiani P, Gurinovich A, Nygaard M, Sasaki T, Sweigart B, Bae H, Andersen SL, Villa F, Atzmon G, Christensen K, et al. 2019. *APOE* alleles and extreme human longevity. *J Gerontol A Biol Sci Med Sci* **74:** 44–51. doi:10.1093/gerona/gly174

Seibel SA, Chou KH, Capp E, Spritzer PM, von Eye Corleta H. 2008. Effect of metformin on IGF-1 and IGFBP-1 levels in obese patients with polycystic ovary syndrome. *Eur J Obstet Gynecol Reprod Biol* **138:** 122–124. doi:10.1016/j.ejogrb.2007.02.001

Simon M, Yang J, Gigas J, Earley EJ, Hillpot E, Zhang L, Zagorulya M, Tombline G, Gilbert M, Yuen SL, et al. 2022. A rare human centenarian variant of SIRT6 enhances genome stability and interaction with Lamin A. *EMBO J* **41:** e110393. doi:10.15252/embj.2021110393

Smith DL Jr, Elam CF Jr, Mattison JA, Lane MA, Roth GS, Ingram DK, Allison DB. 2010. Metformin supplementation and life span in Fischer-344 rats. *J Gerontol A Biol Sci Med Sci* **65A:** 468–474. doi:10.1093/gerona/glq033

Suh Y, Atzmon G, Cho MO, Hwang D, Liu B, Leahy DJ, Barzilai N, Cohen P. 2008. Functionally significant insulin-like growth factor I receptor mutations in centenarians. *Proc Natl Acad Sci* **105:** 3438–3442. doi:10.1073/pnas.0705467105

Tabatabaie V, Surks MI. 2013. The aging thyroid. *Curr Opin Endocrinol Diabetes Obes* **20:** 455–459. doi:10.1097/01.med.0000433055.99570.52

Tan Q, Christiansen L, Bathum L, Li S, Kruse TA, Christensen K. 2006. Genetic association analysis of human longevity in cohort studies of elderly subjects: an example of the *PON1* gene in the Danish 1905 birth cohort. *Genetics* **172:** 1821–1828. doi:10.1534/genetics.105.050914

Tardif JC, Karwatowska-Prokopczuk E, Amour ES, Ballantyne CM, Shapiro MD, Moriarty PM, Baum SJ, Hurh E, Bartlett VJ, Kingsbury J, et al. 2022. Apolipoprotein C-III reduction in subjects with moderate hypertriglyceridaemia and at high cardiovascular risk. *Eur Heart J* **43:** 1401–1412. doi:10.1093/eurheartj/ehab820

Tazearslan C, Huang J, Barzilai N, Suh Y. 2011. Impaired IGF1R signaling in cells expressing longevity-associated human IGF1R alleles. *Aging Cell* **10:** 551–554. doi:10.1111/j.1474-9726.2011.00697.x

The HPS3/TIMI55–REVEAL Collaborative Group; Bowman L, Hopewell JC, Chen F, Wallendszus K, Stevens W, Collins R, Wiviott SD, Cannon CP, Braunwald E, et al. 2017. Effects of anacetrapib in patients with atherosclerotic vascular disease. *N Engl J Med* **377:** 1217–1227. doi:10.1056/NEJMoa1706444

Tian X, Firsanov D, Zhang Z, Cheng Y, Luo L, Tombline G, Tan R, Simon M, Henderson S, Steffan J, et al. 2019. SIRT6 is responsible for more efficient DNA double-strand break repair in long-lived species. *Cell* **177:** 622–638.e22. doi:10.1016/j.cell.2019.03.043

Torres GG, Dose J, Hasenbein TP, Nygaard M, Krause-Kyora B, Mengel-From J, Christensen K, Andersen-Ranberg K, Kolbe D, Lieb W, et al. 2022. Long-lived individuals show a lower burden of variants predisposing to age-related diseases and a higher polygenic longevity score. *Int J Mol Sci* **23:** 10949. doi:10.3390/ijms231810949

Tosca L, Ramé C, Chabrolle C, Tesseraud S, Dupont J. 2010. Metformin decreases IGF1-induced cell proliferation and protein synthesis through AMP-activated protein kinase in cultured bovine granulosa cells. *Reproduction* **139:** 409–418. doi:10.1530/REP-09-0351

Tseng CH. 2012. Diabetes, metformin use, and colon cancer: a population-based cohort study in Taiwan. *Eur J Endocrinol* **167:** 409–416. doi:10.1530/EJE-12-0369

van der Spoel E, Rozing MP, Houwing-Duistermaat JJ, Slagboom PE, Beekman M, de Craen AJ, Westendorp RG, van Heemst D. 2015. Association analysis of insulin-like growth factor-1 axis parameters with survival and functional status in nonagenarians of the Leiden Longevity Study. *Aging (Albany NY)* **7:** 956–963. doi:10.18632/aging.100841

van Heemst D, Beekman M, Mooijaart SP, Heijmans BT, Brandt BW, Zwaan BJ, Slagboom PE, Westendorp RG. 2005. Reduced insulin/IGF-1 signalling and human longevity. *Aging Cell* **4:** 79–85. doi:10.1111/j.1474-9728.2005.00148.x

Vergani C, Lucchi T, Caloni M, Ceconi I, Calabresi C, Scurati S, Arosio B. 2006. I405v polymorphism of the cholesteryl ester transfer protein (CETP) gene in young and very old people. *Arch Gerontol Geriatr* **43:** 213–221. doi:10.1016/j.archger.2005.10.008

Westendorp RG, van Heemst D, Rozing MP, Frölich M, Mooijaart SP, Blauw GJ, Beekman M, Heijmans BT, de Craen AJ, Slagboom PE. 2009. Nonagenarian siblings and their offspring display lower risk of mortality and morbidity than sporadic nonagenarians: the Leiden Longevity Study. *J Am Geriatr Soc* **57:** 1634–1637. doi:10.1111/j.1532-5415.2009.02381.x

Whittington HJ, Hall AR, McLaughlin CP, Hausenloy DJ, Yellon DM, Mocanu MM. 2013. Chronic metformin associated cardioprotection against infarction: not just a glucose lowering phenomenon. *Cardiovasc Drugs Ther* **27:** 5–16. doi:10.1007/s10557-012-6425-x

Zeng Y, Nie C, Min J, Liu X, Li M, Chen H, Xu H, Wang M, Ni T, Li Y, et al. 2016. Novel loci and pathways significantly associated with longevity. *Sci Rep* **6:** 21243. doi:10.1038/srep21243

Zenin A, Tsepilov Y, Sharapov S, Getmantsev E, Menshikov LI, Fedichev PO, Aulchenko Y. 2019. Identification of 12 genetic loci associated with human healthspan. *Commun Biol* **2:** 41. doi:10.1038/s42003-019-0290-0

Zhang WB, Ye K, Barzilai N, Milman S. 2021. The antagonistic pleiotropy of insulin-like growth factor 1. *Aging Cell* **20:** e13443.

Personalized Financial Planning Using Applied Genetics

S. Jay Olshansky,[1,2] Bradley Willcox,[3] Kirk Ashburn,[2] Jeffrey Stukey,[4] and Craig Willcox[5]

[1]School of Public Health, University of Illinois at Chicago, Chicago, Illinois 60612, USA

[2]Wealthspan Financial Partners, Grand Rapids, Michigan 49506, USA

[3]Department of Geriatric Medicine, John A. Burns School of Medicine, University of Hawaii Mānoa, Honolulu, Hawaii 96813, USA

[4]Investment Advisor, Wealthspan Investment Management, Grand Rapids, Michigan 49506, USA

[5]Professor of Public Health and Gerontology, Okinawa International University, Urasoe City, Okinawa 901-2122, Japan

Correspondence: sjayo@uic.edu

Forthcoming advances in geroscience will influence the health span of current and future generations and generate both challenges and opportunities for those approaching or reaching retirement ages. The resulting changes in the life course will influence those reaching stages in life that are commonly associated with retirement. How people plan for that later phase of life is critical—especially given that current approaches to planning are either nonexistent or outdated. In this review, we show how advances in applied genetics can yield valuable information for individuals that are facing the challenges and opportunities that will accompany anticipated advances in geroscience and their unique influence on the life span and health span of current and future generations.

Two of the most important demographic and medical events that have occurred in human history occurred during the last 120 years—the rapid aging of our species (Uhlenberg 2009; Bloom et al. 2015) and life extension brought forth by advances in public health and medicine. Anticipated advances in geroscience have the potential to extend these advances further—with a profound influence on the health span of current and future generations. Survival to older ages is now the norm rather than the exception in most parts of the world—leading to unprecedented opportunities and challenges. By way of illustration, based on death rates prevailing in the United States in 1900, only 39.2% of the babies born in that year were expected to reach the age of 65, 5.5% would reach ages 85+, and 0.25% would survive to ages 100+ (Bell and Miller 2005). Today, survival rates notably improved to 83.9% to ages 65+, 44.0% to 85+, and 3.2% to 100+ (mortality.org). Among those that reached age 65 in 1900, only 13.9% survived to age 85. By 2019, survival to age 85 conditional on having reached age 65, increased to 52.5%.

As a result of these historic events, humanity is now able to experience a much longer and later phase of life with a predictability never before experienced by previous generations. Peter Laslett, in 1991, recognized the importance of this unprecedented survival by labeling it a "fresh map of life" or the "third age" (Laslett 1991). Streeter et al. (2020) recently indicated that a new map of life is needed to accommodate the new reality of regular survival into what used to be when retirement and death occurred, and Ken Dychtwald (Dychtwald and Morrison 2021) emphasized that the world is now experiencing a new version of disengagement/reengagement to and from the workforce that is no longer characterized by a single discrete "retirement" event.

While longer and healthier lives are a welcome respite from a history filled with the tragedy of death that has been common at younger and middle ages, this third age is not without challenges (Brown 2015). Extended survival brings the dual challenge of rising chronic age-related diseases associated with operating our living machines beyond their biological warranty period (Olshansky 2021) and the problem of how to plan, pay for, and properly use those extra years (Sharpe 2021). All of the challenges and opportunities linked to extended survival will be exacerbated by successful efforts to modulate aging through the geroscience interventions described in this article.

In the United States, participation in retirement plans declined in the first two decades of this century during a time when the baby boom cohort was approaching their third age (www.epi.org/publication/the-state-of-american-retirement-savings/). More than one-third of the U.S. population has no retirement savings at all, >60% of those earning <$30 K per yr have not saved anything for retirement, and 38% of the population plans to work past age 65—in part, because they have to fund extra years in retirement (tippinsights.com/36-of-americans-dont-have-any-retirement-savings). In fact, only 44% of workers in the United States participate in a work-related retirement plan, primarily because many employers do not offer retirement plans, and even when they do, the amounts most people save are not even close to ensuring adequate post-retirement living standards (about 70%–80% of income received at age 65) (Ghilarducci et al. 2015).

The COVID pandemic has further challenged retirement decision-making as millions of Amer-

icans retired earlier than expected since the pandemic began (www.aarp.org/work/careers/pandemic-workers-early-retirement), or they began taking early distributions from their retirement accounts because they needed the money (www.accountingtoday.com/news/millions-of-taxpayers-took-early-distributions-from-retirement-accounts-due-to-covid), further jeopardizing their ability to finance the third phase of life. A recent poll by the Commonwealth Fund (www.commonwealthfund.org/publications/surveys/2021/sep/impact-covid-19-older-adults) documented that 19% of the population aged 65 and older in the United States either used up most or all of their savings or had a significant loss in income because of COVID, and among Blacks and Hispanics these percentages were 32% and 39%, respectively.

While better retirement planning requires some knowledge of estimated survival, the life span "calculators" available in the marketplace today are overly simplistic actuarial models that often grossly overestimate or underestimate duration of life because of their reliance on additive algorithms (www.newretirement.com/retirement/longevity-trends-and-life-expectancy-calculators). Additive survival estimation models operate under the premise that risk factors that influence survival operate independent of each other, allowing for the simple addition or subtraction of the survival effects of various mortality-related risk factors relative to a baseline survival estimate for the entire population. One important consequence of using an additive model in a life span calculator is that the life-shortening or life-extending effects of different risk factors are counted more than once. The magnitude of the double or triple counting is influenced by the degree to which the covariates used to estimate survival are correlated with each other. The result is a life span estimate that exaggerates survival prospects by extending the tails of the survival distribution in both directions. This yields an overestimate or underestimate of the true effects of risk factors on life span—an issue made even worse when considering potential life-extending effects of advances in geroscience.

As such, life span calculators based on additive models are most appropriately used for encouraging people to adopt healthier lifestyles by modifying behavioral risk factors. They cannot and should not be used to generate realistic personalized estimates of survival for retirement planning or life insurance underwriting because they are not designed for that purpose. While it is possible to address the problem of additivity by weighting risk factors relative to each other, the creators of commercial life span calculators have no incentive to pursue accuracy and reliability over expediency because the latter is not their goal.

One novel technology that has yet to make its way into the world of life span and health span assessment is to use personal genetic information to generate hyperpersonalized assessments of survival and health as a way to help people plan better for retirement (e.g., financial planning) (Sanese et al. 2019). Empirical evidence supports the use of genetic biomarkers (Brooks-Wilson 2013) to better predict late-age mortality and assess survival and health at the level of individuals from the study of methylation age (Horvath 2013) and telomere length (Cawthon et al. 2003; Bendix et al. 2014). Additional evidence suggests that the FOXO3 (Willcox et al. 2008) and APOE (Sebastiani et al. 2019) genetic polymorphisms exhibit consistent associations with longevity and health in diverse human populations, making them potentially valuable as an additional hyperpersonal longevity assessment tool. As such, applied genetics (AG) holds the potential to become a revolutionary new tool that can help generations across the age structure and their financial planners develop a much more personalized and well justified plan for living life in the third age.

Presented here is a case study of a married couple with an illustration of how assessments of survival and health dynamics using the FOXO3 and APOE genetic polymorphisms, present or absent within these individuals, could be used to help make more informed decisions for retirement planning relative to the use of generic forecasting models, generic assumptions about survival and health, or, as is often the case in financial planning today, no assumptions at all about future health and survival.

Consider the following hypothetical example of a couple that is approaching what is often

thought of as a traditional retirement age in their mid-60s. Presented here is a financial scenario that is commonly observed among higher net worth couples, although AG could be used to augment retirement decisions for people of all socioeconomic backgrounds (Table 1).

WHEN TO RETIRE

Generic recommendations (GRs) on retirement age fall into two categories: (1) the client picks a retirement age based on their personal needs, desires, and job circumstances without any knowledge about or forecasts of personal life span or health span; or (2) the ages of 68–69 are often recommended by an advisor because it offers a higher return relative to full retirement age, but it also allows for an earlier monthly cash flow. The generic assessment of survival shown here also indicates that the female will outlive the male by 2.3 years—an issue that is highly relevant to a decision on when to retire.

AG Recommendation

Data from AG, however, suggest that the female has a higher probability of surviving to age 90 relative to the male because she carries the longevity-enhancing polymorphism of APOE, increasing the chances that the gender gap in survival is likely to exceed 2.3 years, perhaps significantly. The recommendation coming from an advisor with information from AG might include delayed retirement for both spouses to accommodate the possibility that the female could survive more than 2.3 years beyond her partner, and that the female could run out of money given her higher-than-average probability of late-age survival. This approach increases the chances of the female having enough funds to cover her expected additional survival time above and beyond her spouse at an annual level of income consistent with her current standard of living.

WHEN TO DRAW SOCIAL SECURITY

GR provides little guidance on when to draw social security—this is often a decision based on

Table 1. Case study of couple approaching traditional retirement age

	Financial status and demographics		
	Male[a]	Female[a]	Total
Age	63	60	
Assets			$1,000,000[b]
Income	$90,000	$60,000	$150,000[c]
Target income in retirement			75% of current salary
Retirement savings/year	5%	5%	$7500
Home value			$800,000[d]
Withdrawal rate			4%
Genetic profile			
FOX03	No[e]	Yes[f]	
APOE	e4,e4[g]	e2,e2[h]	
Life span, survival, and late-onset AD risk			
Generic life span[i]	83.0	85.3	
Generic survival to age 90[i]	25.3%	35.9%	

[a]Anticipated retirement age of 68.

[b]Accumulated retirement savings.

[c]Fixed annual income.

[d]Mortgage paid off.

[e]People who do not carry the FOX03 genetic polymorphism have an average probability of reaching ages 90+.

[f]Carriers of the FOX03 genetic polymorphism have a 50% greater chance of surviving to ages 90+ relative to average.

[g]Carriers of this version of APOE e4,e4 [C/C] have a 12-fold elevated risk of developing late-onset Alzheimer's disease (AD) and a 61-fold elevated risk of developing early-onset AD.

[h]Carriers of this rare version of APOE have a much lower risk of developing any form of AD, and carriers also have amplified chances of living a long and healthy life—especially when paired with positive carrier status for FOX03.

[i]Based on a generic life table for the total resident population of the United States by gender (www.mortality.org/Country/Country?cntr=USA).

current financial status and anticipated cash flow. In this case, the male is capable of drawing social security at his current age of 63, but the couple is young enough to have time to change their minds if they see that their financial circumstances allow for delays in drawing social security. In other words, in the absence of science-based estimates of life span, most clients have been inclined to begin taking social security well before the maximum age of 70 (crr.bc.edu/wp-content/uploads/2015/05/IB_15-8.pdf).

AG Recommendation

Due to anticipated extended survival for the female from evidence collected through AG, both individuals would be advised to delay drawing social security until the latest possible age, assuming job and cash flow circumstances allows this to occur comfortably. The reason is that the male is carrying a genetic polymorphism that

increases the probability of early-onset and late-onset AD, which would have added costs, and the female has to prepare to fund a remaining period of life that extends for possibly many years beyond her spouse.

LONG-TERM CARE

GR from advisors is not currently based on scientific assessments of health span, so this type of insurance might currently be recommended by advisors based on something other than evidence for or against need.

AG Recommendation

Based on the presence of the APOE e4,e4 genetic polymorphism in the male, it would be appropriate to recommend that only the male take out a long-term care insurance policy. The presence of the APOE e2,e2 and FOX03 genetic polymor-

Cite this article as *Cold Spring Harb Perspect Med* doi: 10.1101/cshperspect.a041206

phisms in the female means there is justification for avoiding the expense of long-term care in her case. Carrying these genetic polymorphisms is not a guarantee of health, longevity, or a need for long-term care, but at least the couple has the ability to make a better-informed decision based on AG.

PORTFOLIO RISK

Many people moving into the retirement phase of life are moving from an accumulation phase to a distribution phase. Aggressively growing assets is no longer the priority; maintaining and protecting accumulated assets becomes critical. Most retirees, and especially females, become more conservative with the level of risk they are willing to take in retirement because of the uncertainty about how much money will be needed (VanDerhei and Bajtelsmit 1995). A generic approach to risk aversion results in lower income replacement in instances where the true prospects for survival are different from those derived through averaging assumptions.

In this hypothetical case, because of the higher-than-average probability that the female will live to ages 90+ based on her assessment using AG, an even more risk-averse set of investment decisions may be justified. Knowledge about the presence or absence of FOX03 and APOE genetic polymorphisms enables this couple to base their chosen level of risk aversion in their portfolio management to a highly personal and scientifically tangible metric, and it yields specific guidance on the magnitude of the risk aversion to consider (e.g., whether to invest in a long-term care policy or guaranteeing income using an annuity).

PRODUCT MIX

Which financial products a client chooses when creating a financial plan can be greatly influenced by the risks they are willing to take and the goals they are trying to accomplish. Someone with a long life span and low risk tolerance may choose to have a smaller amount of their investments allocated to the stock market and may have a more bond-heavy portfolio, or may choose other

alternatives, such as annuities or life insurance. Someone with a small nest egg and long anticipated life span may be comfortable taking more risk—they might decide to have a good portion of their assets in stocks to help grow the pool of assets, so they last as long as possible. Having access to personalized AG makes it possible for clients to make asset allocation and product mix decisions based on personalized assessments as opposed to those based on generic or averaging assumptions.

GENERIC ADVISOR RECOMMENDATION

Financial advisors, without access to AG or other methods of estimating life span and health span, often make investment recommendations for their clients under the simplifying assumption that each spouse will live to somewhere between the ages of 90 and 100 (www.investmentnews.com/how-do-advisors-estimate-a-clients-longevity-80482). While there is a relatively small chance this length of life would actually occur in the real world for most people (25% for average males and 36% for average females in the United States today at the ages of the people presented here), advisors might think of this assumption as a "safe" recommendation because it might guarantee their clients will not run out of money while they are alive. The problem is that the primary goal of financial planning is to enhance the quality of life of their clients *while they are alive*, not plan exclusively to ensure the largest inheritance possible. An advisor recommendation of planning to live to 95 can dampen (often dramatically) the monthly cash flow of the retirees for their remaining years of life for the majority of the population that will not live this long.

Most advisors also use the assumption of a 4% withdrawal rate to provide the income needed for clients throughout retirement (www.schwab.com/resource-center/insights/content/beyond-4-rule-how-much-can-you-safely-spend-retirement), meaning the client can withdraw 4% from their investment account each year. This is assumed to be a "safe" withdrawal rate and will allow the assets to provide the income needed and potentially continue to grow. However, in the hypothetical case study provided here, the typical advisor may not consider long-term care or life insurance as investment vehicles because the simplifying assumption of survival to age 95 precludes the need for such investments. However, an advisor that has access to the results of AG may assume, reasonably, that the husband in this case will require a minimum of 3 years of assistance in a nursing home and likely much more (Genworth cost of care survey 2020: median cost data tables, www.genworth.com/aging-and-you/finances/cost-of-care.html).

OTHER AG-SPECIFIC RECOMMENDATIONS IN THIS CASE STUDY

The result of these new recommendations based on AG is that the wife will likely have all the income she needs throughout her life span to age 92 and still have a sizable amount of money left over. This allows her an opportunity to spend more throughout retirement, if she chooses, or to provide an inheritance to her family and/or give to charity at her death. When this happens, a "positive wealth span" will have been achieved (www.amazon.com/Pursuing-Wealthspan-Revolutionizing-Management-Methuselah/dp/B08DF2FLCJ). This basically means that through sound financial planning based on the use of AG, couples have a greater chance of accomplishing the goal of securing adequate cash flow during their remaining years of life.

AG leads to better information, which leads to more informed planning and a higher probability of achieving a better health and financial outcome.

DISCUSSION

Forthcoming advances in geroscience have the potential to revolutionize health and survival in the coming decades. While radical life extension is not likely, enough changes are forthcoming to warrant the development and use of assessment tools that take into account hyperpersonalized longevity and health assessments of individuals that will enable them to better plan for the changes in life history that geroscience will bring forth.

Two of the most critical pieces of information required for sound retirement planning include an estimate of how long someone is likely to live, and how many of those remaining years of life are likely to be healthy or accompanied by some level of frailty or disability that require additional financial resources. At present, it is rare when either of these personal attributes are measured or used by financial planners as part of retirement planning. If estimated life span is used at all by financial planners, the task often falls on the clients to approximate their own duration of life, or the planner uses averaging assumptions based on generic life tables. Few advisors or retirees have the expertise required to make a judgment on their own anticipated life span, and the use of averaging assumptions guarantees that the vast majority of people being advised are basing their retirement decisions on information known in advance to be false or exaggerated in one direction or another.

It is demonstrated here that AG involving knowledge just about the FOX03 and APOE e2,e3,e4 genetic polymorphisms can be a valuable tool for augmenting science-based estimates of life span and health span derived from personal demographic and health information collected when an advisor meets with their client.

LIMITATIONS

AG in survival estimation is not a guarantee that an individual will live a long or short life, or conversely, that the presence of genetic polymorphisms associated with an expanded or contracted health span will occur as predicted. The proper interpretation of AG in survival analysis for individuals is that the stated statistical probabilities will be observed for the stated proportion of a population that shares a genetic trait. When an individual is informed they carry the FOX03 allele, this should be interpreted to mean they belong to a subgroup of the population that has, for example, a higher chance of surviving to age 90 than noncarriers. Other factors also influence survival such as behavioral risk factors and stochastic events. Regardless, the elevated probability of extended survival associated with carrying the FOX03 allele yields information that the individual did not previously have.

During a wealth management relationship, the final decision on the best course of action for retirement planning will rest with the client, but with the additional information from AG, both the advisor and client have access to powerful predictive information they previously did not have access to. A similar interpretation and decision-making process takes place when AG is used to help women carrying the BRCA mutation (associated with an elevated risk of breast cancer) on how to plan and proceed with their medical care either before or after a cancer diagnosis (Trainer et al. 2010).

CONCLUSIONS

The third phase of life is a new phenomenon in human history, only experienced with regularity by the last few generations. As welcome as the gift of added life may be—manufactured intentionally through advances in public health and medical technology—this new phase of life challenges the financial integrity of social safety nets such as Social Security and Medicare (Sheshinski and Caliendo 2021) and fundamentally transforms modern notions of work and retirement. Advances in geroscience will amplify these challenges and opportunities in the coming decades.

While life past age 65 can be some of the most rewarding and enjoyable years of life as long as health is maintained (Steptoe and Wardle 2012), financial preparedness for survival into the third age has not been practiced routinely in the United States where close to one-third of non-retirees have no retirement savings or pension at all (www.sec.gov/files/retirement-readiness-white-paper.pdf). A similar lack of preparedness exists elsewhere in both developed and developing nations. Furthermore, advanced age itself is often accompanied by an elevated risk of frailty that is associated with the normal aging of our cells and tissues rather than the common risk factors we have grown accustomed to hearing about (e.g., smoking and obesity) (Sprott 2010).

AG offers unique insights into prospective survival and health dynamics that has practical uses for financial planning—especially given the fact that such technology has never before been used to help individuals plan for their retire-

ment. The hypothetical scenarios presented here suggest that AG using carrier status of just the FOX03 and APOE e2, e3, and e4 genetic polymorphisms would likely yield valuable information that advisors and their clients could use to help guide retirement planning. Hyperpersonalized genetic information collected from individuals would likely help individuals and couples experience a "positive wealth span" or at the least a "neutral wealth span," while at the same time lessening the chances of a "negative wealth span" occurring (e.g., running out of money). Using personal genetic information as a supplemental guide to a hyperpersonalized assessment of life span and health span would likely avoid misguided financial advice that could otherwise occur in the absence of a personalized life span/health span assessment.

REFERENCES

Bell FC, Miller ML. 2005. Life tables for the United States Social Security Area 1900–2100. Actuarial Study No. 120, Social Security Administration. https://www.ssa.gov/oact/NOTES/as120/LifeTables_Tbl_6_1910.html

Bendix L, Thinggaard M, Fenger M, Kolvraa S, Avlund K, Linneberg A, Osler M. 2014. Longitudinal changes in leukocyte telomere length and mortality in humans. *J Gerontol A Biol Sci Med Sci* **69A:** 231–239. doi:10.1093/gerona/glt153

Bloom DE, Canning D, Lubet A. 2015. Global population aging: facts, challenges, solutions and perspectives. *Daedalus* **144:** 80–92. doi:10.1162/DAED_a_00332

Brooks-Wilson AR. 2013. Genetics of healthy aging and longevity. *Hum Genet* **132:** 1323–1338. doi:10.1007/s00439-013-1342-z

Brown GC. 2015. Living too long: the current focus of medical research on increasing the quantity, rather than the quality, of life is damaging our health and harming the economy. *EMBO Rep* **16:** 137–141. doi:10.15252/embr.201439518

Cawthon RM, Smith KR, O'Brien E, Sivatchenko A, Kerber RA. 2003. Association between telomere length in blood and mortality in people aged 60 years or older. *Lancet* **361:** 393–395. doi:10.1016/S0140-6736(03)12384-7

Dychtwald K, Morrison R. 2021. *What retirees want: a wholistic view of life's third age.* Wiley, Hoboken, NJ.

Ghilarducci T, Saad-Lessler J, Bahn K. 2015. Are US workers ready for retirement? Trends in plan sponsorship, participation, and preparedness. *J Pension Benefits* Winter: 25–39. Available at https://ssrn.com/abstract=2604299

Horvath S. 2013. DNA methylation age of human tissues and cell types. *Genome Biol* **14:** R115. doi:10.1186/gb-2013-14-10-r115

Laslett P. 1991. *A fresh map of life: the emergence of the third age.* Harvard University Press, Cambridge, MA.

Olshansky SJ. 2021. Aging like Struldbruggs, Dorian Gray or Peter Pan. *Nat Aging* **1:** 576–578. doi:10.1038/s43587-021-00087-7

Sanese P, Forte G, Disciglio V, Grossi V, Simone C. 2019. FOXO3 on the road to longevity: lessons from SNPs and chromatin hubs. *Comput Struct Biotechnol J* **17:** 737–745. doi:10.1016/j.csbj.2019.06.011

Sebastiani P, Gurinovich A, Nygaard M, Sasaki T, Sweigart B, Bae H, Andersen SL, Villa F, Atzmon G, Christensen K, et al. 2019. *APOE* alleles and extreme human longevity. *J Gerontol A Biol Sci Med Sci* **74:** 44–51. doi:10.1093/gerona/gly174

Sharpe DL. 2021. Reinventing retirement. *J Fam Econ Iss* **42:** 11–19. doi:10.1007/s10834-020-09696-7

Sheshinski E, Caliendo F. 2021. Social Security and the increasing longevity gap. *J Public Econ Theory* **23:** 29–52. doi:10.1111/jpet.12477

Sprott RL. 2010. Biomarkers of aging and disease: introduction and definitions. *Exp Gerontol* **45:** 2–4. doi:10.1016/j.exger.2009.07.008

Steptoe A, Wardle J. 2012. Enjoying life and living longer. *Arch Intern Med* **172:** 273–275. doi:10.1001/archinternmed.2011.1028

Streeter J, Leombroni M, Deevy M, Carstensen L. 2020. We need a new map of life. In *Pursuing wealthspan: how science is revolutionizing wealth management* (ed. Olshansky SJ, Ashburn K, Stukey J). Methuselah Books, Ellsworth, IL.

Trainer AH, Lewis CR, Tucker K, Meiser B, Friedlander M, Ward R. 2010. The role of BRCA mutation testing in determining breast cancer therapy. *Nat Rev Clin Oncol* **7:** 708–717. doi:10.1038/nrclinonc.2010.175

Uhlenberg P. 2009. *International handbook of population aging.* Springer, New York.

VanDerhei JL, Bajtelsmit V. 1995. Risk aversion and pension investment choices. Pension Research Council Working Papers 95-5. Wharton School Pension Research Council, University of Pennsylvania, Philadelphia, PA.

Willcox BJ, Donlon TA, He Q, Chen R, Grove JS, Yano K, Masaki KH, Willcox DC, Rodriguez B, Curb JD. 2008. FOXO3A genotype is strongly associated with human longevity. *Proc Natl Acad Sci* **105:** 13987–13992. doi:10.1073/pnas.0801030105

Influence of Aging Science on Global Wealth Management

Michael Hodin

High Lantern Group, New York, New York 10017, USA

Correspondence: mhodin@globalcoalitiononaging.com

Modern longevity transforms long-held assumptions about working, saving, investing, and spending—creating both new opportunities and new challenges for wealth management in the 21st century. To adapt to these shifts, our aging world must evolve its strategies and tools to help people maximize their healthy, productive years, work longer and differently beyond traditional retirement age should they choose to do so, manage caregiving responsibilities, and use a range of tools to plan, save, and invest for longer lives. Employers, policymakers, financial services companies, and individuals can all take steps to enable this new landscape of greater wealth from greater longevity, where people enjoy physical health linked directly to financial health.

Physical health is inextricably linked to financial health (Brown Weida et al. 2020; Bialowolski et al. 2021). Given this simple but profound connection, geroscience advances that expand the average human life span—and, perhaps more importantly, the number of *healthy* years in that life span—have dramatic implications for how people work, live, and manage wealth in our 21st century era of long lives. In a world of more old than young, where more people than ever are living to 90+, we must reshape our assumptions, models, and tools to meet individual and societal financial needs—just as we must reorient healthcare models to enable healthy aging.

Our goal should be a virtuous cycle of longer, healthier lives and greater wealth. However, this requires shifting wealth management to reflect the new dynamics of longevity, such as people's ability and desire to keep working past traditional retirement age, the need to fund those additional years and sometimes decades of life, the growing demand for and costs of caregiving, and the rich financial benefit of healthy aging. These shifts present both new opportunities and new challenges, which demand action from a range of stakeholders—not just the financial services industry, but also policymakers, employers, health systems, families, and individuals.

How we plan and pay for our long lives—generating wealth while keeping costs sustainable—will determine whether widespread prosperity accompanies modern longevity in the 21st century.

SHIFTS: THE NEW FINANCIAL LANDSCAPE IN AN AGE OF LONGEVITY

Today's longevity—enabled by ongoing advances in medicine and public health and about to be influenced by geroscience—reshapes long-held assumptions about working, saving, investing, and spending. Global life expectancy has increased steadily in the past century, with the average global citizen today living approximately 20 years longer than in 1960 (World Bank DataBank 2022, data.worldbank.org/indicator/SP.DYN .LE00.IN). Among the OECD (Organisation for Economic Co-operation and Development) countries and in many advanced economies, it is now normal for an increasing proportion of the population to live for 30 years or more after 60. With this unprecedented longevity comes shifts in people's behaviors, preferences, and needs that our current financial planning and infrastructure must shift to appropriately reflect.

Leaders in the financial services industry are pioneering a new way forward. Lorna Sabbia (Sabbia 2022), managing director of retirement and personal wealth solutions at Bank of America, neatly summarizes the evolving landscape:

> Longer lifespans don't guarantee a financially secure later life, however. If anything, in the absence of significant planning, extreme longevity may make financial security harder to attain. In an effort to change that, a growing number of financial advisory and service providers are turning to a new, more holistic mode of thinking about personal economics. The trend is centered on one key concept: financial wellness.
>
> The main idea behind financial wellness is that individuals can plan for their financial future in a more comprehensive way than in decades past, when they focused primarily on the dollar amounts in their bank or retirement accounts. An emphasis on financial wellness, by contrast, reflects a deeper understanding of where one's money is now and where it will flow in the future, ideally helping individuals meet their short-term needs while they save for their unique mid- and long-term priorities. Wellness is also about establishing healthy behaviors: financially sound savings, investment, and spending practices that will benefit individuals over the course of a long life.

In response, industry leaders like Bank of America are building tools to help individuals ensure their financial wellness, such as free financial education platforms for people at all life stages and tools to track and assess financial wellness throughout life (Better Money Habits 2022, bettermoneyhabits .bankofamerica.com/en; Life Plan 2022, promo

tions.bankofamerica.com/digitalbanking/mobile banking/lifeplan; Financial Wellness for Employees 2022, business.bofa.com/en-us/content/work place-benefits/solutions-and-services/financial-w ellness-for-employees.html).

These kinds of tools can help people to navigate five key shifts brought by modern longevity:

1. People must now pay for lives that may stretch to 100.

   Absent the needed changes to financial planning and wealth management, longer lives can pose significant financial burdens on underprepared individuals. Simply put, people must now find ways to pay for those extra years or decades of life through a combination of working longer, saving more, investing wisely, and minimizing health and care costs. This comes at the same time as the shift away from the 20th century defined benefit plan toward defined contribution plans that place greater responsibility on the individual to plan and maintain lifelong financial wellness.

   Currently, many individuals are concerned that their financial strategies are not keeping up. Globally, just 42% of workers say that "I always make sure that I am saving for retirement" (www.aegon.com/siteassets/ the-new-social-contract-future-proofing-reti rement.pdf). Fully one-third say that they are not currently saving for retirement, and 44% believe that future generations of retirees will be worse off than those currently in retirement (www.aegon.com/siteassets/the-new-social-contract-future-proofing-retirement .pdf).

   Of course, even the assumptions of "working versus retirement" or "retirement saving strategies" rest on outdated 20th century models of work and life. In a world where people have a greater chance than ever to live to ages 90+—with health and productivity into their 60s, 70s, 80s, and beyond—it simply no longer makes sense for many people to enter full retirement in their early 60s, if ever.

2. People can stay healthy and productive for decades beyond traditional retirement age.

Indeed, longer lives are creating new patterns in people's behaviors and preferences for work. Not only are people capable of working for longer, but most now envision a phased transition where they continue working past the traditional retirement age (www.aegon .com/siteassets/the-new-social-contract-futu re-proofing-retirement.pdf). Contrary to long-standing conventional views of retirement, 60 or 65 should no longer represent the most common view of a permanent transition from full-time work to full-time leisure.

Indeed, the majority of workers surveyed globally say that they plan to continue working in some capacity after traditional retirement (www.aegon.com/contentassets/6724d 008b6e14fa1a4cedb41811f748a/retirement- readiness-survey-2018.pdf). This could include shifting to more flexible or part-time hours, taking on consulting or teaching roles, or launching "encore careers" (i.e., entering a new field or kind of job after an initial career). Some older workers seek positions with more flexible hours and ways of working, while others may seek work that is more meaningful and purpose-driven. In one example, almost half of Canadian men between the ages of 60 and 64 chose to reenter the workforce within 10 years of their retirement (Sullivan and Al Ariss 2019). In the United States, nearly one-quarter of workers plan to "never retire," simply continuing to work in the same capacity as they always have (www.usatoday.com/story/ money/2019/07/08/retirement-1-4-dont-plan- retire-despite-aging-workforce/1671687001).

The labor market is currently ripe for this undertapped pool of talent. While ageism and outdated policies have long held back older workers (World Health Organization 2021), organizations may rethink their approach to find the skilled workers that they need. Nearly 70% of employers globally find it challenging to fill open positions (go.manpowergroup. com/hubfs/Talent%20Shortage%202021/ MPG_2021_Outlook_Survey-Global.pdf), and a growing skills gap constrains STEM, manufacturing, and a variety of other sectors. This expands the opportunity for older adults to continue working long past tradi-

tional retirement age—matching both personal preferences and financial necessity.

3. Chronic illness and ageism—not individual preference—prematurely forces many people out of the workforce.

If older adults want to stay in the workforce, what is forcing them out? The answer, sadly, is often ageism or chronic illness. Declining physical health is the most often cited retirement concern among workers around the world, and 39% of current retirees had to leave the workforce sooner than they had planned for these reasons (www.aegon .com/contentassets/6724d008b6e14fa1a4ced b41811f748a/retirement-readiness-survey- 2018.pdf). For this group, their own ill health was the most common reason that they left the workforce, while someone else's ill health was the third most common reason. Yet just one-third of workers have a back-up plan for income if they are forced to stop working prematurely (www.aegon.com/contentassets/ 6724d008b6e14fa1a4cedb41811f748a/retire ment-readiness-survey-2018.pdf).

The second most common reason for premature retirement is job loss—often linked to ageism. According to the United Nations and the World Health Organization, half the people worldwide hold moderately or highly ageist attitudes (www.who.int/teams/social-determi nants-of-health/demographic-change-and-he althy-ageing/combatting-ageism/global-repor t-on-ageism). This directly impacts older workers. According to a ProPublica and Urban Institute analysis, over half of older U.S. workers are laid off or likely forced out of a job at least once (Gosselin 2018).

The financial consequences can be devastating. Just one in ten of these workers ever achieves a level of compensation on par with their earnings before their forced retirement (Gosselin 2018). This ageism—reflected even in the commonly accepted definition for "working age"—calls for a concerted, multistakeholder effort to reshape societal biases.

4. The demand for caregiving is rapidly growing.

Modern longevity is precipitating a major inversion in global population pyramids. OECD countries, in particular, are seeing a transformation of their populations to "more old than young" for the first time, leading to an unprecedented demand for caregiving. By 2030, in the United States, there will be just four potential family caregivers per older adult (The Centers for Disease Control and Prevention 2019). By 2050, Japan's ratio of people ages 15–64 to those over 64, for example, will reach just 1:1 (Kaneda and Tsai 2010).

As the often underappreciated and undermeasured cost of elder care rises concomitantly, the challenge to families and workplaces also grows. Caregiving responsibilities can push middle-aged and older employees to cut back their hours, pass on promotions, or exit the workforce altogether. These impacts can prevent caregivers from maximizing their income and savings in their prime earning years, making the cost trajectory of caregiving even more difficult. The financial impacts disproportionately affect women, who provide the majority of unpaid care around the world (www.unwomen.org/en/news/in-focus/csw61/redistribute-unpaid-work).

5. Health and elder care costs can be the decisive factor in financial well-being.

Healthy aging is not just a health concern but also a financial imperative. With greater longevity comes greater risk of chronic health conditions, such as type 2 diabetes, cancer, and Alzheimer's disease. The costs associated with these conditions reflect some of the highest categories of spending for older adults, families, health systems, and national budgets overall.

In the European Union, an estimated €700 billion, or 70% to 80% of all healthcare spending, goes toward the management of chronic diseases (Seychell 2022). As more people live longer, the amount and complexity of care needed per person will rise as well.

Even in the absence of chronic health conditions, the costs of aging can be overwhelming. A 2019 survey of long-term care services in the United States revealed that the median cost for a private room in a nursing home now exceeds $100,000 per year (www.genworth.com/aging-and-you/finances/cost-of-care.html). Strategies to maximize people's healthy years and address the gaps in the healthcare workforce are therefore a crucial component of managing the financial needs associated with longer lives.

OPPORTUNITIES: HELPING INDIVIDUALS MAXIMIZE THE HEALTH–WEALTH LINK

These shifts define the new landscape for wealth in the 21st century. By updating our assumptions, models, and tools to reflect these dynamics, our societies can seize a range of opportunities to help us stay well, maintain a level of financial security that matches our longevity, and thrive.

Geroscience Advances Are Designed to Embrace Healthy Aging and Maximize Financial Security

Enjoying a healthy, financially secure life depends on expanding "health span" to match our life span. This means maximizing the number of years where an individual is healthy, productive, and largely free from the constraints and costs imposed by chronic disease. The scientific and medical advances of geroscience provide us with the knowledge and therapeutic interventions to achieve an extended health span. Now, individuals need to incorporate these advances into their lifestyles as they begin to emerge, as well as their plans and expectations for their life course.

Work and Learn, Longer and Differently, beyond Traditional Retirement Age

It is past time to "retire retirement." Rather than the outdated learn-work-retire model, societies need to embrace a far more diverse, flexible, and empowering approach to how we use our extra measure of life. That may mean having the choice and financial resources necessary to return to school in middle age, shifting into a coaching or consulting role later in a career, or launching multiple careers throughout the life course, with periods of learning, volunteering, or caregiving in between.

Use a Range of Tools to Plan, Save, and Invest for a Longer Life

Whatever the path, individuals will need to plan for how income, investments, and savings can last longer. They will need updated tools from the financial services industry and their employers, as well as policymakers, who can collaborate to shape offerings for the new financial demands of modern longevity.

Find New Models and Solutions for More Efficient, Equal Caregiving

The need for caregiving is one of the greatest health and financial challenges facing individuals, families, and health systems. To achieve the necessary scale, we need new and more innovative caregiving models that are far more efficient, without placing an undue and unequal burden on family caregivers (the current default in most cases). Developing and scaling these models will not only be critical to manage the direct costs of care—it will also enable more caregivers to remain in the workforce longer, protecting their own lifelong financial wellness and engendering greater social equity.

STRATEGIES: KEY ACTIONS FOR EMPLOYERS, POLICYMAKERS, THE FINANCIAL SERVICES INDUSTRY, AND INDIVIDUALS

Employers, policymakers, the financial services industry, and individuals can all take steps to enable this new landscape of greater wealth from greater longevity. A cross-sector, collaborative approach is essential for achieving the scale of the required changes.

Employers

Employers and the workplace are an ideal center for resources that help people embrace lifelong financial wellness and healthy aging. Organizations that prioritize this approach will stand out in the

talent marketplace and support greater innovation and productivity from multigenerational teams.

Evolve Organizational Culture and Working Models to Enable Older Talent to Stay Longer, with Age-Friendly Workplaces and Options for More Flexible Roles

Older workers are a critical pool of top talent, with deep expertise, decades of experience, proven skills, and a facility for teaching and mentoring. When integrated into a multigenerational workforce, these teams are found to be more productive, innovative, and engaged (The Global Coalition on Aging 2018). Yet, many employers are still not taking proactive steps to recruit, hire, and retain these invaluable workers. This is a missed opportunity for businesses—and a threat to older workers' financial well-being.

Several principles can help employers to attract older workers and build multigenerational teams. First, workplaces should be age-neutral, with an inclusive environment that is free from ageism. This includes both the physical environment, with technologies, facilities, equipment, and services that meet the needs of older workers, and the organizational culture, which should recognize the contributions of all workers. Organizations can also do more to promote lifelong learning and participation, as well as support older workers with healthy aging and their responsibilities as caregivers.

Strengthen Benefits for Employee Caregivers, Including Leave Policies, Care Resources, Planning Tools, and Flexible Work Options

Caregiving for older family members is quickly becoming one of the most important workplace issues of our time. Organizations that proactively support employee caregivers will seize a vital opportunity to attract, hire, and retain top talent, who are looking for these supportive policies as they make employment decisions. Just as support for parents became "table stakes" in the 20th century, support for those caring for older family members will become vital for talent strategy in the 21st century.

Organizations can adopt a range of policies and programs to support caregivers. Inclusive leave policies that can be used for adult care are an important starting point. Forward-looking organizations are also providing employees with free or subsidized care resources, such as care planning, emergency back-up care, and consultations on the legal and financial aspects of care (global coalitiononaging.com/wp-content/uploads/2021/11/GCOA_BAC-Spotlight-on-Caregiving_Employer-Practices-Through-a-Policy-Lens_FINAL.pdf). Flexible work policies, including the rise of remote and hybrid work during the COVID-19 pandemic, can also help employee caregivers balance their professional and familial responsibilities (see Box 1).

Provide Access to Tools that Help Employees Start Saving and Investing Early, Easily Enroll and Increase Contributions, and Plan for the Finances Required for Healthcare

In the era of the 401(k), many workers will turn to their employer for access to tools for saving and investing, as well as the communications and financial literacy to guide wise usage of those tools. Employers take this responsibility seriously—but many can still do more to help support saving and investing for lifelong financial wellness.

The key is not just helping older workers save more but engaging workers of all ages to save throughout their career—from programs helping young workers to invest even while paying off student debt to programs that help middle-aged workers keep saving even amid the expenses of caregiving. Communications can emphasize the importance of saving and investing and underscore the potential high costs of later-life care, while specific planning tools can help to understand and prepare for these scenarios. Where possible, employers can also use "auto-enroll" and "auto-escalate" options to help workers automatically save as their default.

BOX 1. THE IMPACTS AND LESSONS OF COVID-19

COVID-19 has increased the urgency of implementing many of the strategies outlined throughout the literature.

- During the pandemic, many older people left the workforce earlier than they had expected, threatening their long-term financial well-being (Umpierrez 2022).

- The pandemic has also increased the strain on family caregivers and healthcare workers, even as it has led to delays or disruptions in routine care for chronic conditions.

Together, these twin factors threaten to widen the already severe gap between the need and supply for care with sobering financial and healthcare implications.

Further, the COVID-19 pandemic has shown the vital importance of healthy aging, while also generating new burdens, strains, and costs for older adults, caregivers, and health systems. The dramatically higher risk of COVID-19 for older adults, especially those with chronic conditions, demonstrates why a proactive, preventive, and holistic approach to not just managing disease, but promoting health, is so critical in an aging world. This is also a key strategy to avoid costly acute care like hospitalizations, which threaten to generate unsustainably high costs for families, health systems, and societies.

However, the COVID-19 pandemic has also driven new models and innovations at the time when they are needed most.

- The rise of remote and flexible work models can help older workers to continue working in new ways for longer, while also providing vital support to employee caregivers.

- Rapid adoption of telehealth, remote care, and AI-enabled digital health technologies have validated and expanded innovative tools for a "predict and prevent" approach to healthcare.

By embracing these new models, societies can seize new opportunities for health and wealth, while driving a sustainable long-term recovery.

Prioritize Healthy Aging in the Workplace— Pushing beyond Diet and Fitness Campaigns to Include Screening for Common Age-Related Conditions, Adult Immunizations, and Brain Health Campaigns

Organizations can also play a role in helping older workers stay healthy as they age. While fitness campaigns and healthy foods have become fixtures of the workplace, there is significant opportunity to introduce additional offerings that do even more for employees' physical and mental health.

Employers can sponsor screening for common age-related conditions, such as osteoporosis or vision health. Adult immunization campaigns can help to avoid preventable illness and resulting productivity losses for conditions like influenza, pneumonia, and shingles. Brain health efforts can equip older workers to reduce their own risk for cognitive decline, addressing one of the most difficult age-related health challenges.

Policymakers

Policymakers at every level can take action to tailor policies for the emerging landscape of longevity. The most effective policies will be coordinated across sectors and jurisdictions.

Make Health Savings Accounts (HSAs) More Easily Accessible and Enable Auto-Enrollment and Auto-Escalation in Employer-Sponsored 401(k)s and Other Financial Vehicles

HSAs can be a vital tool to help people prepare for the healthcare costs of aging. Policymakers can take action to make HSAs more easily accessible and attractive as a choice for individuals. Additionally, in some geographies, policy changes may be needed to expand the types of expenses that fall within HSA's qualified distributions, such as home care expenses.

As highlighted by the field of behavioral economics, often the most effective "nudge" for wise decisions is to make them the default (Beshears and Kosowsky 2020). In the area of saving and investing, this can be accomplished by defaulting employees into making contributions and escalating those contributions over time. However, in many geographies, policymakers still need to enact policies that enable employers to provide these default options.

Align Policies to Include Different Kinds of Family Caregiving, with Resources, Leave Options, Tax Credits, and Other Support for Those Who Care for Older Adults

As much as employers' caregiving policies need to expand beyond a focus solely on childcare, so too public policies must evolve to reflect the growing number of people who care for older family members.

Ideally, every country should develop and implement a comprehensive national strategy that knits together the different policies, programs, and resources to support family caregivers. This can include paid family leave benefits for all types of caregivers, caregiving "allowances" to help cover the costs of care, tax breaks for those who care for older adults, and easier navigation of resources and support services. Government agencies can also explore multigenerational care services for children and older adults, enabling more efficient and accessible care from a single organization or location.

Support Access to Adult Immunization, Health Screenings, and Telehealth Options

Investment in healthy aging and related innovations can deliver on policymakers' goals and ensure the sustainability of both national and individual healthcare spending. Currently, chronic conditions account for the vast majority of health spending, with costly acute care like emergency room visits and hospitalizations driving much of the cost (www.cdc.gov/chronicdisease/about/costs/index.htm; www.efpia.eu/about-medicines/use-of-medicines/healthcare-systems/introduction). For individuals and families, these emergency costs can devastate financial wellness, especially in someone's later decades. For health systems and national budgets, these costs threaten to become unsustainable as populations age and longer lives become more common.

There are a number of policy tools available. Health systems can drive concerted adult immunization campaigns, addressing low rates of vaccination and avoiding costs, hospitalizations, and deaths. Health agencies can implement nationwide health screenings for conditions like osteoporosis, heart disease, and dementia, helping individuals to receive needed care earlier and avoid health crises. Health systems can also sustain telehealth and remote care options, which can provide care more efficiently and just as effectively in many cases.

For all of these areas, policymakers should adopt a lens that views preventive health measures and healthy aging as an investment in people's physical and financial well-being—ultimately defraying long-term costs.

The Financial Services Industry

Financial services companies can evolve wealth management to reflect the needs and opportunities of longevity. Several actions point a way forward:

Integrate the Needs and Opportunities of Modern Longevity into Financial Planning and Financial Literacy Materials

Financial services companies can play a vital role in alerting employers, families, and individuals to the new financial realities associated with longer lives. There is a particular need for tools that help people learn about, plan for, and assess their financial wellness throughout every stage of life.

For example, Bank of America's Better Money Habits platform offers financial education and tools that can be used by people at any age (bettermoneyhabits.bankofamerica.com/en). Through this platform, people can use the "Life Plan" tool to set and track their financial goals, and the "Financial Wellness Tracker" to assess progress toward those goals.

These kinds of tools, as well as training for financial professionals, should consider those who face greater financial challenges, such as caregivers, women, and people who have exited or are looking to reenter the workforce. These efforts can center on strategies to help people overcome financial disparities and ensure they have the tools they need for financial wellness.

Provide "Financial Gerontology" Training to Prepare Financial Advisors to Provide Skilled Guidance to Older Clients

The financial services industry must equip workers for a growing number of clients in their 70s, 80s, 90s, and beyond. A strictly financial perspective alone is likely insufficient, as health, work, purpose, social connection, and other topics all inform financial well-being, priorities, and decisions.

Financial gerontology training can help to prepare professionals to understand these topics and offer more effective, age-informed counsel. For example, this training might include information on how to help people navigate decisions such as whether to move to a lower-cost community or how to pay for care, as well as how to respond if a client has signs of cognitive decline.

Consider How Plan Design and New Financial Tools Can Help Individuals to Pay for Longer Lives

Modern longevity also has important implications for the assumptions that are effectively "baked in" to 401(k)s and other tools. Traditionally, these models assume that individuals will shift from contributing to spending (or, decumulation) around the time of 20th-century retirement age. However, for many individuals, this assumption no longer holds, as their period of contributions will continue long past traditional retirement age.

Further, there is also a need for tools and materials to help people manage and wisely spend their accumulated savings in their later decades. In many cases, individuals may, in essence, receive their life savings when they retire, but without much guidance on how to effectively manage this sum. These tools for decumulation are a missing piece and an opportunity for leadership in the financial services industry.

Individuals

In the age of longevity, individuals are empowered to live, work, and learn in new ways throughout their lives. Planning for healthy aging and financial security are key to seizing those opportunities.

Consider How to Work, Learn, Save, and Invest across the Course of the Modern Life Span

The policies, tools, and strategies outlined above ultimately aim to empower individuals to take control of their own physical and financial health in today's era of long lives. For all of us as individuals, the first step is recognizing the tremendous opportunities associated with the modern rise in longevity: to explore different jobs and fields, launch second careers, pursue later-life education and training, and, fundamentally, make a bigger impact for longer. While doing this, we can also earn, invest, and save more—positioning us to find greater fulfillment throughout our lives.

Embrace Strategies for Healthy Aging, Including New Findings from the Field of Geroscience

Just as the United Nations and WHO's Decade of Healthy Ageing prompts systemic change, individuals can take concrete, everyday steps to reap the full benefits of modern longevity. Healthy lifestyles, proactive management of chronic conditions, adult immunization, and other steps for healthy aging all have a key role to play. Individuals can also advocate for themselves with providers and health systems, seeking out the kind of proactive, preventive care, further enabled by digital health technologies, that best supports healthy aging. By doing so, as geroscience interventions eventually come online, they will be applied to a healthier population, enhancing their effects.

Plan for the Possibility of Expensive Health and Care Needs

While individuals should strive for healthy aging, we must also plan for the realistic elevated costs of age-related illness. People should consider their backup plan if they are forced to leave the workforce early due to poor health, as well as how they might pay for an extended period of care for themselves or a loved one. This can underscore the importance of proactive planning and saving, as well as prompt more creative thinking about work, life, and care.

Harness Tools for Lifelong Financial Wellness

As policymakers, employers, and the financial services industry update and create new tools, individuals can make sure that they are maximizing the value of these tools. As a starting point, asking human resources professionals and financial services professionals for help can uncover options and benefits that are already available to many individuals. This includes not just financial tools, but also resources for physical and mental health, caregiving support, lifelong learning, career development—in short, all the aspects of life that ultimately shape financial wellness.

CONCLUSION: ACHIEVING WHAT GEROSCIENCE MAKES POSSIBLE

As geroscience transforms the health span of current and future generations, we must enact changes that are just as transformative for our wealth. Together, the actions outlined above offer a pathway to widespread prosperity in a 21st century world defined by healthy longevity.

What could that world look like? It is one where people stay healthy and productive for much longer than ever before, with older workers emerging as a highly valued, sought-after source of talent in a multigenerational workforce. It is one where individuals are planning for the costs of longer lives from the very beginning of their careers, taking advantage of a raft of new financial tools and well-informed financial professionals. It is one where health systems take a predict-and-prevent approach to well-being, helping people to manage chronic conditions and enjoy greater quality of life with better financial well-being.

We all have a part to play in building that world. Now is the time to forge collaborations and take action toward a shared vision for health and wealth in the 21st century.

REFERENCES

Beshears J, Kosowsky H. 2020. Nudging: progress to date and future directions. *Org Behav Hum Decis Process* **161:** 3–19. doi:10.1016/j.obhdp.2020.09.001

Bialowolski P, Weziak-Bialowolska D, Lee MT, Chen Y, VanderWeele TJ, McNeely E. 2021. The role of financial conditions for physical and mental health. Evidence from a longitudinal survey and insurance claims data. *Soc Sci Med* **281:** 114041. doi:10.1016/j.socscimed.2021.114041

Brown Weida E, Phojanakong P, Patel F, Chilton M. 2020. Financial health as a measurable social determinant of health. *PLoS ONE* **15:** e0233359. doi:10.1371/journal.pone.0233359

Gosselin P. 2018. If you're over 50, chances are the decision to leave a job won't be yours. *ProPublica*. https://www.propublica.org/article/older-workers-united-states-pushed-out-of-work-forced-retirement

Kaneda T, Tsai T. 2010. More caregivers needed worldwide for the "oldest old." *Population Reference Bureau*. https:// www.prb.org/resources/more-caregivers-needed-worldwide-for-the-oldest-old

Sabbia L. 2022. Longer lifespans require secure financial futures. *The Boston Globe*. https://www.bostonglobe.com/2022/03/07/opinion/longer-lifespans-require-secure-financial-futures

Seychell M. 2022. Towards better prevention and management of chronic diseases. *European Commission*. https://ec.europa.eu/health/newsletter/169/focus_newsletter_en.htm

Sullivan SE, Al Ariss A. 2019. Employment after retirement: a review and framework for future research. *J Manage* **45:** 262–284. doi:10.1177/0149206318810411

The Centers for Disease Control and Prevention. 2019. Caregiving for family and friends—a public health issue. https://www.cdc.gov/aging/caregiving/caregiver-brief.html

The Global Coalition on Aging. 2018. Guiding principles for age-friendly businesses. https://globalcoalitiononaging.com/wp-content/uploads/2018/06/infographic_guiding-principles-for-age-friendly-businesses.pdf

Umpierrez A. 2022. Pandemic causing older workers to leave workforce earlier than planned. *PLANSPONSOR*. https://www.plansponsor.com/pandemic-causing-older-workers-leave-workforce-earlier-planned

Funding Life-Extension Research

Mehmood Khan

Hevolution Foundation, KAFD, Riyadh 13519, Saudi Arabia

Correspondence: m.khan@hevolution.com

While the worldwide trend in life expectancy continues to increase slightly overall, the trend for the last few decades in developed countries is that more people are spending more years in poor health with multiple chronic comorbidities. These chronic conditions in aging populations consume high proportions of national healthcare budgets. The relatively young field of longevity research, after accumulating insights into the mechanisms of aging and producing dramatic laboratory demonstrations of life extension in some organisms, is entering the translational phase. This phase, through clinical trials, will confirm or refute the "geroscience hypothesis" that drugs can change the trajectory of the processes of aging within cells, and ultimately in living humans. At the same time, traditional funding patterns do not favor such visionary "moonshot" research, which, despite the potential for ultimately providing benefits for everyone, offers little prospect for rapid return on investment and high probabilities for early phase failure. New radical funding strategies incentivizing innovation will have to be called into play.

For fully funding life-extension research, there is no current model. While the goal is surely a grand challenge, one whose achievement can impact every human in the world, it is far from certain that the incentives that fueled the funding of other great medical and technical victories, from the original moonshot to the COVID-19 vaccines, will line up to generate the heat necessary for attracting investors and philanthropic backers to this high-risk venture. The aim of extending healthy human life will need not just highly talented research scientists and clinicians, but also the best minds among risk-tolerant administrators, policymakers, ethicists, and institutions collaborating within entirely new frameworks. It will take a whole society approach. In what follows, we briefly survey serious impediments to success and novel approaches with promise for overcoming all obstacles. We also look at what some key thought leaders have recently contributed to the field.

The time is ripe. Ever since UC San Francisco biologist Cynthia Kenyon doubled a tiny worm's life span by altering a single gene in the 1990s, a newborn field of longevity research has been accumulating insights into the mechanisms of aging. These mechanisms, along with strategies for interdicting them, have arisen from genomics, proteomics, and machine learning and have led repeatedly to dramatic laboratory demonstrations of life extension in worms, mice, monkeys, and other organisms (STAT Reports 2022). The maturing field, now with dozens of companies engaged, is entering the

Cite this article as *Cold Spring Harb Perspect Med* doi: 10.1101/cshperspect.a041208

translational phase with its requisite clinical trials. These trials are poised to confirm or refute the "geroscience hypothesis" that drugs can change the trajectory of the processes of aging within cells, and ultimately in living humans.

The rationale for aging as a target for therapies rather than the specific diseases that have been typically warred against by medical research, the STAT report on "The race for longevity" points out, emerges from important analyses. They show that over the last few decades the proportion of healthy years has remained fairly constant. More people are spending more years in poor health with multiple chronic comorbidities such as heart disease, stroke, diabetes, cancer, arthritis, and chronic obstructive pulmonary disease (COPD). The trend is consistent in developed nations, with estimates showing late-life morbidity consuming 16%–20% of people's lives and more than half of total health spending in the United States (in 2019, the 30% of the population over age 55 accounted for 56% of health spending). Baby boomer annual health care spending is projected to eat up 20% of the economy by 2027.

Basic research into the biologic processes of aging pulls down <1% of the National Institutes of Health (NIH) budget, however. But if it is the aging process itself that creates major vulnerabilities to various diseases, for example through increasingly damaged DNA repair mechanisms, a shift toward much greater spending targeting the breakdown of age-regulating pathways with drugs and other therapies is warranted. New therapies, for example, may be directed toward such targets as telomere attrition, cellular senescence, loss of proteostasis (accumulation of damaged proteins), deregulated nutrient sensing, mitochondrial dysfunction, stem cell exhaustion, and altered intercellular communication.

Putting a focus on the economics of longevity, professor of economics at London Business School Andrew J. Scott compared, in monetary terms, the gains from targeting aging itself compared to efforts to eradicate specific diseases (Scott et al. 2021). His analysis showed that a compression of morbidity that improves health is more valuable than further increases in healthy life expectancy. Scott and colleagues calculated the value of a slowdown in aging that increases life expectancy by 1 yr to be US$38 trillion. Expanding that to 10 yr, the value would be US$367 trillion. The authors noted, "The economic value of gains from targeting aging are large because delaying aging produces complementarities between health and longevity…." The gains in aging, they added, affect a large number of diseases because of the rising prevalence of age-related comorbidities, and create synergies arising from competing risks. "Ultimately, the more progress that is made in improving how we age, the greater the value of further improvements," they concluded.

CURRENT "MOONSHOT" FUNDING MODELS

Complex "moonshots" (e.g., GPS, internet) have generally required mission-driven research models. Traditional government R&D funding has been excellent at moving basic and exploratory science forward. Likewise, industry, especially in developed countries such as the United States, United Kingdom, Europe, and Japan, have made tremendous contributions to bringing products and services to market by leveraging R&D that is nearly or already at translational stages. These countries have excelled at combining multiple technologies and discoveries to deliver products and services and platforms, for example, computer hardware and software, laboratory equipment, diagnostics, and therapeutics (COVID vaccines being the most recent). In the latter case, biotech and pharmaceutical companies leveraged fundamental virology R&D performed and/or funded by the U.S. government (DARPA/NIH, etc.).

With a grand mission that is at once very specific (the aging process), but also enormously broad and complex in terms of its many aspects, it is easy to see that unprecedented levels of coordination and collaboration that are multi-sectional, multi-institutional, and multinational will be called into play—for the research itself and its funding. Today's funding from government focuses fundamentally around individual researchers/scientists, especially those with an established track record. Among the unintended consequences of this funding pattern is relatively advanced age among government-funded researchers. In an NIH posting by Michael Lauer from 2021 (Lauer 2021), the mean age of NIH-funded researchers receiving support on a first NIH R01 award for Principal Investigators both for those self-identifying as men or as women increased from 40 yr in 1995 to 44 in 2020. For MDs, the mean age increased from 41 to 46 yr. With this trend, new entrants are selected against in the competition for funding and with them their potentially groundbreaking new and novel ideas and their perhaps nontraditional disciplines and approaches.

At the same time, the distribution of the vast majority of government funding is focused within the countries and regions providing the funds (e.g., NIH/NSF, Europe, United Kingdom, Japan, and, more recently, China and India). As a result, collaborations are limited and the ability to source the best ideas from around the world is curtailed, and some scientists, especially those early in their careers, are compelled to migrate to where the work is, hence causing local brain drain.

The private sector does provide significant R&D funding. In the United States, total private sector funding exceeds total government funding. As in the case of Airbus, funding can come from sources crossing national boundaries. This scope of funding belongs to late-stage, translational research related to specific products, services, and platforms, with the intent of maintaining market competitiveness.

Historically, there have been exceptions, for example, Bell Laboratories, and more recently, Google. They are few. Also rare is R&D conducted at pre-competitive stages aimed at furthering a field or solving an industry-wide challenge. When technical breakthroughs or first mover success does occur, the market becomes dominated by one or two players (e.g., software systems, social media, e-commerce, commercial aircraft manufacturers, etc.). In this manner, collaboration and pre-competitive sharing and R&D funding for commercial research are all further limited.

In theory, the Pharma and Biotech sectors could devise a way to legally share information or otherwise collaborate on the safety of therapeutics while still competing on efficacy. Sharing safety data, for example, could save time, energy, and resources with the effect of accelerating innovation and shortening the path to market. The result would be safer therapies, avoidance of unnecessary duplication of research, and avoidance of the worst-case instance of uncovering serious safety issues in the post-marketing period.

Nonprofit funding has remained relatively modest compared to public and private sources, and has been directed toward small-scale projects. While the Gates Foundation and Wellcome Trust do represent exceptions, their grants are often spread rather thin across too many fields and are not directed specifically toward grand challenges offering demonstrable scientific benefits. Nonprofits often have a sharper focus on a specific disease (e.g., diabetes, cystic fibrosis, rare diseases, and other conditions). Their missions may include important advocacy work or R&D devoid of commercial interest—although recently this has changed, with royalties or other commercial returns directed to the nonprofit itself. These changes, with their potential for conflicts of interest and mission primacy issues, are not without impact on the perceived roles of not-for-profit organizations.

GAME-CHANGING TECHNOLOGIES

The advent of highly sophisticated communications technologies that offer new dimensions for worldwide conferencing and collaborations is raising questions about the basic infrastructures of research. For example, consider R&D laboratories operated remotely via robotics, dispensing with the need for researchers to have in-house brick and mortar laboratories. When, as the metaverse develops, collaborations cross geographic regions and nations using laboratories "in the cloud," how will they (the laboratories and the researchers) be funded? How will the collaborations be conducted and funded and how will the rewards be shared? A period of rapid change awaits us. Just as technologies are scaling and being democratized across the developing world, seemingly leapfrogging across developmental stages, so could R&D and academic research. Questions loom about training for acquiring the required skills that science demands—skills for design and analysis versus physically carrying out a specific methodology and conducting the experiments. Models for basic bench, preclinical, and clinical research will change, along with their funding. This journey has already started.

FUNDING COLLABORATIONS AND COMBINATIONS

Today, while governments, nonprofits, venture capital, and public markets all fund R&D, they tend to fund at usually distinct phases of the R&D continuum (i.e., Basic [biology] → Disease [pathophysiology] → Target → Preclinical → Clinical → Market). Investment is also necessary for the development of tools (e.g., molecular probes and biomarkers) and the creation of standards in parallel with the above stages. While institutions like the U.S. NIST (National Institutes of Standards and Technology) perform a critical role in standardizations and metrics, quite frequently development of molecular tools or biomarkers falls between the cracks. In the field of aging and geroscience, this remains a largely unmet need, one that remains mostly unfunded by any sector. Research at the clinical stage, at times, and especially with recent aging trials, does not fall neatly into the purview of any single government agency, as witnessed in the TAME (Targeting Aging with Metformin) trial debacle (see below). The private sector does not see itself as having a role here because investor expectations do not incentivize funding of clinical trials of inexpensive generics or even never-marketed, off-patent, or patent-expired molecules.

Funding policies and patterns will have to be revamped. Among the prominent needs:

- Remove barriers to combining sources of funding from different sectors.

- Incentivize multinational collaborations and funding.

- Invite new disciplines and younger scientists from both developed and developing countries.

- Disconnect, where appropriate, R&D funding from the teaching mission of institutions. More equitable, direct means of funding teaching need to be established.

- Global communications and remote laboratories can facilitate collaborations between senior scientists/faculty and junior scientists. Newly arising questions regarding intellectual property/ownership/authorship will have to be sorted out.

When the aspiration is on a "moonshot" scale with potential to be as disruptive as the creation of the internet or GPS technology, the challenge becomes one of funding an "open-source" approach while allowing competitors to engage in creation of in-market applications out of late-stage R&D. It is noteworthy that with the development of COVID vaccines, for example, Oxford and AstraZeneca saw their role as one of serving societal needs and agreed to zero-net profit/royalties.

Today we recognize and celebrate the "star/hero scientist," and author of the first landmark published paper. In truth, frequently the data and breakthroughs cannot be reproduced or validated independently, often because of lack of funding or incentives to conduct such research. Furthermore, getting a validation study funded is difficult, as is getting one published in high-profile journals. This also inhibits progress.

Questions arise: Could a focused research organization (FRO) or ideally a network of FROs be created, funded, governed, and coordinated to move the field of aging forward? Could such a network be designed, managed, and funded across geographies and sectors, but still with minimal bureaucracy?

What role can prizes (like the $10 million Ansari XPrize) play in creating incentives toward innovation?

SUPPORTIVE/PRELIMINARY DATA

Today's funding often presupposes the existence of supportive/preliminary data, pushing investigators to generate data *before* getting funded ("use past grants to generate data for future applications"). The question then becomes, "How can we fund early-stage ideas, even without proof-of-concept data to generate and support early hypotheses?"

Could ARPA-H (Advanced Research Projects Agency-Health) be a model for this ecosystem or an ARPA-Aging model for funding the discovery/development/application/and implementation of research stages? Could it offer a model that answers the often-voiced concern of recent years in the scientific community that R&D funding processes have become too conservative, and in effect encourage only incremental advances in science and technology.

How then can high-risk, high-reward (HRHR) R&D be incentivized? The problem is inherent in the U.S. National Institutes of Health (NIH) HRHR definition. It states that such research tests "ideas that have the potential for high impact, but that may be too novel, span too diverse a range of disciplines, or be at a stage too early to fare well in the traditional peer review process" (Packalen and Bhattacharya 2018). A report published in 2021 (Machado 2021) exploring this question, "Quantitative indicators for high-risk/high-reward research," identified four main categories of HRHR funding mechanisms:

1. Funding mechanisms specifically designed to support HRHR research and that are supporting such research as a primary goal.

2. Funding mechanisms that have HRHR research as their primary mission within a broader set of objectives.

3. Funding mechanisms in which supporting HRHR research is a secondary goal or an important consideration in the proposal evaluation process.

4. Funding mechanisms geared toward supporting scientific research with multiple possible goals including advancing scientific knowledge, achieving economic outcomes, or advancing societal outcomes, although there are no clear criteria for fostering HRHR research.

The main funding sectors are government, nonprofit/philanthropy, venture capital/financial markets, corporations, and prizes (e.g., the XPrize). For their engagement with HRHR research, key contextual factors and policies play an important role. Political support for risk-taking and commitment for the long term, for example, was found to be both the most important factor and the most challenging. Also, research institution tenure and promotion and advancement policies, powerful incentives for researchers (especially early-career ones), favor conservative research projects that are more likely to be accepted for publication. These institutions, to encourage HRHR research, will have to reconsider these human resource policies. To effect such changes, they will have to actively promote and favor consideration of a "riskiness" factor of a research project or portfolio. In addition, a specific revision of tenure and promotion practices in the direction of rewarding risk-taking and providing seed or bridge funding for HRHR research is needed. The "how" question, in this regard, does stand in sharp outline. The report did not identify a "one-size-fits-all" funding approach, but did state in no uncertain terms the consequences of ignoring the problem: "… failure to encourage and to support research on risky, 'out-of-the-box' ideas may jeopardize a country's longer-term ability to innovate and compete economically, to harness science toward solving national and global challenges, and to contribute to the progress of science as a whole."

Another report, "Energizing and employing America for a brighter economic future" (National Research Council 2007), produced at the request of the U.S. Congress back in 2007, identified factors contributing to eroding U.S. competitiveness in the global economy, and named a decline in support for "high-risk or transformative research," particularly in the physical sciences, engineering, mathematics, and information sciences. The trend, it said, increases the likelihood that breakthrough, "disruptive" technologies, the kinds of discoveries that yield huge returns, will not be found locally in the United States. Similar concerns have been articulated in

Europe and Japan about their own research establishments.

Listing factors fostering R&D timidity, Machado's OECD report included the sense that because funding agencies spend public dollars, they need to show results promising societal benefit and technological breakthroughs. Also, scientific review panels, perceiving the same pressure, reward lower risk, higher certainty projects. Third, influential individuals or parties with vested interests may undermine avenues of original research.

What does constitute worthy HRHR research? Canada's New Frontiers in Research Fund (2018) program sought research that is interdisciplinary, international, fast breaking, and high risk, and looked for projects going in unique directions, challenging current paradigms, and deepening understanding of complex and challenging issues. Also, the program included bringing new disciplines together to solve existing problems and/or taking current frameworks, methods, and techniques and developing or adapting them.

The OECD report devised the following as a working HRHR definition: "High-risk, high-reward (HRHR) research is research that (1) strives to understand or support solutions to ambitious scientific, technological, or societal challenges; (2) strives to cross scientific, technological, or societal paradigms in a revolutionary way; (3) involves a high degree of novelty; and (4) carries a high risk of not realizing its full ambition as well as the potential for high, transformational impact on a scientific, technological, or societal challenge."

The OECD report listed three categories of funding mechanisms, with the first being dedicated HRHR research programs with supporting HRHR research as their primary goal. These programs are in the minority, the OECD report authors noted, mentioning U.S. (Defense Advanced Research Projects Agency [DARPA]), French, and UK examples.

The second category program has, within a broader objective set, supported HRHR research as part of its primary mission. The U.S. National Science Foundation's RAISE program, for example, aims at supporting bold, interdisciplinary projects. RAISE requires two or more intellectually distinct disciplines to be incorporated within a research project.

With the third category of research funding mechanisms, supporting HRHR research is a secondary goal or an important consideration for the proposal's evaluators. Examples of this most common mechanism were from Europe, the United States, Ireland, Poland, and Norway, with Norway's ENERGIX program aimed at energy breakthroughs that may produce major leaps forward.

A potential fourth category of funding mechanism is geared toward supporting research with multiple possible goals (i.e., advancing scientific knowledge, achieving economic outcomes, or advancing societal outcomes). Here, also, researchers are encouraged to pursue high-risk or potentially transformative approaches.

NONGOVERNMENTAL FUNDING OF HRHR

Although the larger part of HRHR funding comes from governmental sources, other organizations and especially private foundations, because they are under fewer restrictions, can play an important role. They have more freedom in how they define their objectives and achieve them and fewer or less stringent financial accountability requirements. With more freedom, they may better tolerate risk and projects delving into unchartered territory. They may also choose to support specific scientists rather than specific projects, and may provide grants over a longer time period. The OECD report mentions Howard Hughes Medical Institute (HHMI) (www.hhmi.org) as a pioneer in placing "big bets" on people rather than projects. At the opposite pole, targeting ideas rather than people, the Danish Lundbeck Foundation has based some funding on anonymous proposals, forcing reviewers to focus on the project's apparent merit.

The strategy of presenting specific challenges and dangling financial prizes for their achievement has gained currency in recent years. In the United States, the practice, as a spur to innovation, gained congressional legislative support in 2010. One clear advantage, outside of the potential successes generated, is that government does not foot the bill for the "also rans." They can still gain patents and commercially useful insights. Also, by specifying the desired result but not the way to get there, process innovation may be a valuable byproduct.

The OECD report specifically identifies DARPA, the XPrize Foundation, and Ireland's Future Innovator Prize as users of incentivizing prizes and as being HRHR research oriented. The last example represents a hybrid experiment, with first-stage winners getting a small grant, and later-stage winners getting larger ones.

The portfolio approach, which tries to balance high-risk and reliable financial return projects, has become attractive to program managers and policymakers. It strives to forestall the politically difficult situation of having a very high percentage of no-breakthrough projects by spreading the risk. It allows differing selection processes and, at the national/strategic level (or even multinational level), enables the acceptance of mission-oriented, higher risk use of public funding.

LONG-TERM STRATEGIC FUNDING

While the need to show tangible results works against patience and risk tolerance among government policymakers, there are notable examples of successful HRHR research. Among them in the United States, the National Science Foundation's funding for LIGO (the Laser Interferometer Gravitational Wave Observatory), two laser-based scientific facilities designed to verify the existence of the gravitational waves predicted by Albert Einstein about a century back. At the project onset in the late 1980s, gravitational wave detectors had not yet been designed and failure risks were substantial. The verification did not occur until 2015, and numerous threats to the project's funding in intervening years had to be overcome. International support for CERN's building and operation of the Large Hadron Collider (LHC) faced similar challenges; its discovery

of the Higgs boson and the expanding of the understanding of the universe that both LIGO and LHC delivered justified the risk tolerance and patience.

These examples, however, are the exception. The OECD report authors devised a novelty indicator that quantifies the "riskiness" of a research project or portfolio and the level of knowledge of field combination in "more exploratory risky ways" in journal articles, allowing researchers, research managers, and others to adjust risk to an appropriate level. They found that in the years 2005–2017, more than half of all articles scored 0 or 1 for novelty, with few scoring very high (10 or higher). The countries with more articles scoring among the top 10% were the Netherlands, Switzerland, and Denmark followed by the United States and the United Kingdom. The analysis also showed that these countries were the ones scoring very high in terms of scientific impact measured through numbers of article citations. Also, from a long-term perspective, the novelty indicator is positively associated with citations. The overall citation performance of highly novel articles is not initially elevated, but it increases over time, often becoming substantially superior over longer time spans. For research project portfolios, inclusion of high novelty research can potentially help balance risk and reward. In the case of targeting and increasing healthy life spans, the potential return-on-investment (ROI) is massive, as Andrew J. Scott demonstrated.

Many worthy projects, stated Adam Marblestone et al. in a recent article in *Nature* (Marblestone et al. 2022), wither or fail to get launched because they do not fit neatly into categories attractive to venture capitalists, academic laboratories, or start-up firms—especially in the instance of projects that would create public goods, for example, data sets or tools valuable for making research faster and easier. "These engineering improvements do not fulfil teaching requirements or provide the papers or pizzazz that both senior academics and their trainees need to propel their careers." Such midscale projects that enable research and are typically overlooked could be taken up by FROs with full-time scientists, engineers, and executives, and funding at the US$20–$100 million level over ~5 yr. They would pursue definite milestones, such as improving by tenfold a measurement system or gathering pre-specified quantities of data. But unlike the grand, charismatic LHC at CERN, Human Cell Atlas, Hubble Space Telescope, or ENCODE (encyclopedia of DNA elements) in data collection, the FRO model would support a stream of smaller, easier-to-launch projects. First efforts have, as proposed products, high-throughput brain-mapping techniques, tools for engineering non-model microorganisms, and analysis of aging interventions in mice. In a few years, it will be clearer whether the FRO model accelerates neuroscience, synthetic biology, and longevity research in a manner similar to how Bell Labs, Xerox PARC, and other U.S. corporate laboratories merged fundamental research with large-scale product development (examples include laser printers, photovoltaic cells in solar panels, the programming language C++, transistors, etc.) in the second half of the twentieth century. More recently, Alphabet's subsidiary Google DeepMind developed an algorithm for predicting protein folding. Today, though, most industry laboratories cannot pursue projects for which near-term commercial objectives are not apparent. Those that do make sure that what they learn remains proprietary. We propose that funding precludes such secrecy, but with means devised to preserve commercial advantages for the research authors. Otherwise, as with proposed sharing of safety data among pharmaceutical researchers, efforts are duplicated and progress at the scientific community/national/global levels is slowed. Finding practical ways to democratize advancing knowledge and discoveries while incentivizing individual initiative needs priority consideration.

DARPA, held widely as an example of institutional innovation, identifies very specific technologic needs and assembles research groups to meet them. The U.S. government has created DARPA variants to address energy- (ARPA-E) and intelligence-related projects (IARPA).

Some research institutions are set up to take on government- or industry-sponsored applied engineering projects. SRI International in Menlo Park, CA, the Fraunhofer Society Institutes in Germany, and the European Innovation Council Accelerator are examples. Permanent institutes independent from academia such as the Allen Institute for Brain Science in Seattle, Washington, and the Janelia Research Campus (Ashburn, Virginia) of the Howard Hughes Medical Institute, through large-scale data collection, have developed broadly used tools. Similarly, the Allen Institute has established tools that are easily standardized for mapping gene expression in the mouse brain. The stated goal of Marblestone et al. is to develop a playbook model for FROs allowing them to get technologies or data sets deployed rapidly for use across the research community. They want to support an ecosystem of small- to midscale projects less suited for academia and other organizations. An FRO might develop a technology *and* demonstrate that independent laboratories can implement it. FROs use time-bound milestones and strong project management but are not bound to academic publishing.

In terms of structuring, Marblestone et al. suggest that semi-permanent project manager/administrator groups can be matched with scientific staff at the outset to create a focused scientific leadership team. Alternatives to academia's ladder or the potential financial rewards of start-ups will have to find their strong career progression models. Experience and experimentation will have to refine the FRO model. Marblestone et al. conclude, "We and others hope to develop the model to a point at which governments could set goals to fund a certain number of FROs each year, confident that, although some will fail, others will make research more powerful and efficient."

A *Science* article published last year on the ARPA-H opportunities (Collins et al. 2021) often came to similar conclusions about bold research ideas that may fall through the cracks between the traditional NIH support for incremental, hypothesis-driven research and commercial support for return-on-investment-driven research. These traits may be seen as fatal to potential funders: too risky, too expensive, too time-consuming, too "applied," calling for too much complex multiparty coordination, not enough near-term market opportunity, and too broad a scope. Further, bold ideas around creating platforms, capabilities, and resources helpful across research on many diseases do not attract the attention of potential funding sources.

The authors add that consideration of a project's impact on health ecosystem inequities is generally ignored in the private sector as well. Finding or creating the levers for funding the democratization of technologies for the benefit of all is a present challenge.

A WORD ABOUT FAILURE

The path necessary for coordinating multiple entities and individuals working toward a "moonshot"-type goal has to skirt along and sometimes across many institutional and even cultural boundaries. Nobility of purpose does not inoculate against all such obstacles that crop up along the way. The debacle experienced around the TAME trial of metformin stands out in sharp outline in the narrative of the previously cited STAT report ("The race for longevity"). When in the late 1990s serendipitous observations that cancers, heart attacks, dementia, and Alzheimer's disease were reduced in patients taking metformin, a safe and "dirt cheap" drug, versus those receiving other diabetes medications attracted serious attention among clinical researchers. Nir Barzilai, the Albert Einstein College Institute for Aging Research director, went into action. He had been interested in testing drugs to extend human "health span," and metformin seemed to be an excellent candidate, good enough to attract, for the first time in history, a National Institutes of Aging grant to conduct a clinical trial that targets aging. The plan was to track 3000 elderly individuals over 5 yr to see whether metformin would forestall cardiovascular disease, cancer, cognitive decline, and mortality.

The biggest obstacle to Barzilai's plan appeared to be the FDA, because federal regulators at the FDA recognize only the "one disease, one drug" model for approvals. Aging, not being a disease, was precluded from FDA paths forward in clinical testing. But when Barzilai and a group of top-tier school academics met with the FDA, to everyone's considerable surprise, the agency agreed to the plan in 2015—leaving *only* the funding, $30–$50 million, to be addressed. But with metformin being a generic drug, pharmaceutical funding was ruled out. The NIH offered about $9 million to identify aging process biomarkers, but Barzilai's supposition that the rest would be granted by philanthropists and philanthropic organizations proved to be incorrect. And it has stayed incorrect for roughly the last 8 yr, despite the view by some that TAME could be paradigm shifting and create a biotech framework that could be followed into the future by others. While Barzilai still believes that TAME will happen "because it has to happen," James Peyer, CEO of Cambrian Biopharma, called the TAME story "a particularly tragic one," and noted, "It should almost be done by now."

LEAPING PAST LIMITATIONS

Given the limitations on HRHR research funding imposed by commercial and political entities and academia, which groups have the freedom and means to, as Regina E. Dugan and Kaigham J. Gabriel put it in "Changing the business of breakthroughs" (Dugan and Gabriel 2022) "… take an unconventional and optimistic view of what's possible in order to act on behalf of future generations?" Who can see beyond borders, disciplines, and barriers and change the way science is done (and funded)? At this time, according to Dugan and Gabriel, it is independent philanthropy that can drive a network of diverse contributors toward a common goal and that can create the necessary structures while deploying and synchronizing resources. "… [I]ndependent philanthropy can step into this void. And at a time when humanity is in urgent need of action, philanthropy can act quickly, without concern for election cycles or the lengthy process of realigning political will and global economic incentive structures."

Pointing to the recent example of the development of the mRNA vaccines and of the culture fostered by DARPA, they urge that visionary programs with goals greater than any one individual and aimed at breakthroughs need to move quickly, generate a sense of momentum, and have the agility to create cross-discipline collaboration and a unity that pushes past obstacles. While DARPA was designed to serve U.S. strategic interests, Dugan and Gabriel are certain that its model can be adjusted in the service of increasing the number and pace of revolutionary breakthroughs around global challenges. For that, national boundaries, distinctions around basic versus applied research, life sciences versus physical sciences, and perhaps, most critically, between public versus private funding have to be dissolved in the service of a higher good. At the same time, progress toward clearly defined goals must be testable and measurable.

Dugan and Gabriel hold out as an example their organization's (Wellcome Leap) model. Wellcome Leap is a new entity established in 2020 to tackle huge global challenges in health. It hires experienced leadership teams with a mandate to "stack the odds in favor of breakthroughs." To build a sense of urgency and team momentum, it uses a master funding agreement that allows funding of individuals in days or weeks instead of months or a year. Not requiring a consensus process for evaluating proposals helps create more diverse teams of early- and late-career researchers from diverse quarters—a method that elevates young investigators. Further, the use of contracts rather than grants favors risk tolerance. Staged decision-making regarding going forward allows off-ramps for unproductive lines of work.

The question they are most often asked, Dugan and Gabriel note, is about how they choose programs. Citing Donald Stokes' *Pasteur's Quadrant* (Stokes 1997), they choose "use-inspired research"—research that is mission-driven—aimed at new capabilities or specific problems. It calls for advancement of science to create new solutions, and avoids pure curiosity-driven basic science that lacks a target application.

As we look to the future, AI, neural networks, machine learning, and evolution of the metaverse will require large learning data sets. It will require especially those data sets linking molecular laboratory data to phenotypic data from real-world, large, and diverse populations in their "living" environments if we are to understand and intervene in aging.

CONCLUDING REMARKS

Funding will have to come from a combination of government, private, and likely nonprofit sources collaborating in complementary areas. Ownership, the need for a focus on the common good, ethics, inclusivity, and the remediation of inequities all count as critical issues demanding that attention be directed to them proactively. These are key links to funding that successfully attain the scale and duration that this grand vision will inevitably demand.

THE NEED FOR TRUST

Finally, consumer and citizen perception is an increasingly important aspect that all stakeholders, including funding agencies from all sectors, will have to address if science—especially the field of aging/geroscience—is to have a societal license to operate. We need the trust of society.

REFERENCES

Collins FS, Schwetz TA, Tabak LA, Lander ES. 2021. ARPA-H: accelerating biomedical breakthroughs. *Science* **373:** 165–167. doi:10.1126/science.abj8547

Dugan RE, Gabriel KJ. 2022. Changing the business of breakthroughs. *Issues Sci Technol* **38:** 70–74.

Lauer M. 2021. Long-term trends in the age of principal investigators supported for the first time on NIH R01–equivalent awards. National Institutes of Health, Bethesda, MD. https://nexus.od.nih.gov/all/2021/11/18/long-term-trends-in-the-age-of-principal-investigators-supported-for-the-first-time-on-nih-r01-awards

Machado D. 2021. Quantitative indicators for high-risk/high-reward research. OECD Science, Technology and Industry Working Papers, No. 2021/07. OECD Publishing, Paris. https://doi.org/10.1787/675cbef6-en

Marblestone A, Gamick A, Kalil T, Martin C, Cvitkovic M, Rodriques SG. 2022. Unblock research bottlenecks with non-profit start-ups. *Nature* **601:** 188–190. doi:10.1038/d41586-022-00018-5

National Research Council. 2007. Energizing and employing America for a brighter economic future. *Committee on Prospering in the Global Economy of the 21st Century: An Agenda for American Science and Technology.* National Academy of Sciences, Washington, DC.

Packalen M, Bhattacharya J. 2018. Does the NIH fund edge science? Working Paper 24860. National Bureau of Economic Research, Cambridge, MA. http://www.nber.org/papers/w24860

Scott AJ, Ellison M, Sinclair DA. 2021. The economic value of targeting aging. *Nature Aging* **1:** 616–623. doi:10.1038/s43587-021-00080-0

STAT Reports. 2022. The race for longevity: how scientists—and industry—are seeking to extend healthy lives. https://reports.statnews.com/products/race-for-longevity?variant=39820067405927

Stokes DE. 1997. *Pasteur's quadrant: basic science and technological innovation.* Brookings Institution Press, Washington, DC.

Crowdfunding and Crowdsourcing of Aging Science

Keith Comito

Lifespan Extension Advocacy Foundation, Seaford, New York 11783, USA

Correspondence: keith@lifespan.io

Crowdsourcing is a term that describes a method of distributed effort by which a goal is accomplished by a large group of people, typically initiated by a public call-to-action and is a portmanteau of the words "crowd" and "outsourcing" coined in 2005. Crowdfunding is the practice of funding a project or venture via crowdsourced financial contributions. Crowdsourcing and crowdfunding have been used to advance scientific progress for hundreds of years, with the frequency and scale of their use rapidly increasing during the twenty-first century, thanks to the advent of the internet and the mainstream adoption of related connective technologies. The field of aging research has uniquely benefited from this trend, with the emergence of multiple communities and platforms designed to coordinate gerontology funding and research collaboration. Furthermore, the recent widespread adoption of blockchain technology is also creating powerful new opportunities to crowdfund and crowdsource aging research specifically.

Crowdsourcing (Estellés-Arolas and González-Ladrón-de-Guevara 2012), and its financially focused subtype "crowdfunding" (www.merriam-webster.com/dictionary/crowdfunding) have been used since the early eighteenth century to further scientific goals, with one of the earliest documented instances being of the British government offering a public monetary prize for the best way to measure a ship's longitudinal position in 1714 (Dawson and Bynghall 2012).

The emergence of the internet in the late twentieth century greatly expanded the scale and scope of crowdsourcing to assist in scientific endeavors. Notably, the launch of SETI@home in 1999 (setiathome.berkeley.edu), which allowed owners of personal computers to volunteer otherwise unused computing power to aid in the search for extraterrestrial frequency emissions, marked a milestone in mainstream awareness of crowdsourcing. This was followed in regard to biology specifically with projects such as Foldit in 2008 (fold.it), which involved over 57,000 participants helping to discover the topology of native protein structures through playing an online protein-folding puzzle game (Markoff 2010).

This type of crowdsourcing, in which every individual participant involved contributes to the final work collectively, differed from earlier "inducement prize" strategies, in which a reward is offered to any individual or group that can accomplish a stated goal. One such prize notable in the field of aging research is the Methuselah Mouse Prize, or Mprize, which was created by

Cite this article as *Cold Spring Harb Perspect Med* doi: 10.1101/cshperspect.a041209

the Methuselah Foundation (www.mfoundation
.org) in 2003 to reward breakthroughs in the
increase of maximal life span and successful rejuvenation in mice (Bailey 2004), and directly
inspired by the 1714 Longitude Prize (Dawson
and Bynghall 2012).

Crowdfunding in its modern conception became truly mainstream with the launch of online
platforms specifically dedicated to the distributed
collection of funds, such as Indiegogo in 2008
(www.indiegogo.com) and Kickstarter in 2009
(kickstarter.com). While general solicitation of
donations via the Web, such as that currently
employed by many longevity-focused organizations such as the SENS Research Foundation
(www.sens.org) and International Longevity
Alliance (www.ilc-alliance.org), can rightly be
considered a form of crowdfunding; the term
typically denotes the use of such dedicated platforms.

More recently, startup investment listing
websites such as AngelList (angel.co) and equity-based investment platforms such as WeFunder (wefunder.com) have emerged, facilitated by
regulations such as Title III of the 2012 JOBS
Act's Regulation CF (CROWDFUND Act 2012)
in the United States, which came into effect May
16, 2016.

Furthermore, recent developments in blockchain technology (Wikipedia 2022a), first imple-
mented in the form of the digital currency Bitcoin
in 2008 (Nakamoto 2008) and extended with pro-
grammable "smart contracts" in 2014 via the
Ethereum blockchain (Buterin 2014), are facilitating new forms of decentralized funding and
collaboration. The fact that several pioneers of
this new technology are vocal supporters of life
extension research, coupled with the powerful capabilities of the technology itself, are laying the
ground for exciting developments in the crowdsourcing of aging research in the near future.

CROWDFUNDING VERSUS TRADITIONAL FUNDING APPROACHES—BRIDGING THE "VALLEY OF DEATH"

Fundraising in the field of aging biotechnology
presents unique and specific challenges, and this
can make crowdfunding particularly attractive

for researchers and entrepreneurs seeking to advance their projects. Beyond typical challenges
acquiring grant funding due to high competition for limited resources (Alberts et al. 2014;
National Institutes of Health 2022a), for example, receiving grants for early-stage studies into
the mechanisms of aging is especially arduous.
Directly addressing the root causes of human
aging is still a paradigm-shifting idea, and, as
such, government allocations for such research
are below that of various end-stage diseases,
such as cancer and Alzheimer's (National Institutes of Health 2022b).

Crowdfunding provides a viable alternative
to this traditional funding approach, because,
while it can take many years and millions of
dollars to fully bring a potential therapy to market (Mullin 2014), completing early-stage proof-
of-concept research can often be accomplished
with amounts crowdfunding can raise. There is
also an additional benefit in that crowdfunding
presents a lower bureaucratic barrier-to-entry as
compared to the traditional grant application
process, which can often be challenging. All
that is required with most crowdfunding platforms is that the campaign creators comply
with the crowdfunding platform's stated terms
of service and privacy policy, the same as with
many other websites. With decentralized crowdfunding approaches, such as those facilitated by
blockchain technology, the barrier-to-entry can
be reduced to the effort required to create a cryptocurrency wallet and solicit support on social
media.

With regard to acquiring investment capital,
aging research projects also have unique difficul-
ties to overcome as compared to other sectors. It
is typical for investors to wish to maximize return-on-investment (ROI) as rapidly as possible,
and the long-time horizons involved in aging
research therapies have historically made traditional investment in such projects difficult
(McCaslin 2018). A successful round of crowdfunding and consequent delivery of basic research goals can serve to de-risk such investment
possibilities in the eyes of potential investors.

Rather than being a competing source of
funding in relation to grants and investment
capital, crowdfunding can, in fact, be a synergis-

tic one. In the case of grants, for example, it can expand opportunities if the applying team is able to demonstrate traction by having secured additional sources of funding (Instrumentl 2022), and crowdfunding can be one such source. In the case of investment, a successful crowdfunding campaign not only raises capital to help deliver proof-of-concept results, but also allows the research team to demonstrate they are capable of conveying the details of their work successfully enough to gather public support—both of which can serve to de-risk further investment.

Importantly, crowdfunding platforms can also serve as a hub for the investment community, with platform administrators actively working to connect successful project teams with interested investors, catalyzing follow-on funding that can take the crowdfunded project beyond the basic research phase. As an example, specific to aging research, the nonprofit organization Lifespan Extension Advocacy Foundation (LEAF) has assisted teams that have run successful campaigns on its crowdfunding platform Lifespan.io (www .lifespan.io) acquire additional investment capital for their projects by matching them with a network of investors—coordinated by LEAF—that are specifically interested in rejuvenation biotechnology projects (Lifespan.io 2022b).

In these ways, crowdfunding can fill a novel and vital role in building a bridge across the so-called investment "valley of death" (Wikipedia 2022b) and help therapies that can delay or ameliorate the diseases of aging reach the public as quickly as possible.

CROWDFUNDING PLATFORMS AND THEIR USE TO FUND AGING SCIENCE

When it comes to dedicated crowdfunding platforms, it is typical to display available projects in a campaign-style structure, where users may contribute funds via various payment methods, such as credit card processors, PayPal, or cryptocurrencies, toward achieving a specific goal amount to be reached by a specified deadline date.

In some campaigns, the specified goal amount must be reached before the deadline for any funds to be transferred—so called "all-or-nothing" campaigns—while some platforms al-

low transfer of donated funds regardless of whether the specified goal amount has been reached—so called "flexible funding" campaigns. In either case, such contributions can take the form of pure donations, with no additional reward, or be incentivized by the campaign creators via items or experience-based rewards that are of perceived value proportional with the amount contributed—typically delimited by discrete reward levels. Crowdfunding platforms usually take a small percentage of raised funds as a fee in exchange for hosting campaigns on their website.

Crowdfunding platforms are intrinsically social in nature, allowing contributors to share campaigns with their friends and colleagues, as well as showcase their own contributions for the purpose of incentivizing others to do likewise. While this capability to readily enlist additional supporters can be of great use to various scientific endeavors, aging science projects have been historically underrepresented on general crowdfunding platforms such as Kickstarter and Indiegogo. For example, of over 550,000 projects launched (Kickstarter 2022a), Kickstarter's project search function returns zero aging research projects for relevant search terms such as "longevity," "life extension," "biology," "gerontology," and other related phrases. This absence may be partially accounted for by Kickstarter policies that prohibit the involvement of genetically engineered organisms in projects (Geere 2013), as well as any projects "claiming to diagnose, cure, treat, or prevent an illness or condition (whether via a device, app, book, nutritional supplement, or other means)" (Kickstarter 2022b). While Indiegogo does not share these same explicit restrictions regarding biotechnology projects, there have been only a few campaigns hosted on the service involving aging science, which have reached significant funding goals, such as a 2013 project aiming to test a combination of geroprotective drugs in mice (Wuttke 2013), and a 2015 project to create a longevity-focused cookbook (Konovalenko 2015).

Another reason for the comparative shortage of aging science projects on platforms such as Kickstarter and Indiegogo may be the comparative lack of popularity of such projects in relation to those in other categories such as gaming, tech, and fashion (Wikipedia 2022c). The team composition of scientific projects also rarely includes strong dedicated marketing teams to surmount this, and even promising scientific campaigns are typically underfunded on these platforms (Rider 2016).

Possibly in response to some of these issues, in 2012 multiple crowdfunding platforms dedicated specifically to the support of scientific projects were launched, such as Microryza, later rebranded as Experiment (2022a), Walacea, later rebranded as Crowd.Science (2022a), and Petridish (2022).

While platforms such as these have raised funds for a variety of projects, the amounts raised on a per-project basis have historically been well below the amounts usually required for aging research projects—with the average amount raised by a project on Experiment being approximately $4000 (Experiment 2022b), and the average amount raised by a project in the health campaign category on Crowd.Science being less than $8500 (Crowd.Science 2022b). In comparison, other sources of funding available to credible biology research projects, such as SBIR and STTR grants in the United States (Small Business Innovation Research 2022), typically offer funding in the hundreds of thousands.

It is worth noting that aging science projects have appeared with negligible frequency on these platforms. For example, only one such project has been listed on Experiment.com, namely, a 2015 campaign aimed at developing various physiological biomarkers for age (reaction times, sense of touch, etc.), and determining which testing techniques provide the most useful results (Small and Hoekstra 2016). Petridish.org did not list any such projects and the site was discontinued in 2015.

CROWDFUNDING PLATFORMS SPECIFICALLY FOR AGING RESEARCH

In 2015, the 501(c)(3) nonprofit organization LEAF launched the crowdfunding platform Lifespan.io dedicated specifically to funding aging science projects. Unlike preexisting platforms, Lifespan.io only runs campaigns for a few proj-

ects each year, with each campaign project passing a thorough evaluation process by LEAF's board of directors and scientific advisory board. Furthermore, LEAF provides each project direct assistance in terms of graphics and video creation, campaign text editing, and PR support in the form of various social media, marketing, and outreach initiatives. This strategy has proven successful, with 100% of the nine campaigns hosted thus far on Lifespan.io successfully raising their goal amounts, and the average amount raised per project being greater than $65,000. Another distinguishing characteristic of Lifespan.io is its ability to raise funds for for-profit initiatives in a manner that is potentially tax-deductible for United States citizens, by serving as a fiscal sponsor (Wikipedia 2022d) for initiatives concordant with its nonprofit mission. Platforms administered by for-profit companies such as Kickstarter and Experiment are incapable of fiscal sponsorship in this manner.

Projects funded on Lifespan.io include research projects from teams such as those at Harvard Medical School and the SENS Research Foundation, as well as projects focused on developing biomarkers of aging (Lifespan.io 2022a). In 2017, Lifespan.io also began to host campaigns designed to collect recurring monthly donations, similar in functionality to the art patronage crowdfunding platform Patreon (www.patreon.com). It has thus far used this functionality to raise funds for its own continued operations, as well as other operations of LEAF (Lifespan.io 2022c). The most recent campaign on Lifespan.io was one to support the first large-scale placebo-controlled clinical trial to determine the effects of rapamycin on human longevity, and this was completed in May of 2021 raising a total of $182,838 (Fig. 1; Lifespan.io 2022d).

EQUITY CROWDFUNDING FOR AGING RESEARCH

In addition to donation-based crowdfunding, there also exists equity-based investment platforms, which can rightly be considered a form of crowdsourced investment or crowdfunding, such as WeFunder, StartEngine (www.startengine.com), and Republic (republic.co), as

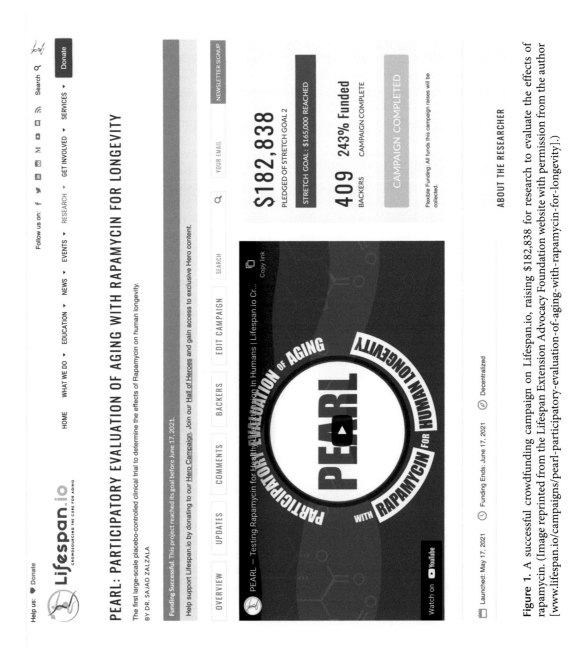

Figure 1. A successful crowdfunding campaign on Lifespan.io, raising $182,838 for research to evaluate the effects of rapamycin. (Image reprinted from the Lifespan Extension Advocacy Foundation website with permission from the author [www.lifespan.io/campaigns/pearl-participatory-evaluation-of-aging-with-rapamycin-for-longevity].)

well as startup investment listing websites such as AngelList. While such platforms can be used to support aging science, to date there have been few examples of their use for this purpose, with the investments search function of StartEngine (2022), for example, returning zero results when searching for terms relating to aging research, and the analogous search function of WeFunder (2022a) returning only a handful of results, including one pertaining to the development of biomarkers for aging (WeFunder 2022b) and one pertaining to the testing of identified drug candidates for aging reversal (WeFunder 2022c).

This dearth of listings may be due in part to the newness of equity-based crowdfunding generally, and the related regulatory landscape surrounding this type of investment having yet to fully settle (Wikipedia 2022e). In a stated effort to reduce startup fundraising friction and streamline compliance with regulations that currently exist, such as SEC general solicitation rule 506 (c) (U.S. Securities and Exchange Commission 2022), in 2020 AngelList launched a rolling fund mechanism (AngelList 2022a) by which fund managers can fundraise publicly and continuously, via a quarterly subscription model (AngelList 2022b). Of the 84 rolling funds currently listed in AngelLists's rolling fund explorer, several are explicitly focused on funding biotechnology and health startups, and one listing—Healthspan Capital Rolling Fund—is specifically focused on funding longevity biotechnology seed companies specifically (AngelList 2022c).

CRYPTOCURRENCY AS A CROWDFUNDING MECHANISM FOR AGING SCIENCE

One of the most promising recent developments regarding crowdfunding for aging science is the advent of widespread adoption of cryptocurrency. Transaction analysis made possible by public blockchain technology shows that by the end of Q2 2021 global adoption of cryptocurrency had grown by more than 2300% since the end of Q3 2019 (Chainalysis 2021), and a November 11, 2021 Pew Research Center poll finds that 86% of Americans are familiar with cryptocurrencies such as Bitcoin and Ethereum, with 16% of these respondents having invested, traded, or used cryptocurrency themselves (Pew Research Center 2021). This adoption, coupled with the emergence of new cryptocurrency philanthropy platforms such as Endaoment (2022a) and The Giving Block (thegivingblock.com), augments existing crowdfunding initiatives with increased transaction flexibility and creates additional channels by which donors can support aging science projects. The Giving Block, for example, showcases an impact index fund—a method that allows donations to be spread across nonprofits of a particular type—specifically for health-related charities (The Giving Block 2022), and Endaoment has recently created a similar vehicle specifically for supporting life extension–related charities (Endaoment 2022b).

Blockchain technology has also facilitated the creation of hitherto unseen methods of crowdfunding and passionate communities of individuals dedicated to using them to fund public goods (Wikipedia 2022f) such as increased healthy life spans. A prominent example of this is Gitcoin (2022a), a community and crowdfunding platform founded in 2017, which employs quadratic funding—a unique donation-matching system pioneered by Ethereum cofounder Vitalik Buterin in which a large pool of matching funds rewards projects in a manner that proportionally and quadratically scales with increasing levels of small donor support and public engagement (Buterin et al. 2018). Since launching, Gitcoin has raised over 61 million dollars for public goods (Gitcoin 2022b), which includes projects focused directly on aging science (Gitcoin 2022c). In December of 2021, Gitcoin also began launching fundraising rounds specifically dedicated to longevity, such as its GR12 Longevity Cause Round, which raised over $450,000 for a variety of aging science projects curated by the aging science organizations VitaDAO and Lifespan.io (Fig. 2; Hill 2021a).

Blockchain technology also creates additional financial mechanisms by which funding can be raised for aging science projects. One such mechanism is reflection, by which a cryptocurrency smart contract can transfer a defined percentage of all transactions to a specific wallet or divided among several receiving wallets. Transhuman Coin (www.transhumancoin.finance) is one

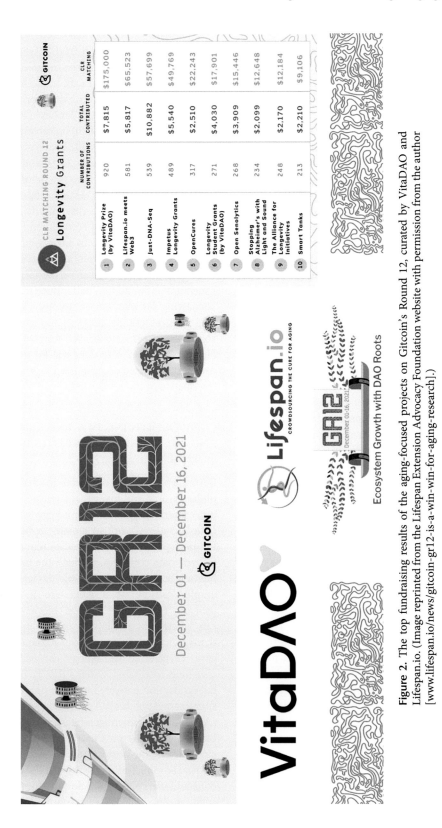

	NUMBER OF CONTRIBUTIONS	TOTAL CONTRIBUTED	CLR MATCHING
1 Longevity Prize (by VitaDAO)	920	$7,815	$175,000
2 Lifespan.io meets Web3	581	$5,817	$65,523
3 Just-DNA-Seq	539	$10,882	$57,699
4 Impetus Longevity Grants	489	$5,540	$49,769
5 OpenCures	317	$2,510	$22,243
6 Longevity Student Grants (by VitaDAO)	271	$4,030	$17,901
7 Open Senolytics	268	$3,909	$15,446
8 Stopping Alzheimer's with Light and Sound	234	$2,099	$12,648
9 The Alliance for Longevity Initiatives	248	$2,170	$12,184
10 Smart Tanks	213	$2,210	$9,106

Figure 2. The top fundraising results of the aging-focused projects on Gitcoin's Round 12, curated by VitaDAO and Lifespan.io. (Image reprinted from the Lifespan Extension Advocacy Foundation website with permission from the author [www.lifespan.io/news/gitcoin-gr12-is-a-win-for-aging-research].)

such cryptocurrency, in which 2% of all Transhuman Coin token (or THC) transactions are reflected to all holders of the coin, with charities focused on aging science being significant holders of the coin, and thus receiving a significant percentage of such reflections.

Another mechanism used to fundraise for aging science projects is token airdrops—a process that involves cryptocurrency token creators freely distributing cryptocurrency tokens to wallet addresses that fulfill specific conditions. A prominent example of this occurred in July of 2021, when the launch of the PulseChain cryptocurrency (pulsechain.com) used donations to the SENS Research Foundation as part of its airdrop conditions (SENS Research Foundation 2021), leading to over 20 million dollars being raised—approximately four times the annual revenue that the SENS Research Foundation historically receives (Hill 2021b)—in only a few days' time.

In addition to facilitating new models of philanthropy, cryptocurrency has also made possible new types of crowdsourced investment, particularly via the construction of decentralized autonomous organizations, or DAOs (Wikipedia 2022g)—entities whose governance is coordinated using cryptocurrency tokens that confer voting powers regarding the DAO's operations, and in which contributions from members toward the organizational goals of the DAO may be internally compensated with additional tokens. A notable example of this is VitaDAO (2022), an aging science-focused DAO that launched in 2021 and works to accelerate progress in the longevity space via collectively funding research and digitizing related intellectual property in the form of a particular type of nonfungible cryptocurrency token, or NFT (Wikipedia 2022h). Tools have also emerged that facilitate the creation of investment-focused DAOs, such as Syndicate.io (2022), which allows a group of up to 99 participants—be they accredited or non-accredited investors—to pool their capital and vote as a group on where to invest those funds. Other DAOs, such as LongevityDAO (www.longevitydao.net), adopt a fundraising approach using NFTs that is more widespread in use as compared to the unique IP-NFT mechanism employed by VitaDAO, namely,

creating and selling an art-based NFT series and directing the proceeds to charity.

It is also worth noting that interest in aging science has been coupled with blockchain technology since its inception, with, for example, notable cypherpunk Hal Finney (Wikipedia 2022i)—creator of the first reusable proof-of-work system (Wikipedia 2022j), receiver of the first Bitcoin transaction in 2009, and possibly Bitcoin's pseudonymous creator, Satoshi Nakamoto (Wikipedia 2022k)—expressing interest in life extension and being cryogenically frozen by the Alcor Life Extension Foundation (2014) after his death in 2014 due to amyotrophic lateral sclerosis (ALS). This common thread continues to the present, with blockchain pioneers such as Ethereum cofounder Vitalik Buterin publicly advocating for increased funding of life extension research (Milova 2018a), and it is reasonable to assume this unabashed support from key blockchain opinion leaders will be a powerful driver of increased decentralized support for aging science in the near future.

CROWDSOURCING IN AGING RESEARCH AND THE PROMISE OF DECENTRALIZED SCIENCE

Beyond providing additional mechanisms of philanthropic and investment-related fundraising, current advances in technology with regard to decentralized work are creating opportunities for new paradigms of crowdsourcing. Decentralized data collection through the use of mobile applications and wearable devices, for example, can be of a great use in research projects where physiological biomarker data can function as a reliable proxy for age-related damage, as with Parkinson's or Alzheimer's disease. Large-scale technology companies have also built integrated systems that facilitate this data collection natively into their products. One such example of this is Apple's ResearchKit SDK (Apple 2022), which facilitates the collection of biomarker data from a user's iPhone, as well as streamlining the bureaucratic elements of clinical trial administration such as patient informed consent form collection. Additionally, platforms such as Zooniverse (www.zooniverse.org) are building off of the earlier work of projects like Foldit through organizing projects where crowdsourced citizen scientists can participate in structured tasks such as image pattern recognition—tasks that can be useful to life science research projects directly and/or by providing "ground truth" data to train related machine learning classifiers (Ponti and Seredko 2022).

Blockchain technology has also become instrumental in the fast-growing movement to decentralize science in general, colloquially referred to as DeSci (Hamburg 2022), with a variety of DAOs emerging to leverage modern tools such as smart contracts, cryptocurrency tokens, and NFTs to improve aspects of science such as research reproducibility, cooperation, data standardization, interoperability, and privacy. Lab-DAO (2022a), for example, provides a marketplace protocol that allows members of the LabDAO community to exchange computational services with each other (LabDAO 2022b). ResearchHub (www.researchhub.com) allows users to collaborate on scientific research, similar to what GitHub has done for software engineering, and rewards users with a DAO governance token, ResearchCoin, for uploading new content to the platform, discussing research, and other activities. It contains a hub specifically dedicated to longevity research (ResearchHub 2022). Another example is CureDAO (2022), which is creating an open-source health data storage, interoperability, and analysis platform to discover how millions of factors like foods, drugs, and supplements affect human health.

The advent of such organizations and systems opens pathways for new models of clinical trials—those where therapy administration and data collection is crowdsourced by the patients themselves, while still ensuring proper compliance with data privacy regulations such as HIPAA (US Health Insurance Portability and Accountability Act 1996) and the UK Data Protection Act (www.legislation.gov.uk/ukpga/2018/12/contents). The ability to acquire data from many participants in a uniform manner can also circumvent challenges inherent to traditional clinical trials, such as competition over limited patient pools (Gelinas et al. 2017). Furthermore, such systems also have a unique abil-

ity to drive research into potential therapies lacking a traditional profit motive, due to lack of patentability for example, as patients themselves can provide incentive via crowdfunding and/or data sharing. Indeed, several organizations have already begun moving in this direction, such as Open Longevity (openlongevity.org) in Russia, and OpenCures (www.opencures.org) in the United States. Lifespan.io has also announced, via project campaigns on Gitcoin, plans to conduct decentralized clinical trials designed to test nonpharmacological interventions for dementia (Gitcoin 2022d,e), as well as the forthcoming intersection of this work with blockchain gaming ecosystems, NFTs, and infectious disease detection (Enjin 2022).

PUBLISHED RESEARCH RESULTING FROM CROWDFUNDING

While the recency in widespread use of crowdfunding and decentralization to support aging research means that many endeavors benefiting from such approaches are still ongoing, it is important to note that multiple projects that have been supported by related mechanisms are already leading to published research.

The MitoSENS Mitochondrial Repair Project (Lifespan.io 2022e), for example, the first crowdfunding campaign to launch on Lifespan.io on August 17, 2015, resulted in a 2016 publication demonstrating the nuclear expression of two mitochondrial genes: ATP6 and ATP8 (Boominathan et al. 2016). Another example is NOVOS (2022a), a nutraceutical company emerging from the Lifespan.io/Longevity Investor Network ecosystem, recently announcing the results of two in vitro studies—conducted by Ichor Life Sciences and the Aging Research Laboratories at Newcastle University—which demonstrate a significant reduction in DNA damage in irradiated human cells versus control cells and a senescence-mitigating effect in human cells, respectively (NOVOS 2022b).

Additionally, crowdfunded trials to study the long-term effects of nicotinamide mononucleotide (NMN) in mice (Lifespan.io 2022f), to determine the effects of rapamycin on human longevity (Lifespan.io 2022d), and to understand the effect of exercise in relation to rapamycin consumption (YouTube 2022) are currently underway and expected to produce related publications.

CROWDSOURCING AS CATALYST FOR ADVOCACY AND INCREASED PUBLIC FUNDING

When considering the impact of crowdfunding and crowdsourcing in hastening the progress of aging science, it is important to acknowledge downstream effects such as raising public awareness and support regarding the feasibility and societal benefits of increased healthy human life spans (Goldman et al. 2013). The highly visible nature of such initiatives, and the ease with which related successes can be shared on social media and news outlets, makes them a powerful method of engaging an increasing percentage of the population. This in turn can build societal pressure for increased funding from governments and international organizations to be directed toward aging science.

Additionally, the direct involvement inherent to crowdfunding and crowdsourcing initiatives promotes an understanding of, and sense of direct agency in, the progress of aging science among the public. This can serve to preemptively address common concerns the lay person might have regarding the work of the field, such as the fear that successful breakthroughs will lead to a protracted period of frailty, rather than a prolonged period of health (Hill 2017), or that the benefits of such work will only apply to the rich (Bagalà 2017). The latter concern, for example, is directly mitigated by the public dissemination of information inherent to crowdfunding campaigns, especially if project creators are obligated to make the results of their project freely available and open access (Wikipedia 2022l), as is the case for all projects on Lifespan.io.

An illustrative example of the capability of crowdsourcing to catalyze change at the national level is the work of The Jimmy Fund (www.jimmy fund.org/about-us/about-the-jimmy-fund), a charity founded by early cancer-research advocates in 1948 to raise awareness and funds from the public. Using the story of one particular boy as a

focal point, The Jimmy Fund made use of radio broadcasts, marathons, and telethons to raise millions of dollars for cancer research during a time when financial support was otherwise scarce. This growing public support was then leveraged to launch bold initiatives such as letter-writing campaigns to members of the United States congress and commissioning full-page advertising spreads in popular newspapers that implored the Nixon administration to act. These tactics proved successful and, in 1971, resulted in the passage of the National Cancer Act (Wikipedia 2022m), also known as the "War on Cancer," eventually leading to billions of dollars allocated by the United States government to cancer research—far beyond the funding initially raised directly by The Jimmy Fund itself.

This example of The Jimmy Fund has been explicitly referenced by the founders of LEAF (Comito 2016) as a model to emulate regarding the use of crowdfunding for research as a catalyst to greatly increase government funding and public support for aging science. Putting this into practice, LEAF has leveraged success in crowdfunding over $750,000 for aging science projects (Lifespan.io 2022a) to build a significant following on social media platforms such as *Facebook* (140,000+) and *YouTube* (3,250,000+), produce a highly trafficked online news outlet on the subject of aging research (Lifespan.io 2022g), orchestrate interviews and appearances on mainstream news outlets like *Fox News* and *The Young Turks* (Lifespan.io 2022h), and collaborate with other *YouTube* celebrities to create videos that have informed and engaged tens of millions of viewers (Lifespan.io 2022i). In 2021, LEAF announced the formation of the Alliance for Longevity Initiatives (A4LI) (Hill 2022) the first 501 (c)(4) organization founded in the United States with the express goal to advance legislation and polices that will increase the healthy human life span (Alliance for Longevity Initiatives 2022). Notably, the A4LI itself benefited from crowdfunding during the Gitcoin GR12 Longevity Cause Round (Gitcoin 2022f), completing the demonstration of a clear virtuous circle of crowdfunding and advocacy.

Crowdsourcing has also started to play a role in catalyzing change at the international level.

A clear example of this involves the World Health Organization's 2019–2023 "General Programme of Work" (World Health Organization 2022), a 5-year action plan on global health that included no specific prioritization dedicated to aging or age-related disease in its original draft. In response to this, a coalition of organizations and aging science advocates launched a letter-writing campaign to the World Health Organization (Milova 2017), which was successful in bringing about the addition of these priorities to the forthcoming Programme of Work (Milova 2018b).

CONCLUDING REMARKS

While crowdfunding and crowdsourcing have been used throughout history to advance scientific goals, recent technological advances in regard to decentralized work and collaboration are creating powerful new mechanisms to fund and conduct scientific research on a massive scale. This has particular relevance to aging science, both because consequent advances in areas such as biomarkers are uniquely suited to serve this field of work, and because many pioneers who are spearheading new and popular forms of such approaches have publicly made overcoming age-related disease a top priority.

As shown by various initiatives through time —from the 1714 Longitude Prize (Dawson and Bynghall 2012), through to The Jimmy Fund, SETI@home, Foldit, and modern initiatives facilitated by blockchain technology—crowdfunding and crowdsourcing have the ability to drive scientific progress in ways both direct and indirect. The power of such initiatives to engage, incentivize, and inspire the public has been shown to not only catalyze funding and the acquisition of needed data to support aging science, but also to improve the public perception of the field generally, and make the ground fertile for favorable policy change at the national and international levels. In this way, crowdsourcing and crowdfunding are vital driving forces to accelerate the development of aging science, supporting individual research projects and engendering societal conditions that will bring increased positive attention and funding into the field in general.

Humanity has possessed the desire to overcome the diseases and disabilities of aging since the dawn of recorded history (Wikipedia 2022n), and the time has never been more appropriate for us to come together as a species, as a crowd, and leverage our shared capabilities to accomplish this most ancient and noble of goals.

REFERENCES

Alberts B, Kirschner MW, Tilghman S, Varmus H. 2014. Rescuing US biomedical research from its systemic flaws. *Proc Natl Acad Sci* **111:** 5773–5777. doi:10.1073/pnas .1404402111

Alcor Life Extension Foundation. 2014. Hal Finney becomes Alcor's 128th patient. https://www.alcor.org/2014/12/ hal-finney-becomes-alcors-128th-patient

Alliance for Longevity Initiatives. 2022. Let's live better for longer. https://a4li.org

AngelList. 2022a. Introducing rolling funds. https://www .angellist.com/blog/rolling-venture-fund-launch

AngelList. 2022b. Rolling funds. https://www.angellist.com/ start-rolling

AngelList. 2022c. Healthspan capital rolling fund. https:// angel.co/v/back/healthspan-capital-rolling-fund

Apple. 2022. Building tools to advance research and care. https://www.researchandcare.org

Bagalà N. 2017. Will increased lifespans be only for the rich? Lifespan.io. https://www.lifespan.io/news/only-the-rich

Bailey R. 2004. Methuselah mouse. *Reason*, August 18. http:// reason.com/archives/2004/08/18/methuselah-mouse

Boominathan A, Vanhoozer S, Basisty N, Powers K, Crampton AL, Wang X, Friedricks N, Schilling B, Brand MD, O'Connor MS. 2016. Stable nuclear expression of ATP8 and ATP6 genes rescues a mtDNA complex V null mutant. *Nucleic Acids Res* **44:** 9342–9357.

Buterin V. 2014. Ethereum whitepaper: a next-generation smart contract and decentralized application platform. https://ethereum.org/en/whitepaper

Buterin V, Hitzig Z, Weyl EG. 2018. Liberal radicalism: a flexible design for philanthropic matching funds. *SSRN*. http://dx.doi.org/10.2139/ssrn.3243656

Chainalysis. 2021. The 2021 Global Crypto Adoption Index: worldwide adoption jumps over 880% with P2P platforms driving cryptocurrency usage in emerging markets. https://blog.chainalysis.com/reports/2021-global-crypto- adoption-index

Comito K. 2016. Life extension: how to reach a societal turning point—talk by Keith Comito at D.N.A. Conference. Lifespan.io. https://www.lifespan.io/news/life-extension- how-to-reach-a-societal-turning-point

CROWDFUND Act. 2012. H.R. 3606. https://www.govinfo .gov/content/pkg/BILLS-112hr3606enr/pdf/BILLS-112h r3606enr.pdf

Crowd.Science. 2022a. Together we can fund science that benefits all of us. https://crowd.science

Crowd.Science. 2022b. Health. https://crowd.science/campaigns/category/health

CureDAO. 2022. A community-owned platform for the precision health of the future. https://www.curedao.org

Dawson R, Bynghall S. 2012. *Getting results from crowds.* Advanced Human Technologies, San Francisco, CA.

Endaoment. 2022a. Your nonprofit now accepts any cryptocurrency, delivered as dollars. https://endaoment.org

Endaoment. 2022b. Life extension fund. https://app.endaoment.org/life

Enjin. 2022. The Enjin room, ep. 15: rewriting medical science with crypto and NFT funding. https://enjin.io/blog/the-enjin-room-ep-15

Estellés-Arolas E, González-Ladrón-de-Guevara F. 2012. Towards an integrated crowdsourcing definition. *J Inf Sci* 38: 189–200. doi:10.1177/0165551512437638

Experiment. 2022a. Help fund the next wave of scientific research. https://experiment.com

Experiment. 2022b. Community statistics. https://experiment.com/stats

Geere D. 2013. Kickstarter bans project creators from giving away genetically-modified organisms. *The Verge*, August 2. https://www.theverge.com/2013/8/2/4583562/kickstarter-bans-project-creators-from-giving-GMO-rewards

Gelinas L, Lynch HF, Bierer BE, Cohen IG. 2017. When clinical trials compete: prioritizing study recruitment. *J Med Ethics* 43: 803–809. doi:10.1136/medethics-2016-103680

Gitcoin. 2022a. Millions in open source project funding. https://gitcoin.co

Gitcoin. 2022b. Funding for open source software. https://gitcoin.co/results

Gitcoin. 2022c. Explore grants. https://gitcoin.co/grants/explorer/?sort_option=-amount_received&grant_tags=Longevity

Gitcoin. 2022d. Lifespan.io meets Web3—Crowdsourced clinical trials, inverse quadratic funding, and you! https://gitcoin.co/grants/3998/lifespanio-meets-web3-crowdsourced-clinical-trial

Gitcoin. 2022e. Stopping Alzheimer's with light and sound. https://gitcoin.co/grants/3853/stopping-alzheimers-with-light-and-sound

Gitcoin. 2022f. The alliance for longevity initiatives. https://gitcoin.co/grants/3945/the-alliance-for-longevity-initiatives

Goldman DP, Cutler DM, Rowe JW, Michaud PC, Sullivan J, Peneva D, Olshansky SJ. 2013. Substantial health and economic returns from delayed aging may warrant a new focus for medical research. *Health Aff (Millwood)* 32: 1698–1705. doi:10.1377/hlthaff.2013.0052

Hamburg S. 2022. A guide to DeSci, the latest Web3 movement. Future. https://future.com/what-is-decentralized-science-aka-desci

Hill S. 2017. Why a longer life does not mean longer decrepitude. https://lifeboat.com/blog/2017/10/why-a-longer-life-does-not-mean-longer-decrepitude

Hill S. 2021a. Gitcoin GR12 is a win-win for aging research. Lifespan.io. https://www.lifespan.io/news/gitcoin-gr12-is-a-win-win-for-aging-research

Hill S. 2021b. PulseChain Airdrop raises $20m for SENS. Lifespan.io. https://www.lifespan.io/news/pulsechain-airdrop-has-raised-20m-for-sens-research

Hill S. 2022. Creating political action to increase healthy human lifespan. Lifespan.io. https://www.lifespan.io/news/creating-political-action-to-increase-healthy-human-lifespan

Instrumentl. 2022. What are matching grants? Grant writing 101. https://www.instrumentl.com/blog/what-are-matching-grants

Kickstarter. 2022a. Stats. https://www.kickstarter.com/help/stats

Kickstarter. 2022b. Prohibited items. https://www.kickstarter.com/rules/prohibited

Konovalenko M. 2015. Longevity cookbook. Indiegogo. https://www.indiegogo.com/projects/longevity-cookbook

LabDAO. 2022a. Open tools accelerate progress. https://www.labdao.xyz

LabDAO. 2022b. What is the LabExchange? https://docs.labdao.xyz/lab-exchange/what_is_openlab

Lifespan.io. 2022a. Research. https://www.lifespan.io/crowdfunding

Lifespan.io. 2022b. The longevity investor network. https://www.lifespan.io/longevity-investor-network

Lifespan.io. 2022c. Join us: become a lifespan hero! https://www.lifespan.io/campaigns/join-us-become-a-lifespan-hero

Lifespan.io. 2022d. PEARL: participatory evaluation of aging with rapamycin for longevity. https://www.lifespan.io/campaigns/pearl-participatory-evaluation-of-aging-with-rapamycin-for-longevity

Lifespan.io. 2022e. MitoSENS mitochondrial repair project. https://www.lifespan.io/campaigns/sens-mitochondrial-repair-project

Lifespan.io. 2022f. Can NMN increase longevity? https://www.lifespan.io/campaigns/can-nmn-increase-longevity

Lifespan.io. 2022g. Your #1 source for life extension news. https://www.lifespan.io/news-main

Lifespan.io. 2022h. Lifespan.io in the popular press. https://www.lifespan.io/about-press

Lifespan.io. 2022i. The Lifespan.io video series. https://www.lifespan.io/video-series

Markoff J. 2010. In a video game, tackling the complexities of protein folding. *The New York Times*, August 4. https://www.nytimes.com/2010/08/05/science/05protein.html

McCaslin T. 2018. James Peyer: navigating the "biotech valley of death." *Geroscience*, January 9. http://geroscience.com/biotech-valley-of-death

Milova E. 2017. Does the WHO five year plan leave healthy aging out of the picture? Lifespan.io. https://www.lifespan.io/news/does-who-five-year-plan-leave-healthy-aging-out-of-the-picture

Milova E. 2018a. Vitalik Buterin: the best thing to donate money to is the fight against aging. Lifespan.io. https://www.lifespan.io/news/vitalik-buterin-the-best-thing-to-donate-money-to-is-the-fight-against-aging

Milova E. 2018b. World Health Organization puts the elderly back in the picture. Lifespan.io. https://www.lifespan.io/news/world-health-organization-puts-the-elderly-back-in-the-picture

Mullin R. 2014. Cost to develop new pharmaceutical drug now exceeds $2.5B. *Scientific American*, November 24. https://www.scientificamerican.com/article/cost-to-develop-new-pharmaceutical-drug-now-exceeds-2-5b

Nakamoto S. 2008. Bitcoin: a peer-to-peer electronic cash system. https://bitcoin.org/bitcoin.pdf

National Institutes of Health. 2022a. NIH success rates. https://report.nih.gov/funding/nih-budget-and-spending-data-past-fiscal-years/success-rates

National Institutes of Health. 2022b. Estimates of funding for various research, condition, and disease categories (RCDC). https://report.nih.gov/funding/categorical-spending

NOVOS. 2022a. Younger for longer. https://novoslabs.com

NOVOS. 2022b. Study: NOVOS' ingredients support healthy DNA and modify senescent cells. https://novoslabs.com/press-release-new-study-results-on-novos-ingredients

Petridish. 2022. Fund science and explore the world with renowned researchers. https://web.archive.org/web/20140103100244/petridish.org

Pew Research Center. 2021. Nearly nine-in-ten Americans say they have heard at least a little about cryptocurrency, and 16% say they have ever invested in, traded or used one themselves. https://www.pewresearch.org/fact-tank/2021/11/11/16-of-americans-say-they-have-ever-invested-in-traded-or-used-cryptocurrency/ft_2021-11-11_cryptocurrency_01

Ponti M, Seredko A. 2022. Human-machine-learning integration and task allocation in citizen science. *Humanit Soc Sci Commun* 9: 48. doi:10.1057/s41599-022-01049-z

ResearchHub. 2022. Longevity. https://www.researchhub.com/hubs/longevity

Rider T. 2016. DRACO may be a cure for all viral infections. Indiegogo. https://www.indiegogo.com/projects/draco-may-be-a-cure-for-all-viral-infections-science-health

SENS Research Foundation. 2021. PulseChain airdrop. https://www.sens.org/pulse-chain-airdrop

Small E, Hoekstra A. 2016. Which human physical aging biomarkers validate genetic and biochemical aging reversal success? Experiment. https://experiment.com/projects/which-human-physical-aging-biomarkers-validate-genetic-and-biochemical-aging-reversal-success

Small Business Innovation Research. 2022. About the SBIR and STTR programs. https://www.sbir.gov/about/about-sbir

StartEngine. 2022. Invest in StartEngine. https://www.startengine.com/explore

Syndicate.io. 2022. Turn any wallet into a web3-native investing DAO. https://syndicate.io

The Giving Block. 2022. Impact index fund: health and medicine. https://thegivingblock.com/impact-index-funds/health-medicine

US Health Insurance Portability and Accountability Act. 1996. Pub. L. No. 104-91 Stat. 1936. https://www.govinfo.gov/content/pkg/STATUTE-110/pdf/STATUTE-110-Pg1936.pdf

U.S. Securities and Exchange Commission. 2022. General solicitation—Rule 506(c). https://www.sec.gov/education/smallbusiness/exemptofferings/rule506c

VitaDAO. 2022. We're democratising longevity. https://www.vitadao.com

WeFunder. 2022a. Explore. https://wefunder.com/explore/all

WeFunder. 2022b. AgeMeter test is emerging validation standard for major emerging aging reversal industry. https://wefunder-staging.com/agemeter

WeFunder. 2022c. A pharmaceutical company dedicated to treating aging and age-related disease. https://wefunder.com/gerostate.alpha

Wikipedia. 2022a. Blockchain. https://en.wikipedia.org/wiki/Blockchain

Wikipedia. 2022b. Venture capital. https://en.wikipedia.org/wiki/Venture_capital

Wikipedia. 2022c. List of highest-funded crowdfunding projects. https://en.wikipedia.org/wiki/List_of_highest_funded_crowdfunding_projects

Wikipedia. 2022d. Fiscal sponsorship. https://en.wikipedia.org/wiki/Fiscal_sponsorship

Wikipedia. 2022e. Equity crowdfunding: regulation. https://en.wikipedia.org/wiki/Equity_crowdfunding#Regulation

Wikipedia. 2022f. Public good (economics). https://en.wikipedia.org/wiki/Public_good_(economics)

Wikipedia. 2022g. Decentralized autonomous organization. https://en.wikipedia.org/wiki/Decentralized_autonomous_organization

Wikipedia. 2022h. Non-fungible token. https://en.wikipedia.org/wiki/Non-fungible_token

Wikipedia. 2022i. Hal Finney (computer scientist). https://en.wikipedia.org/wiki/Hal_Finney_(computer_scientist)

Wikipedia. 2022j. Proof of work. https://en.wikipedia.org/wiki/Proof_of_work

Wikipedia. 2022k. Satoshi Nakamoto. https://en.wikipedia.org/wiki/Satoshi_Nakamoto#Hal_Finney

Wikipedia. 2022l. Open access. https://en.wikipedia.org/wiki/Open_access

Wikipedia. 2022m. War on cancer: National Cancer Act of 1971. https://en.wikipedia.org/wiki/War_on_cancer#National_Cancer_Act_of_1971

Wikipedia. 2022n. Epic of Gilgamesh. https://en.wikipedia.org/wiki/Epic_of_Gilgamesh

World Health Organization. 2022. *Thirteenth general programme of work, 2019–2023*. World Health Organization, Geneva. https://www.who.int/about/what-we-do/thirteenth-general-programme-of-work-2019---2023

Wuttke D. 2013. I am a little mouse and I want to live longer! *Indiegogo*. https://www.indiegogo.com/projects/i-am-a-little-mouse-and-i-want-to-live-longer

YouTube. 2022. Dr. Brad Stanfield—my rapamycin longevity trial is ready! https://www.youtube.com/watch?v=DVLqJWATYF0

The Funding Channels of Geroscience

Stephanie Lederman

Executive Director, American Federation for Aging Research (AFAR), New York, New York 10018, USA

Correspondence: stephanie@afar.org

This review examines the interconnected channels of government, individual, and corporate funding for geroscience. A sometimes-slow flow of federal and philanthropic funding over 50 years is now becoming sufficient to understand how the processes of aging drive disease. The amount has not yet been enough to push the benefits of geroscience into new therapeutics, but that is poised to change. Prominent billionaires, venture capitalists, and new foundations are investing billions in researching approaches for preventing, delaying, or curing the chronic diseases of older people; major pharmaceutical companies are poised to join them once the Food and Drug Administration qualifies aging as a treatable condition. The coming decade could see considerable progress, not only in the science but also in the creation of fresh nonprofit and for-profit funding streams.

Funding for aging research, even after the arrival of the more cutting-edge term, "geroscience," has not been easy to come by. Only now, half a century after efforts to understand the basic biology of aging began in earnest, has enough been invested and enough research completed to create a sense of cautious optimism that therapeutics to extend our healthy life spans may be only a few years away.

At first, the slow pace of funding was difficult to understand. Why would there not be universal support for efforts to assure we remain in top health, free of debilitating illness or disease, for much longer in our lives? Who would not want to use science to find ways to make our health span almost as long as our life span?

It has taken a long time to rebut the skeptics of aging science—and build a critical mass of government, philanthropic, and industry support for these efforts—partly because the public has lacked a clear understanding of what the field was accomplishing and what it is capable of achieving. Some have asserted our work is a waste of time and money, because they believe the aging process is immutable and so there is nothing meaningful that can be done to slow its debilitating effects (Peterson 1999). Others have insisted the success of our work would do more harm than good, because significantly increasing the population of older people would exacerbate the world's problem of too many people chasing too few resources, rattling society, and causing economic havoc (Vaiserman and Lushchak 2017).

Answering those arguments is easy for anyone reading this collection. A rapidly expanding body of scientific evidence shows that the effects of aging can be delayed in a broad range of species, probably including humans, meaning there are likely to be more ways to keep people healthy much longer in life. And a world populated by older people who are healthy and independent would be much less expensive for governments, and much more productive for the economy, than a world where a disproportionate share of older people is sick and reliant on others for care. A landmark study in 2021 concluded, in fact, that increasing healthy life expectancy in the United States by just one year would add an astonishing $38 trillion to the American economy over time, boosting the gross domestic product by 3.5% annually (Scott et al. 2021). Other research has found that people who live to be 100, the iconic milestone for a long and healthy life, have significantly compressed morbidity, the time at the end of life conscribed by illness or disability (Ismail et al. 2016). This means they get to live until their final days without sickness or debilitation, then simply die of "natural causes."

Fortunately, the tide of misperception and disinterest about the benefits of aging research is turning, and signs of strengthened interest in funding have started to flourish, spurred in part by a generational shift among the U.S. governmental, philanthropic, and entrepreneurial leadership. The potential promise of geroscience was a "tough sell" in the past few decades to the thought leaders of the baby boom generation for many reasons, including a necessary focus on more immediately pressing problems. But, consciously or not, they may have collectively concluded that any breakthroughs promising to extend our lives would come too late to benefit them. But the shifting of the balance of power to generation X and the millennials, with decades of life ahead of them and much more confidence in science and technology, is part of what creates this time of cautious optimism (Fry 2020).

Government and philanthropic funding is supporting a considerable pipeline of research into the biology of aging. The coming decades should see considerable and demonstrable progress, not only in the science but also in the creation of new funding streams—mostly flowing through for-profit enterprises. A burgeoning list of startup biotechnology companies has already invested billions in potential treatments for the diseases of aging and will hopefully be joined in the next few years by the pharmaceutical behemoths, who would be more inclined to invest heavily if and when the Federal Food and Drug Administration is persuaded to recognize that slowing the effects aging could be achieved with interventions.

At that point, corporate America will likely take the lead for financing the acceleration of scientific advances in geroscience, and then pay to conduct the translational research required to bring the benefits of our work into the lives of millions across the globe.

THE FUNDERS: A REVIEW

The funding "ecosystem" that pays for aging science—an interconnected network of government agencies, biotechnology and pharmaceutical companies, and individual and foundation philanthropists—started to germinate more than a half a century ago and has been expanding ever since.

Government on the Ground Floor

The pivotal moment in the origin story of aging research funding was December 1971, when the White House Conference on Aging, a once-a-decade summit on aging policy, recommended the creation of the National Institute on Aging (NIA) (www.nia.nih.gov/about/history). Congress did so 3 years later (PL 93-296: www.govtrack.us/congress/bills/93/s775), and the NIA opened in the fall of 1974 with a mission to improve the health and well-being of older adults through federally supported research. It is now one of 27 centers and institutes within the National Institutes of Health, an arm of the Department of Health and Human Services. The NIA's overall budget has been growing rapidly—to $4.26 billion in fiscal 2022 (appropriations report: www.congress.gov/117/crpt/hrpt96/CRPT-117hrpt96.pdf) marking a 38% increase in just 4 years (NIA budget summary: www.nia.nih.gov/about/budget/fiscal-year-2021-budget#applang). But this is for researching all matters related to aging, and for many years congresses and presidents have made Alzheimer's disease and related dementia NIA's top priority; current law dictates that 80% of the agency's budget go to that endeavor (appropriations report: www.congress.gov/117/crpt/hrpt96/CRPT-117hr pt96.pdf, p. 131).

In addition, a decade ago saw the launch of the Trans-NIH Geroscience Interest Group, which seeks to stimulate interest and involvement throughout the agency in the basic science of aging (www.nia.nih.gov/gsig). The group now includes 21 of the 27 NIH centers, and by one estimate their cumulative funding for research focused on the basic biology of aging amounted to about 1% of the NIH budget in 2019, or $382 million (Leung and Kennedy 2019). Such an amount underscores how the federal government has been by far the largest funder of geroscience to date.

The Trans-NIH Geroscience Interest Group has also hosted three summits for scientists, advocates, and funders, conducts annual meetings on the NIH campus outside Washington, and hosts regular smaller workshops and meetings on topics of interest to the geroscience community.

That the NIH would act as a "convener" in this way suggests the science of aging is rising within the federal funding hierarchy. But there is still plenty more the federal government could do, starting with making much more detail available about its spending in the field.

The Foundational Foundations

The first significant philanthropic effort to focus on the biology of aging was launched in 1965 by successful commodities trader Paul F. Glenn, who chose to honor his grandparents by starting the Glenn Foundation for Medical Research. By the time Glenn died in 2020, he had endowed the foundation in perpetuity, and it had funded more than $100 million in research, mainly at the nine academic institutions hosting Glenn Centers for the Biology of Aging Research.

The other visionary philanthropist at this time was Irving S. Wright, MD, who founded the American Federation for Aging Research in 1981, a decade after the conclusion of his successful career as a cardiologist. He decided too little was being done to address the future clinical care needs of baby boomers, and that the best way was with funding to persuade talented scientists and physicians to pursue careers in research on aging. In the ensuing four decades, AFAR has raised almost $200 million from individuals, businesses, and other nonprofits, and used the money to support more than 4300 scientific investigators. In 2021, AFAR made 66 grants totaling $4.5 million.

Tech Billionaires Step In

The belief that science and technology can help us live longer and healthier has been of great interest to Silicon Valley culture since its beginning (Friend 2017), and the main benefactors of geroscience in the past two decades have been well-known technology entrepreneurs.

Larry Ellison, cofounder of what is now called the Oracle Corp., the world's second biggest software company, created the Ellison Medical Foundation in 1997, and it awarded nearly $430 million in the subsequent 15 years. Its executive director estimated more than 80% went to investigate the biology of aging (Leuty 2013), but that vein of funding was stopped without explanation in 2013.

The move seemed all the more surprising because it came just after Google cofounder and CEO Larry Page announced the launch of Calico—short for the California Life Company—a research and pharmaceutical business focused on studying the aging process and accompanying diseases (Miller and Pollack 2013).

Now under the umbrella of Google holding company Alphabet, since 2014 Calico has been in a partnership with AbbVie, a biopharmaceutical spinoff by Abbott Laboratories. Each firm has so far agreed to invest $1.75 billion in a shared effort to discover, develop, and bring to market therapies for patients with age-related diseases (press release: news.abbvie.com/news/press-releases/abbvie-and-calico-announce-second-extension-collaboration-focused-on-aging-and-age-related-diseases.htm?_ga=2.103653766.762962550.1658510688-100783079.1658510687).

The New Philanthropists

The collaboration between Calico and AbbVie, recently extended through 2030, underscores the fundamental division of labor in the world of American geroscience, with businesses focused almost entirely on the high-risk, high-reward enterprise of finding treatments or cures for specific diseases. (One modest exception to this has been Pfizer, which has donated $3.3 million to AFAR for basic research.) The federal government, foundations such as AFAR, and philanthropies have remained focused on critically needed research into the underlying biology of aging, which could someday form the basis of the entrepreneurs' work.

Several significant new nonprofit players joined the funding arena in 2021, including The Astera Institute (astera.org) and the Impetus Grants (impetusgrants.org).

A consortium of biotech founders, clinicians, and longevity research institutions announced the Longevity Science Foundation, which says its commitment is to distribute more than $1 billion in a decade "to research, institutions and projects advancing healthy human longevity and extending the healthy human lifespan to more than 120 years."

But that generosity looks to be outstripped, by an order of magnitude, by the Hevolution Foundation, established by royal decree in Saudi Arabia and headquartered in Riyadh. Hevolution is reportedly planning to allocate at least $1 billion annually in pursuit of its vision "to incentivize healthspan science across disciplines and borders for the benefit of all" (www.nist.gov/director/vcat/biography-dr-mehmood-khan). Directing the spending will be CEO Mehmood Khan, MD, a former chief scientific officer at PepsiCo, and Felipe Sierra, PhD, who was the director of the NIA's Division of Aging Biology until 2020.

A Surge of Investment

Prominent billionaires and venture capitalists, meanwhile, pushed investment in longevity biotechnology into the billions for the first time in 2021. More than $2 billion was raised by such companies in more than 40 deals, according to *Longevity.Technology*, a news site for the ballooning industry, and more than a dozen of them were for more than $100 million (Newman 2021).

The year got off to a headline-grabbing start in January. After reportedly raising at least $270 million from investors including Amazon founder Jeff Bezos and Russian-born billionaire tech investor Yuri Milner, Altos Labs announced its startup with plans to create research operations in the Bay Area, Britain, and Japan and a mission to pursue biological reprogramming technology that can "restore cell health and resilience to reverse disease, injury, and the disabilities that can occur throughout life" (altoslabs.com).

And in March, German investor Christian Angermayer announced that two of the most prominent American longevity scientists, David Sinclair and Peter Attia, would take the helm of his new $200 million Frontier Acquisition Corp. Another German billionaire, Michael Greve, said he would invest more than $300 million in startups focused on life span extension. New U.S. venture capital funds focused on slowing aging that raised $100 million or more included Korify Capital, Apollo Health Ventures, and the Maximon Longevity Co-Investment Fund.

INVESTING IN PEOPLE

The world of aging research and geroscience has long been underpopulated. Work toward breakthroughs in the basic science of aging has been constrained by a limited pool of scientists willing to devote themselves to this work. There has not been a steady supply of early-stage, proof-of-concept clinical trials, and that has been a bottleneck in the development of geroscience interventions. And a critical barrier to the world of translation has been the scarcity of investigators with the combined training and expertise in clinical research, caring for older adults, and the aging biology that is essential to leading these trials.

While an abundance of biologists, biochemists, and physicians are eager to take high-paid positions doing research for pharmaceutical companies, there remains a persistent shortage of investigators making their careers in the world of academic research—not only because the compensation is generally less than in industry, but also because there have not been that many places offering opportunities for scientists to run their own laboratories.

By the Private Sector

While federal government spending that persuades people to start and stay in the aging sciences is as old as the National Institute on Aging's start in 1974, philanthropic efforts to increase and improve the geroscience workforce got off the ground in 1988. That is when the John A. Hartford Foundation created the Centers of Excellence in Geriatric Medicine and Geriatric Psychiatry, which paid for improved geriatrics teaching in medical schools on the expectation that doing so would increase the roster of physicians who take on investigations in aging science from the outset of their careers (Reuben et al. 2017). The initiative is widely credited with strengthening the national network of geriatrics programs (Isaacs et al. 2019), and has been a major driver of increased prestige for the field.

The John A. Hartford Foundation also took the lead in 1994, along with the Atlantic Philanthropies and several other foundations and nonprofits, in launching the Paul B. Beeson Physician Faculty Scholars in Aging Research Program. Named for an American infectious disease physician-scientist, it made $450,000 grants over 3 years—sufficient funds to entice a fresh cadre of physician-scientists to devote their energies to the field, not only by developing breakthrough research but also by mentoring and steering others into the field.

The Ellison Medical Foundation, created by Oracle Corp. cofounder Larry Ellison, also made major efforts to improve the aging research workforce by supporting the work of both first-time and senior investigators during a 15-year run that ended in 2013.

The Beeson awards were entirely foundation-funded for a decade, at which time the NIA added its support. This public–private partnership allowed the awards to grow for several years to as much as $800,000 over 5 years. With the program flourishing, the John A. Hartford Foundation and Atlantic Philanthropies have since wound down their support. The NIA is now the sole funder, with AFAR organizing the annual meetings.

Private support for building the workforce in the basic biology of aging has faded for much of the past decade, leaving AFAR as the main philanthropic player through a portfolio of programs, which offer a ladder of opportunity to support scientists to get established in the field and then remain for their careers, with $4.5 million in grants annually available for medical students, graduate students, postdoctoral fellows, and junior and senior faculty.

The American Aging Association, a prominent biogerontology nonprofit known as AGE, also dedicates resources to geroscience career development.

By the Public Sector

To be sure, however, the future of a robust aging research workforce is securely in the hands of the federal government. Academic research centers also play an important role, with both public and private funding, providing scientists with salaries, laboratory space, infrastructure, materials, and other support.

The National Institutes of Health delivers almost all this money, principally through the National Institute on Aging but with some grants allocated by the other arms of the NIH that focus on diseases that affect older people such as the National Cancer Institute and the National Heart, Lung, and Blood Institute.

The five main categories of NIH grant opportunities are coded by letters that do not always correspond exactly to the type of work getting funded. Whereas F is for fellowships, for example, a curious K is used for career development awards, grants made available usually for scientists already committed to specialized aspects of study (The Beeson awards fall into this category.) But there are also T grants (for training), including NIA awards to senior researchers willing to mentor newcomers to the aging field, and NIA grants to train medical students and postdoctoral fellows in aging science.

R is for research, and one category of NIA research grants is designed to whet the appetites of early career investigators for the field of geroscience. Known by the acronym GEMSSTAR (Grants for Early Medical or Surgical Specialists' Transition to Aging Research), this money goes to early-career oncologists, neurologists, rheumatologists, anesthesiologists, nephrologists, emergency medicine physicians, and others with an interest in research leading them to subspecialize in older patients.

Beyond these grants to launch and sustain individuals' careers in aging science, the NIA has several programs designed to enhance the workforce through collaboration, by fostering team approaches and by incubating cooperation among research institutions.

One fruitful effort has been the NIA Center Programs, providing more than 100 awards to institutions across the country. This includes the Nathan Shock Centers of Excellence in the Basic Biology of Aging (nathanshockcenters.org/about-the-centers) with the Pepper Older Americans Independence Centers (www.peppercenter.org), which focus on research and research career development on maintaining or restoring independence in older persons. But workforce development also happens at the Alzheimer's Disease Centers, the Resource Centers for Minority Aging Research, Roybal Centers for Translation Research in the Behavioral and Social Sciences of Aging, and the Centers on the Demography and Economics of Aging.

In 2018, the NIA started the Research Centers Collaborative Network, managed by AFAR and Wake Forest School of Medicine, to advance aging research by bringing different research groups and disciplines together.

The newest NIA effort, started in 2021, is the Translational Geroscience Network (www.gerosciencenetwork.org), a collaboration of researchers looking at clinical interventions that target fundamental mechanisms of aging to delay, prevent, or treat age-related diseases and disabilities as a group, instead of one at a time. The Translational Geroscience Network includes eight institutions across the United States (www.gerosciencenetwork.org). At this point, government and philanthropic support to create and preserve the workforce appears solid. The challenge ahead will be to prevent too many of these scientists, whose work remains foundational in the field, from leaving academic research for the shinier laboratories and more financially lucrative positions sprouting in the booming world of for-profit translational science.

INVESTING IN DISCOVERIES

The most important place in the world of pharmaceuticals is what the drug developers themselves ruefully call "the valley of death"—the long path, filled with scientific uncertainties and regulatory complexity, they must navigate to transform a discovery at the laboratory bench into a medicine taken at the bedside. Those who decide to finance such journeys must embrace their high-risk, high-reward nature and accept that many research insights will get "lost in translation" and never become therapeutics.

And the creation of drugs targeting the fundamental mechanisms of aging comes with far greater challenges than developing medicines to treat a particular illness (Le Couteur et al. 2022). That is because, unlike a disease, multiple biological pathways and processes get altered in every organ and tissue as we get older, and this cascade of change begins with the simple passage of time but is also affected by our genetics and environment. And yet an enormous and fast-growing roster of enterprises is working to develop treatments that retard or reverse the aging process, or ward off the chronic diseases of aging.

The National Institute on Aging now has nearly 100 people working for its Translational Gerontology Branch, where the drug design and development branch describes itself as working on medicines "that improve brain function and/or forestall the neurodegenerative process in age-related neurodegenerative disorders" (www.nia.nih.gov/research/labs/tgb).

More importantly, more than 100 biotech firms are now developing therapies to increase health span and life span, according to the news site *Longevity.Technology*, with new ones seemingly announcing themselves every week (longevity.technology/about-us).

One sign of the industry's rapid maturation was the creation in 2021 of its own trade group, The Longevity Biotechnology Association (longevitybiotech.org).

At the moment, these businesses seem to be making some of their biggest bets on these four therapeutic approaches to preventing, delaying, minimizing, or even curing the chronic diseases of aging:

Cite this article as *Cold Spring Harb Perspect Med* doi: 10.1101/cshperspect.a041210

- *Cell reprogramming* (Mosteiro et al. 2016): By "turning on" a handful of genes, almost any of our body's cell types—liver cell, skin cell, lung cell, brain cell—can be transformed in the laboratory to resemble the type of stem cell from which all our cells originated. Such cellular reprogramming may also restore many aspects of youthful cell function.

- *Senolytics* (Tchkonia and Kirkland 2018): Senescent cells are those too old and damaged to replicate and repair aging tissue, and they also can degrade surrounding tissue. A new category of drugs aims to selectively induce the death of senescent cells, and by clearing our bodies of them improve our overall health.

- *Caloric restriction* (de Cabo and Mattson 2019): Intermittent fasting, which reduces daily calorie intake without sacrificing nutrition, is seen as a straightforward way to extend healthy life span. For those unable to go without eating for more than half a day, therapeutics are being developed to mimic fasting's beneficial effects.

- *Young blood* (Conboy et al. 2003): It has been speculated for centuries that the blood of young people has substances capable of revitalizing older adults. Research now shows that blood of young mice rejuvenates the damaged heart, brain, and muscle of older mice—launching a major scientific search for the molecules involved.

The next step, which is detailed below, would be persuading the Food and Drug Administration that aging is its own indication for therapeutics—a regulatory breakthrough that would catalyze a surge of translational investment by the big pharmaceutical companies.

LOOKING AHEAD

The world of geroscience funding has entered the 2020s at a crucial juncture.

One could plausibly argue that the amount spent by the government, philanthropists, investors, and corporations has created a metaphorical glass half full: The funding has been sufficient for us to understand how the processes of aging drive chronic illnesses—and to set the stage for a new generation of investment in transformational treatments allowing us to live healthier lives for many additional years. But one could also argue the glass remains frustratingly half empty: The amount spent to date has not generated any blockbuster announcement and has not been enough to push the benefits of geroscience from the laboratories into our lives through a wave of new therapeutics.

The best way forward, of course, is to fill the vessel to the brim! To do so, it will be essential to prevent money from being wasted on the sketchy scientific meanderings of hucksters promising some magical path to the fountain of youth. Instead, strengthening and evolving the pipeline of research in the biology of aging, while supporting the efforts to translate that science into medicines targeting aging and age-related disease, is crucial.

Funding a robust pipeline of biomedical research into the processes of aging is what will generate the only reliable building blocks for a "gerofuture" filled with vitality and longevity for millions—by developing interventions that target the "hallmarks" of aging with the promise of delaying or preventing the onset of the most common age-related diseases or conditions.

In 2021, AFAR convened a trio of GeroFutures Think Tanks; an international gathering of two dozen experts from the biotech, biology, philanthropy, and private sectors explored opportunities and gaps in geroscience research, therapeutics, and collaboration and wrestled with tough questions about the main challenges and most promising areas of the work (GeroFutures Think Tanks report: www.afar.org/imported/Cover_G eroFuturesThinkTankReport_November2021-1 .jpg).

The need for better collaboration between private and research sectors, within the United States and internationally, along with the need for interdisciplinary research on aging, stood out. And inadequate funding was most often cited as the top barrier to those things happening. Aging research does not have as high a profile among many other governments' funding agencies as it does for the National Institutes of Health, but investments around the world remain inadequate to make the world of aging research attractive to young scientists. And so, the panelists called for a new wave of government, philanthropic, and industry funding to create research information clearinghouses and networks of collaborating laboratories, possibly on several continents, to generate a critical mass of researchers from different disciplines working together.

Private sector investors in geroscience have different priorities. They are keenly interested in discoveries with promise for a payoff in the near future. Work on biological aging clocks and biomarkers are of particular importance now, because understanding the pace of aging will not only increase opportunities for therapeutics but also unlock more investment opportunities. Research confirmed by multiple laboratories independently is also attractive to investors, as are discoveries that point toward a practical clinical path for addressing aging—in other words, finding an intervention that not only targets an existing disease but also looks to slow aging processes and affect the underlying biology of aging.

The surest way to stimulate research and development investment would be for the Food and Drug Administration to approve "aging" as an "indication"—meaning that the process of getting older is a medical condition, which, on its own, qualifies for treatments with FDA-approved medicine. Such an FDA ruling would dramatically shorten the time it takes transformative interventions to gain approval and reach the people who need them.

Moving forward with what is known as the TAME (Target Aging with Metformin) Trial would be a critical first step, because this project aims to provide proof-of-concept that the biology of aging can be targeted through therapeutic interventions. A campaign is nearing completion to raise $50 million to conduct clinical trials at 14 research institutions, involving more than 3000 people aged 65–79. The trial will test for 6 years whether taking the common diabetes drug Metformin delays the development or progression of such age-related chronic diseases as heart disease, cancer, and dementia. (The NIH's Geroscience Network recommended Metformin for such a trial because of its proven safety profile and low cost.)

If the answer is "yes," as the trial's leader, AFAR's Scientific Director Nir Barzilai, MD, expects, that would provide the FDA with a strong rationale to open its regulatory doors and approve aging as its own indication. Biotech entrepreneurs and legacy pharmaceutical companies alike, and associated tranches of private and public investors, would then be incentivized to invest money into developing transformative interventions—because therapeutics to combat aging could gain FDA approval and reach the public in dramatically shortened time.

There are other challenges besides the long wait for the FDA's green light.

The world of aging research is populated by intensely smart people doing a wide range of promising research on provocative theories, and those scientists have drawn attention from a wide array of wealthy people, well-invested foundations, deep-pocketed entrepreneurs, major businesses, and the federal government. But those funders are still not putting enough money behind the work.

But this combined community of the funders and the funded does not speak with a single and unified voice about its priorities, and neither has it developed a cohesive group of leaders. To that end, a nascent communications and lobbying effort is developing. And its first modest if important goal has been to persuade congress, as part of its annual budget process, to get the NIA "to convene a meeting of experts across NIH, other relevant federal agencies, academic researchers, and the private sector to set a research agenda for the field" (Proposed FY 2023 National Institute on Aging appropriations bill report language, via American Federation for Aging Research: www.nia.nih.gov/sites/default/files/2022-03/nia-congressional-justification-2023.pdf.)

Another more miasmic but perhaps more immediate challenge is presented by the burgeoning anti-aging industry, which in recent decades has expanded far beyond the highly profitable and centuries-old world of selling age-obscuring cosmetics. Now, a raft of startups has been investing in purportedly scientific efforts to develop mechanisms that stop if not reverse the aging process—promising they are near the cusp of discovering the twenty-first century version of the Fountain of Youth, mentioned in myths since the fifth century BCE as a spring with waters that would restore to youth all who drank or bathed in it. In the interim, there is already a $1 billion-a-year American market in "nutraceuticals," sometimes called "bioceuticals." These foods, or products made from foods, are marketed as having physiological benefits or providing protection against chronic disease—and those claims and related products go largely unregulated, because the products exist in the same FDA category as dietary supplements and food additives.

Beyond the potential disappointment for consumers, of course, is the evident "brand confusion" that many Americans have when trying to distinguish between those peddling pseudoscience and those doing the science-based research into the biology of aging. Skepticism about all efforts to combat aging then tends to tarnish the legitimate as well as the illegitimate, and too often that has caused potentially rich veins of funding from wealthy individuals to dry up. Not helping the situation is the reality that some scientists who have distinguished themselves by producing serious research have developed products for businesses on the wrong side of the anti-aging divide.

These challenges, while significant, are nevertheless surmountable—and they will be surmounted fastest, and most triumphantly, when four decades of funding is rewarded with a headline-worthy discovery at the laboratory bench being translated for the bedside.

REFERENCES

Conboy IM, Conboy MJ, Smythe GM, Rando TA. 2003. Notch-mediated restoration of regenerative potential to aged muscle. *Science* **302:** 1575–1577. doi:10.1126/science.1087573

de Cabo R, Mattson MP. 2019. Effects of intermittent fasting on health, aging, and disease. *N Engl J Med* **381:** 2541–2551. doi:10.1056/NEJMra1905136

Friend T. 2017. Silicon Valley's quest to live forever. *The New Yorker* (March 27, 2017). https://www.newyorker.com/magazine/2017/04/03/silicon-valleys-quest-to-live-forever

Fry R. 2020. Millennials overtake baby boomers as America's largest generation. *Pew Research Center*. http://pewrsr.ch/2FgVPwv

Isaacs S, Jellinek PS, Fulmer T. 2019. The John A. Hartford Foundation and the growth of geriatrics. *Health Aff (Millwood)* **38:** 164–168. doi:10.1377/hlthaff.2018.05297

Ismail K, Nussbaum L, Sebastiani P, Andersen S, Perls T, Barzilai N, Milmay S. 2016. Compression of morbidity is observed across cohorts with exceptional longevity. *J Am Geriatr Soc* **64:** 1583–1591. doi:10.1111/jgs.14222

Le Couteur DG, Anderson RM, de Cabo R. 2022. Can we make drug discovery targeting fundamental mechanisms of aging a reality? *Expert Opin Drug Discov* **17:** 97–100. doi:10.1080/17460441.2022.1993818

Leng S, Kenndy B. 2019. International investment in geroscience. *Public Policy & Aging Report*. https://doi.org/10.1093/ppar/prz024

Leuty R. 2013. As Google's Calico targets aging, Ellison foundation opts out, leaving researchers in the lurch. *San Francisco Business Times*. https://www.bizjournals.com/sanfrancisco/blog/biotech/2013/12/larry-ellison-foundationaging-calico.html?page=all

Miller CC, Pollack A. 2013. Tech titans form biotechnology company. *The New York Times*. https://bits.biogs.nytimes.com/2013/09/18/google-and-former-genentech-chiefan nounce-new-biotech-company/

Mosteiro L, Pantoja C, Alcazar N, Marión RM, Chondronasiou D, Rovira M, Fernandez-Marcos PJ, Muñoz-Martin M, Blanco-Aparicio C, Pastor J, et al. 2016. Tissue damage and senescence provide critical signals for cellular reprogramming in vivo. *Science* **354:** aaf4445. doi:10.1126/science.aaf4445

Newman P. 2021. Longevity Investment 2021: From seed to SPAC. Longevity.Technology. https://longevity.technology/longevity-investment-2021-from-seed-to-spac/

Peterson P. 1999. *Gray dawn: How the coming age wave will transform America and the world.* Times Books, New York.

Reuben DB, Kaplan DB, van der Willik O, Brien-Suric NO. 2017. John A. Hartford Foundation Centers Of Excellence program: history, impact, and legacy. *J Am Geriatr Soc* **65:** 1396–1400. doi:10.1111/jgs.14852

Scott AJ, Ellkison M, Sinclair DA. 2021. The economic value of targeting aging. *Nat Aging* **1:** 616–623. doi:10.1038/s43587-021-00080-0

Tchkonia T, Kirkland JL. 2018. Aging, cell senescence, and chronic disease: emerging therapeutic strategies. *JAMA* **320:** 1319–1320. doi:10.1001/jama.2018.12440

Vaiserman A, Lushchak O. 2017. Implementation of longevity-promoting supplements and medications in public health practice: achievements, challenges and future perspectives. *J Transl Med* **15:** 160. doi:10.1186/s12967-017-1259-8

The Role of the National Institute on Aging in the Development of the Field of Geroscience

Felipe Sierra[1] and Ronald A. Kohanski[2]

[1]Hevolution Foundation, Riyadh 13519, Saudi Arabia

[2]Division of Aging Biology, National Institute on Aging, National Institutes of Health, Bethesda, Maryland 20814, USA

Correspondence: f.sierra@hevolution.com

The conceptualization of the field of geroscience, which began about 10 years ago, marks, together with the publication of "The hallmarks of aging" (see López-Otín C, Blasco MA, Partridge L, Serrano M, Kroemer G. Cell 153: 1194–1217, 2013), a significant watershed in the development of aging research. Based on a very simple and commonly accepted premise, namely, that aging biology is at the core the most significant risk factor for all chronic diseases affecting the elderly, geroscience became possible because of earlier significant developments in the field of aging biology. Here we describe the origins of the concept, as well as its current status in the field. The principles of geroscience provide an important new biomedical perspective and have spawned a significantly increased interest in aging biology within the larger biomedical scientific community.

THE EARLY DAYS

It is often said that advances are accelerated by people being in the right place at the right time. We were lucky to be the Director and Deputy Director of the Division of Aging Biology (DAB) at the National Institute on Aging (NIA) in the first two decades of this century, a time of extraordinary advances in the field of aging biology research. Indeed, at the end of the twentieth century, the field had switched from being primarily descriptive and focused on physiology and disease, to a more mechanistic field driven by molecular and genetic approaches. A major shift had already occurred as a result of two initiatives driven by the NIA: the Longevity Assurance Genes (LAG) initiative request for applications (RFAs) issued in 1992 (initially called "Genetic and Molecular Basis of Aging"), and the creation of the Interventions Testing Program (ITP) in mice (Warner et al. 2000; Miller et al. 2007; Nadon et al. 2008). The former was envisioned to answer the question, "How much of aging is inherited?" from the observation that long life in humans was something of a family trait. The latter hoped to create a bridge between research on mechanisms in animal models and ways to extend healthy life in humans. Early work primarily in *Caenorhabditis elegans* and funded by the LAG initiative had dispelled the idea that the genetics of aging would be too complex to be deciphered, as several individual genes capable of extending life span were identified in rapid succession. That in turn led to the identification of metabolic and regulatory pathways whose modification by genetic, pharmacological, or dietary means allowed significant extension of life span in laboratory organisms ranging from yeast to mice. These findings represented a watershed in the field that spurred the interest of other scientists who began to see aging as an interesting frontier and field of study (for review, see Lithgow 2013). In 2009, the publication from the ITP indicating that rapamycin could significantly extend life span in genetically heterogeneous mice was again a major turning point in the field (Harrison et al. 2009). However, at the time the LAG was initiated, I was among those who had never been interested in aging but, while working at Nestlé in Switzerland, saw an opportunity where I could add my own grain of sand to the burgeoning field.

So, in 2002, right in the middle of this initial wave of activity in the field, I was lucky to join the NIA as a Program Officer in charge of the cell biology portfolio of the DAB. Ron Kohanski joined in 2005, coming from Mount Sinai School of Medicine by way of Johns Hopkins and having worked in the biochemistry of insulin receptors and their developmental functions in fruit flies (Song et al. 2003), to establish a portfolio on stem cell aging, which in 2005 was a little-explored area of aging research. Moreover, fortune would have it that Huber Warner, then Director of the Division, decided to retire just a few years later. Reluctantly, I acquiesced to the pressure of friends and colleagues, applied for the position, and indeed became the Director of the DAB in April 2006, and soon after chose Ron to be Deputy Director. The positions allowed us a much broader overview of the field and soon we became concerned that the goal of aging research seemed to be greater life span rather than our real objective, which is better health at older ages. Indeed, with the exception of a few so-called "immortalists," most investigators—and most of the human population—are in tune with improving the quality of life as we age. Accordingly, one of our earliest efforts leading the DAB was to introduce into the field the concept of "health span," the proportion of our lives that we live "in good health." Of course, the concept was not new and had been discussed

extensively in demographic circles (e.g., see Olshansky et al. 2006; Crimmins 2015), but it was nevertheless a difficult concept to introduce among experimentalists: while life span is a binary measurement (dead or alive), health span is much more complex, and indeed, while the concept itself is relatively easy to grasp, there is still to this day no accepted definition of the term as a quantifiable entity. We pushed for acceptance of the term during an early summit organized by the DAB as a way to collect the current wisdom of the field, and the proceedings were published in 2009 (Sierra 2009, and other articles in the same journal issue). Slowly over the next few years, the concept did take hold and it is now well used by the research community, despite lacking a simple pragmatic definition.

Health span represents the core of what later became geroscience, and as we worked to deliver lectures and propositions on the subject, we became more attracted to the idea that aging biology is the major risk factor for the development of diseases. Of course, this is by no means a novel concept, the idea being as old as humanity (Gruman 1966), and it had been espoused in the modern era of biogerontology as early as 1956 (McKay et al. 1956). But what many in the field came to realize was that understanding the basic biological mechanisms of aging had advanced enough to think about tackling diseases from that angle. The basic concept then forming was that directly addressing the biology of aging would be a much more efficient way of preventing or delaying the chronic diseases that affect the elderly population. Eventually I wrote a first draft of a "manifesto," which was shared with a few scientists in the field. That effort received no more than modest support, saying basically that the idea was good, but the status quo—emphasizing life span—would lessen its utility. But as leaders of the DAB, there was some chance of being seen as differing in our perspective from much of the research community, while being part of it! So, at this point, I shared my ideas with Ron Kohanski, and through several coffee-soaked discussions at the Starbucks across the street from our office, we refined the ideas and arguments and became ready to present them to Richard Hodes, the NIA Director, to see whether he would support them. For the record, it is important to state that, from this point on, Ron and I shared responsibility (or blame) for the development of geroscience at the National Institutes of Health (NIH).

But there was one sticking point that still needed to be addressed: If we were to develop a new strategy in biomedicine, we needed a catchy name for it. An obvious idea was to follow the example of some other successful disciplines that had provided an overarching conceptual framework to handle hitherto independent (yet related) fields. "Neuroscience" came to mind, and from then, the term "geroscience" was a likely choice. There was a catch, however; a few years earlier Gordon Lithgow from the Buck Institute had used the term in the title of one of his NIH grants, which was indeed focused on the same concept: aging is the main risk factor for multiple diseases. Yet, the name was perfect, so Gordon was contacted, and he agreed we could borrow the term!

Years later, a PubMed search revealed an even earlier use of the term, in 2005, by the team of Don Ingram and George Roth, who had created a company called GeroScience Inc. (Roth 2005; Roth et al. 2005). Among the earliest publications referring to geroscience as its own term, and in the sense that is currently understood mentioned "the nascent field of geroscience [which] is only beginning to inform oncology of the relationship between cancer and ageing" (Benz and Yau 2008) and an opinion piece about the language used to explain research on "life extension" in which geroscience was mentioned in passing (Settertsen et al. 2009). The first time the term appears in a publication from NIH program staff is in a couple of 2013 papers by NIA program officers (Howcroft et al. 2013; Sierra and Kohanski 2013). Nevertheless (and perhaps to the chagrin of Don and George), I have often started talks about geroscience by showing a photo of Gordon Lithgow, followed by a view of the inside of a Catholic church; the idea being "Gordon introduced me to the term, but I had the pulpit," which comes back to the beginning: being in the right place at the right time. In short, the concept of geroscience entered the mainstream before the term itself took hold.

In late 2011 or early 2012, we presented the concept and the idea to Richard Hodes, the NIA Director. He was immediately very supportive and saw the potential for a transformative approach that would have implications far beyond the NIA. He suggested that we convene a selected group of NIH institute directors to gauge their possible level of enthusiasm. That was an extraordinary meeting; we got together at The Cloisters in the NIH Campus, and Richard was the one who presented the idea, with me standing alongside. The excitement was palpable, with the most vivid memory being Dr. Anthony Fauci (National Institute of Allergy and Infectious Diseases [NIAID] Director) barely being able to remain seated, so excited was he about the concept. But what happened next was astonishing: The Institute directors were very enthusiastic and asked "What's next?" Having expected some reluctance and misgivings from scientists outside the aging field, we had honed over several months the pros and cons, supporting arguments, and conceptual aspects of developing geroscience, but how to proceed to bring the ideas into fruition was still to be formulated! So, in haste, I suggested that we form a trans-NIH working group to map the next steps. Thus was born the GeroScience Interest Group (GSIG) (the S was necessary because the acronym GIG was already in use by the Genetics Interest Group) (Sierra and Kohanski 2017). Enthusiastic volunteers were recruited from 20 of the NIH institutes and centers, and we started meeting monthly. We decided that the first joint activity should be a relatively small workshop focused on inflammation, since this was an easy pick for a transversal mechanism that increases with aging (inflammaging) and is suspected to play a role in multiple chronic diseases and conditions that interested other NIH institutes. The meeting took place September 6–7, 2012, and publication of the proceedings (Howcroft et al. 2013) was an important step toward establishing geroscience in the research community. By the time of this workshop, it was already becoming obvious that the concept had taken root in the research community and interest was growing, so the next step was a more ambitious geroscience summit. Manuel Serrano was among the participants in the inflammation workshop, and his presentation introduced us to the now famous "hallmarks of aging" figure (from López-Otín et al. 2013). This was very satisfying because at the time we were already in the midst of developing the agenda for the geroscience summit, and the similarities between the hallmarks and the scientific sessions we had in mind became evident, so we knew we were within the mainstream of thought on aging.

The first Geroscience Summit was a 2-day meeting at the NIH Campus on October 30–31, 2013, with financial support from several outside organizations and, perhaps more importantly, featured an opening lecture by the NIH Director, Francis Collins, and a closing address by Richard Hodes, NIA Director. Their endorsement of geroscience as a concept was crucial for further development of the field, and the proceedings were published in *Cell* in November 2014 (Kennedy et al. 2014), just about a year after the seminal paper by López-Otín et al. (2013) describing the hallmarks of aging (López-Otín et al. 2013). Importantly, there was significant encouragement from NIH leadership and supportive language in congressional bills (e.g., www.congress.gov/11 1/crpt/srpt66/CRPT-111srpt66.pdf), and, over the years, efforts by several NIH institutes were made to target some funds to selected topics in geroscience through RFAs, in addition to funding primarily through investigator-initiated applications to advance geroscience research. The field prospered, also facilitated by the generous support of organizations such as the Glenn Foundation, the Alliance for Aging Research, American Federation for Aging Research, and the Gerontological Society of America, among others. Recently, the NIH leadership has, in fact, supported major common fund programs highly relevant to geroscience in several dimensions, including, for example, the Molecular Transducer of Physical Activity program—exercise improves health—and the Cellular Senescence Network—addressing one of the major hallmarks of aging (Roy et al. 2020; Sanford et al. 2020). Of note, when we say there were limited funds specifically for geroscience in the NIH budget, the support from NIH leadership cannot be underestimated; certainly, there is power in money, but there is also power in lending the support of a prestigious organization, and the support from NIH was there-

fore crucial to the development of the field. More specifically, the freedom we were accorded to pursue the goals of geroscience was an invaluable asset that facilitated the development of the field.

THE CURRENT STATUS OF THE FIELD

Much has changed since the early days of 10 years ago. The field of geroscience has exploded and much has been gained through the creation of multiple consortia (some still active, others having lived their useful lives), working groups within multiple science organizations, creation of a dedicated journal, additional summits and workshops, etc. But those are a mix of administrative and scientific advances, and it is fair to consider the role that geroscience has—or has not—played over the past 10 years to advance healthier aging.

To start, the science of aging biology and field geroscience have definitely increased in volume of publications. How much of this increase is really due to the advent of geroscience is difficult to assess. Since the initial goal of the trans-NIH GSIG was to encourage other institutes beyond the NIA to consider aging as a risk factor for their diseases of interest, an analysis was done in 2017 (the fifth anniversary of the creation of GSIG) to assess whether funding for aging research at NIH institutes other than the NIA had increased. Figure 1 indicates a significant doubling that encompasses multiple NIH institutes, but again, geroscience is not the only NIA effort aimed at funding aging research by other institutes.

Perhaps more important than this is the fact that there have been important shifts in the last decade in terms of the scientific focus of geroscience. Indeed, the entire field was initially promoted within the Division of Aging Biology of the NIA, and thus the focus was entirely on how the biology of aging could contribute to increase our armamentarium against the chronic diseases of old age. Because of the early focus on diseases, soon after its inception, the concept attracted the interest of the Division of Geriatrics and Gerontology within the NIA, and, more recently, the other divisions (Neuroscience and Behavioral and Social Research) are engaging actively in support of geroscience. This is a very positive development that has increased the range of subjects

Cite this article as *Cold Spring Harb Perspect Med* doi: 10.1101/cshperspect.a041211

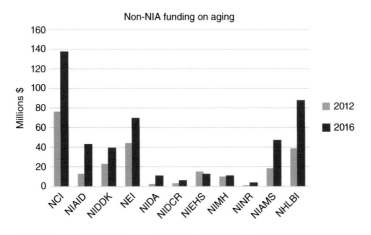

Figure 1. Increase in funding on "aging" in several National Institutes of Health (NIH) institutes, between 2012 (blue) and 2016 (red), corresponding to the first 5 years of functioning of the trans-NIH GeroScience Interest Group (GSIG). (NIA) National Institute on Aging. Chart created from data derived from The Research, Condition, and Disease Categorization Process in an NIH RePORT (report.nih.gov/funding/categorical-spending/rcdc).

being investigated, from aging biology-based new therapies for Alzheimer's to how behavioral issues affect the biology of aging. Yet in parallel, there have been important shifts in focus within the core group of biology of aging researchers that took upon themselves the mantle of geroscience. Indeed, the early definition of geroscience, as stated in Wikipedia as well as early publications, was as "an interdisciplinary field that aims to understand the relationship between aging and age-related diseases." The focus thus was on how the biology of aging could help combat diseases. However, it was clear from the beginning that what distinguishes geroscience from geriatrics is that geriatrics deals with disease treatment, while geroscience is at its core a preventative approach, and that led to a feeling that the focus should move away from diseases, per se. In fact, aging biology research encompasses much more than just "disease susceptibility," and the focus of geroscience expanded to also include so-called "conditions" of the elderly: those functional losses such as frailty and fatigability that, while not considered to be diseases, nevertheless play an important role in the loss of quality of life that often accompanies advanced ages. So, the focus of geroscience is shifting gradually away from diseases and focusing more on functions that support quality of life. This in turn led inexorably to a new focus on the role of aging biology on frailty,

but since frailty is a late stage often accompanied by disease, in the last few years there have been important efforts to move even earlier in the causative chain, to the study of resilience. Indeed, the loss of resilience may start rather early in midlife, and if we could develop appropriate measurements of resilience, preventative interventions could be applied much earlier. Alas, we have found the same roadblocks as with the early efforts on health span; it has been very difficult to develop widely accepted methods to measure resilience, so again we find ourselves in a situation where an easy-to-grasp concept crashes against the reality of a difficult practical measurement.

In addition to these conceptual shifts, a major change has occurred precisely because the field is maturing and advancing at an accelerating pace, so in recent years considerable effort is being put into translating the research in animal models to the human population. As a result, what started as a theoretical construct (addressing aging biology may be more productive in our war against disease than addressing each disease individually) has now garnered the latest scientific advances to start making inroads into addressing health issues in humans. Indeed, when geroscience started there were significant data in animal models, but work in humans was just a distant goal for the future. At the time of this writing, significant efforts are being made to bring so-called geroprotectors such as rapamycin derivatives, NAD boosters, and senolytics into the clinic. Some of these have been successful, others less so, but most efforts are still focused on treating specific diseases. Both "treating" and "specific diseases" represent a deviation from the major tenets of geroscience as they stand in 2022, but efforts at "preventing" and "multimorbidity" (the more accurate domains where geroscience could play a role) are finding difficult regulatory and funding barriers. A major effort focused on "true geroscience" was generated at a meeting of the DAB-funded Geroscience Network, held in 2014 in Spain. One result of these discussions was the development of the TAME trial concept (targeting aging with metformin), a proposal for a placebo-controlled clinical trial that reflects the goals of geroscience (Barzilai et al. 2016). While far from being the only approach, two geroscience principles related to possible expectations about clinical trial inputs and outcomes were laid out in that publication, which are (1) one pharmacological agent may impact multiple pathways and hallmarks of aging, and (2) multiple conditions of aging might be impacted in parallel (in effect, testing the geroscience hypothesis).

In summary, the field of geroscience is still evolving and growing, further demonstrating a healthy capacity to incentivize research in diverse fields. The support of the NIH, both administratively and through funding, has been key to the development of the field in its early stages, and this support is expected to continue and grow as the field shows success in its mission of using knowledge derived from aging biology to improve the quality of life of the elderly population.

ACKNOWLEDGMENTS

The opinions expressed in this article are those of the authors and are not to be construed as those of the Hevolution Foundation nor the National Institute on Aging.

REFERENCES

Barzilai N, Crandall JP, Kritchevsky SB, Espeland MA. 2016. Metformin as a tool to target aging. *Cell Metab* **23:** 1060–1065. doi:10.1016/j.cmet.2016.05.011

Benz CC, Yau C. 2008. Ageing, oxidative stress and cancer: paradigms in parallax. *Nat Rev Cancer* **8:** 875–879. doi:10.1038/nrc2522

Crimmins EM. 2015. Lifespan and healthspan: past, present, and promise. *Gerontologist* **55:** 901–911. doi:10.1093/geront/gnv130

Gruman GJ. 1966. A history of ideas about the prolongation of life: the evolution of prolongevity hypotheses to 1800. *Trans Am Philos Soc* **56:** 1–102. doi:10.2307/1006096

Harrison DE, Strong R, Sharp ZE, Nelson JF, Astle CM, Flurkey K, Nadon NL, Wilkinson JE, Frenkel K, Carter CS, et al. 2009. Rapamycin fed late in life extends lifespan in genetically heterogeneous mice. *Nature* **460:** 392–395. doi:10.1038/nature08221

Howcroft TK, Campisi J, Louis GB, Smith MT, Wise B, Wyss-Coray T, Augustine AD, McElhaney JE, Kohanski R, Sierra F. 2013. The role of inflammation in age-related disease. *Aging* **5:** 84–93. doi:10.18632/aging.100531

Kennedy BK, Berger SL, Brunet A, Campisi J, Cuervo AM, Epel ES, Franceschi C, Lithgow GJ, Morimoto RI, Pessin JE, et al. 2014. Aging: a common driver of chronic diseases and a target for novel interventions. *Cell* **159:** 709–713. doi:10.1016/j.cell.2014.10.039

Lithgow GJ. 2013. Origins of geroscience. *Public Policy Aging Rep* **23:** 10–11. doi:10.1093/ppar/23.4.10

López-Otín C, Blasco MA, Partridge L, Serrano M, Kroemer G. 2013. The hallmarks of aging. *Cell* **153:** 1194–1217. doi:10.1016/j.cell.2013.05.039

McKay CM, Pope F, Lunsford W. 1956. Experimental prolongation of the life span. *Bull NY Acad Med* **32:** 91–101.

Miller RA, Harrison DE, Astle CM, Floyd RA, Flurkey K, Hensley KL, Javors MA, Leeuwenburgh C, Nelson JF, Ongini E, et al. 2007. An aging interventions testing program: study design and interim report. *Aging Cell* **6:** 565–575. doi:10.1111/j.1474-9726.2007.00311.x

Nadon NL, Strong R, Miller RA, Nelson J, Javors M, Sharp ZD, Peralba JM, Harrison DE. 2008. Design of aging intervention studies: the NIA interventions testing program. *Age (Omaha)* **30:** 187–199. doi:10.1007/s11357-008-9048-1

Olshansky SJ, Perry D, Miller RA, Butler RN. 2006. In pursuit of the longevity dividend. *Scientist* **20:** 28–36.

Roth GS. 2005. Caloric restriction and caloric restriction mimetics: current status and promise for the future. *J Am Geriatr Soc* **53:** S280–S283. doi:10.1111/j.1532-5415.2005.53489.x

Roth GS, Lane MA, Ingram DK. 2005. Caloric restriction mimetics: the next phase. *Ann NY Acad Sci* **1057:** 365–371. doi:10.1196/annals.1356.027

Roy AL, Sierra F, Howcroft K, Singer DS, Sharpless N, Hodes RJ, Wilder EL, Anderson JM. 2020. A blueprint for characterizing senescence. *Cell* **183:** 1143–1146. doi:10.1016/j.cell.2020.10.032

Sanford JA, Nogiec CD, Lindholm ME, Adkins JN, Amar D, Dasari S, Drugan JK, Fernández FM, Radom-Aizik S, Schenk S, et al. 2020. Molecular transducers of physical activity consortium (MoTrPAC): mapping the dynamic responses to exercise. *Cell* **181:** 1464–1474. doi:10.1016/j.cell.2020.06.004

Settersten RA Jr, Fishman JR, Lambrix MA, Flatt MA, Binstock RH. 2009. The salience of language in probing public attitudes about life extension. *Am J Bioeth* **9:** 81–82. doi:10.1080/15265160903320521

Sierra F. 2009. Biology of aging summit report. *J Gerontol A Biol Sci Med Sci* **64A:** 155–156. doi:10.1093/gerona/gln069

Sierra F, Kohanski R. 2013. Geroscience offers a new model for investigating the links between aging biology and susceptibility to aging-related chronic diseases. *Public Policy Aging Rep* **23:** 7–11. doi:10.1093/ppar/23.4.7

Sierra F, Kohanski R. 2017. Geroscience and the trans-NIH geroscience interest group, GSIG. *GeroScience* **39:** 1–5. doi:10.1007/s11357-016-9954-6

Song J, Wu L, Chen Z, Kohanski RA, Pick L. 2003. Axons guided by insulin receptor in *Drosophila* visual system. *Science* **300:** 502–505. doi:10.1126/science.1081203

Warner HR, Ingram D, Miller RA, Nadon NA, Richardson AG. 2000. Program for testing biological interventions to promote healthy aging. *Mech Ageing Dev* **115:** 199–207. doi:10.1016/S0047-6374(00)00118-4

Index